Dao of Chinese Medicine

DONALD E. KENDALL

DAO OF CHINESE MEDICINE

UNDERSTANDING AN ANCIENT HEALING ART

OXFORD
UNIVERSITY PRESS

OXFORD
UNIVERSITY PRESS

Oxford University Press is a department of the University of Oxford.
It furthers the University's objective of excellence in research, scholarship,
and education by publishing worldwide in

Oxford New York

Auckland Bangkok Buenos Aires Cape Town Chennai
Dar es Salaam Delhi Hong Kong Istanbul Karachi Kolkata
Kuala Lumpur Madrid Melbourne Mexico City Mumbai Nairobi
São Paulo Shanghai Taipei Tokyo Toronto

Oxford is a registered trade mark of Oxford University Press

Published in the United States
by Oxford University Press Inc. New York

First published 2002
This impression (lowest digit)

5 7 9 10 8 6 4

British Library Cataloguing in Publication Data
available

Library of Congress Cataloging-in-Publication Data
available

ISBN 978-0-19-592104-5

Printed in Hong Kong
Published by Oxford University Press (China) Ltd
18th Floor, Warwick House East, Taikoo Place, 979 King's Road, Quarry Bay,
Hong Kong

Dedicated to the ancient Chinese physicians,
and subsequent practitioners,
whose genius gave the world the great treasure of Chinese medicine.

Contents

Preface

The ancient art of Chinese medicine, with its herbal, needling (acupuncture), nutritional, heating, and physical therapies, some dating back to the third millennium BCE, provides viable, effective health care options for patients here at the beginning of the third millennium of the common era. As more is known about Chinese medicine in the West, an increasing number of practitioners train in its application, while interest from the public continues to rise dramatically. The movement toward alternative approaches to conventional medicine started in earnest during the 1960s and 1970s in the United States and Western Europe, where until then conventional medicine had basically been the only health care option available. By the end of the 1980s so many Americans were seeking alternative health care that in 1991 Congress mandated the National Institutes of Health (NIH) to set up an Office of Alternative Medicine, which was renamed the National Center for Complementary and Alternative Medicine in 1998. It was not until the publication of a *New England Journal of Medicine* article (Eisenberg et. al.: 1993) that the sheer number of patients involved was recognized: between one- and two-thirds of all patients in the United States were using some form of alternative or complementary therapy, including Chinese medicine and acupuncture. It was estimated that up to 13 billion dollars were being spent annually in the United States alone on nonconventional treatment. An updated study in the *Journal of the American Medical Association* (Eisenberg et. al.: 1998) shows a continuation of this trend, with estimated out-of-pocket expenses in the United States for alternative therapies in 1997 reaching 27 billion dollars, comparable to the out-of-pocket expenses for mainstream physician services.

It may seem ironic, given the incredible scientific advances in Western medicine since the 1950s, that people are seeking alternative solutions to their health care needs. Part of the problem may lie in the fact that many of the highly technical treatment approaches of conventional care are heroic in nature, and applied in only the most dire and life-threatening situations. Another factor may be the public's awareness of the potential harmful side effects of some pharmaceuticals, and their corresponding desire to try something that is perceived as safer. Perhaps the main reason we pursue alternative therapies is that human disease has changed little in the past five thousand years. It is true there have been incredible reductions in infectious diseases thanks to improved hygiene, sanitation, and vaccination over the years, but the main health hazards that faced the ancient Chinese are still prevalent throughout the world at the beginning of the twenty-first century. The Chinese recognized that so-called civilization was contrary to natural living, and brought with it certain strains and stresses, which they called "the dust"—possibly a reference to the dusty conditions of overcrowded ancient cities. The treatment for stress was known as "wiping away the dust."

The risks to health are much the same today, and include the physical and emotional stress caused by living in large complex societies, overcrowding, adverse environmental factors, air pollution, poor water quality, bad eating habits, overeating, alcohol and drug use, smoking, lack of exercise, overwork, and poor sleeping habits. As a consequence, heart disease, cancer, diabetes, infertility, impotence, asthma, allergic disorders, gastrointestinal and urogenital disorders, acute and chronic pain, arthritis, rheumatism, anxiety, and depression, among others, are widespread. These diseases represent the general malaise of civilization, and no single medical approach can solve all these problems for all people. Chinese medicine has survived for many centuries for the very reason that it has been effective in addressing a wide range of human ailments, including those mentioned above.

Western interest in Chinese medicine and acupuncture has increased steadily since the 1960s and 1970s; some countries now license practitioners specifically trained in this medical art. In the year 2001, while some areas of the United States do not yet permit its practice—except by conventionally trained medical doctors—most states do allow independent practitioners. A great debate has ensued over the past decade in the United States whether Chinese medicine, or at least acupuncture, needs to be recognized as a valid medical procedure. In 1997, some 175 years after acupuncture was first introduced in America, the NIH issued a Consensus Statement (No. 107; 1997 Nov 3–5; 15 (5): 1–34), which recognizes acupuncture as a useful therapeutic intervention for a wide range of conditions. However, it also notes that there are many inconsistencies in the research design of acupuncture studies, revealing the major problem that has plagued Chinese medicine since its inception in the West four hundred to five hundred years ago. Incomplete source material and poor translations have muddled the story of Chinese medicine since it was first introduced in the West.

Accurately translating Chinese into Western languages, including Latin, was and still is a challenge because the context of spoken and written Chinese, especially that of the ancient written form, is often misunderstood. Chinese is more context-sensitive than most other languages. For this reason many early and present translations are flawed. If the reader understands the context of the sentence, paragraph, or chapter, or understands the context of the subject presented—even though an abbreviated form or a substitution for the Chinese term in question may be used subsequent to its first full reference—the true meaning can be discerned. The critical point is to understand in what context the key terms are used; without this, there is little chance of translating Chinese correctly or consistently.

Jesuit missionaries in the fifteenth century were the first to bring Chinese medicine, including acupuncture, to Europe. The first text on the subject was written in Italy in the 1500s, based on information gathered from people who had traveled to the Orient. The earliest first-hand Western account of Chinese medicine was provided by the Dutch physician Willem ten Rhijne in 1683, based on his two-year stay in Japan. He reported that the Chinese emphasized the circulation of blood and vital air (*qi*, 气) through the vascular system, and that Chinese physiology involved blood vessels and nerves. Ten Rhijne interpreted the Chinese concept of environmental or pathogenic factors (*xie*, 邪) that affect the internal body as "airs" penetrating the body. From this he incorrectly concluded that Chinese medicine was essentially the same as the empirical ancient Greek concepts of Hippocrates and Galen that were held in disrepute during his time. Equating Chinese medicine with the outdated Greek ideas persisted in the West until the 1930s. Then in the 1930s and 1940s the Chinese character for air (qi), or vital air, was inaccurately interpreted as "energy," while the Chinese vascular system was replaced with "meridians." These interpretations led to a whole new concept of Chinese medicine. These fundamental errors have been responsible for much misdirection in trying to understand the reality of Chinese medicine, and in the setting of design research protocol to verify its basic theories.

After the energy-meridian idea was popularized, ten Rhijne's report about the involvement of nerves and blood vessels in Chinese physiology was considered erroneous, and little thought was given to the physiological basis of Chinese medicine. The great discoveries of the ancient Chinese physicians, including blood circulation, organization of the cardiovascular system, somatovisceral relationships (communication between the external body and the internal organs), internal organ systems, immune system function, and the organization of the musculoskeletal system, were obscured. Once modern research was applied to understanding how acupuncture works, it became obvious that the mechanisms do not involve mysterious energy circulation, but involve extremely complex physiological mechanisms that can be described in Western terms. This research is continuing. To date, the bioenergetics involved is explained in terms of modern science by individuals who have been awarded Nobel prizes for their efforts. Chinese medicine is best characterized as physiological, or perhaps functional, medicine.

The purpose of this text is to present the true story—the way or *dao* (道)—of Chinese medicine, so that its basic premise, including its physiological mechanisms, can be viewed in Western terms. The confusion introduced by the energy-meridian theory stimulated a movement in the medical community to discard Chinese medical theory and reinvent acupuncture so it could be explained simply in Western terms. However, before throwing out such a vitally important medical theory as that represented by Chinese medicine, it is the author's hope that time is given to understand this great medical treasure and evaluate it on its true basis. As a health care strategy, Chinese medicine can be considered an alternative or an integral therapy, but it is a primary health approach that is part of world or global medicine. It is essential that the world's population has access to all proven medical strategies and is not limited to only one dominant approach. The best of all therapeutic strategies must be a part of world medicine, but with the caveat that all approaches need a common basis of explanation, as represented by modern science.

This text represents a dedicated labor extended over many years, including research, teaching, and clinical practice, to bring light to understanding Chinese medicine. Much of this information was compiled for teaching classes on all aspects of Chinese medicine. Many students have improved their clinical applications because this material gave them a better grasp of Chinese medicine and its real-world physiology. They have admonished the author, over the years, to get this information into print so they can show their patients and medical colleagues that Chinese medicine is scientifically grounded. The task of summarizing the ideas, theories, and mechanisms of Chinese medicine into one volume has been a definite challenge. For this task the author received many helpful suggestions, but two individuals expended considerable effort to review much of the information, and gave recommendations to help make the information more understandable. Therefore the author is pleased to acknowledge the important contribution of Stephen L. Paine and Christiane W. Christ. In addition, the author is deeply grateful and indebted to both Anastasia Edwards, the commissioning editor, whose sage advice and support made this book project possible, and to Carey Vail, whose superb editing skills brought clarity to the original text.

The overall goal of this text is to provide information on Chinese medicine that allows individuals to make rational decisions when seeking alternative or integrative strategies to address their health concerns. This text also provides information for scholars, students, practitioners, medical doctors, researchers, and others interested in detailed theories and applications of Chinese medicine. Those who are intrigued by Asian culture will find the story of Chinese medicine, and its contribution to medical history, a fascinating tale.

Donald E. (Deke) Kendall, 2001

1

In Search of the Dao

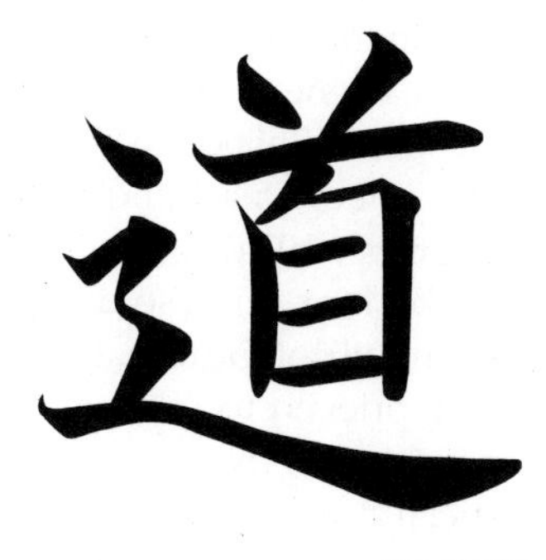

Dao: The Way

> Reducing medical information to basic principles is like collecting items in a bag. When the bag is full but not bound, the information spills out and is lost. When the study of medical materials is completed, but not summarized into principles, it cannot be applied to obtain marvelous success.
>
> Yellow Emperor, *NJLS 48 (Obeying the Taboos)*[1]

The history of Chinese medicine, from its early beginnings five thousand years ago to the present, reveals a truly fascinating story. Details are largely unknown outside of Asia, except for knowledge of a needling therapy called acupuncture[2] in the West (Ma, J.: 1983). The use of herbal remedies also represents a significant aspect of Chinese medicine, and information on the rich heritage of Chinese herbs is becoming increasingly available. A special heating method called moxibustion is also commonly used, alongside other treatment methods (Chapter 5). Chinese medical theories are founded on anatomical and physiological knowledge derived by the ancient physicians (Chapter 3). Blood circulation (Chapter 10), and a rudimentary grasp of the immune system, was understood more than two thousand years before it was in the West. The ancient Chinese also described the internal organs and other anatomical features, including the entire vascular (Chapters 9 and 11) and muscular (Chapter 12) systems. An elementary comprehension of the brain, spinal cord, and nerves was established, with mention of vascular and neural connections to the heart, eyes, and optic nerves. No details, however, were provided on specific peripheral nerves. It was observed that propagated sensations (PS) could be provoked along pathways associated with vessel and muscle distributions, possibly involving the nervous system.

Perhaps long before the Chinese developed their understanding of physiology, they studied the influence of the solar seasons, the five annual climatic phases, and the six prevailing weather conditions on farming and survival throughout each year. These studies represented their geophysical model that was applied to explain most relationships in the physical world (Chapter 6), including those involving health, disease, and human physiology (Chapter 3).

Chinese medicine and acupuncture have been employed in many Western countries since the 1930s; however, the first European exposure occurred four hundred to five hundred years ago. Reports from China and Japan were sporadic from the early contacts up to the 1930s, giving rise to infrequent periods of interest in Europe. Two or three decades lapsed between each wave of new information about Chinese culture and its medicine. Early reports were based on data gathered by Jesuit missionaries, diplomats, tradesmen, and a few physicians who actually traveled to China or Japan. Some reports were based only on interviews with people who had visited the Orient. Willem ten Rhijne (1647–1700), a Dutch physician stationed in Japan for two years, provided the initial first-hand report on Chinese medicine and acupuncture in 1683 (Carrubba and Bowers: 1974).

Ten Rhijne's curiosity was aroused by four Chinese diagrams he had acquired, showing small spots on the human body, arranged longitudinally along the surface. These spots represented locations that are needled, pricked to release a few drops of blood, heated by moxibustion, cupped, massaged, or stimulated by other physical means to cure disease. To the Chinese, the spots depict superficial nodes or critical junctures (*jie*, 节) formed where collateral branches (*luo*, 络)[3] of deeper distribution blood vessels (*jing*, 经)[4] supply the body surface. Distribution vessels are the main arteries and veins of the body, and ten Rhijne was informed that vessels involved related nerves as well. The superficial nodes were recognized not simply as anatomical structures, such as skin, flesh, muscles, and bones, but involved afferent and efferent neural properties (Chapter 3). Hence, nodes represent neurovascular concentrations of fine vascular structures and related nerves. As shown in Chapter 14, these nodes require neural and vascular participation in order to function. A slight depression or cavity, called *xue* (穴), *xuewei* (穴位), or *xuedao* (穴道), is often detected by lightly moving the index finger along the skin overlying a node location. Schnorrenberger (1996) prefers to use the term foramen (a small opening through which nerve fibers and corresponding vessels distribute) for the Chinese word xue. Lee and Cheung (1978) refer to nodes as loci, while many books now just call them points, but this nomenclature gives these locations a static connotation.

Eventually the nodes were called acupoints,[5] and the pathways formed by connecting the points together were referred to as meridians in the West. Ten Rhijne noted that his diagrams involved blood vessels, and the Chinese practitioners he met in Japan had constructed hydraulic machines to demonstrate how blood continuously circulates through the body. Replacing the blood vascular system with nonexistent meridians is the single greatest translation error to befall Chinese medicine. This was further complicated by Western translations of the word for air (*qi*, 气) breathed in from the atmosphere as some form of unexplainable energy. Palos (1963) reports that the character qi was formerly known to mean air or breath, but conventional medical science calls it energy. He gives no explanation to justify this amendment. Using qi to mean energy and xuewei to mean point are considered "the two most important mistranslations" by Schnorrenberger (1996), both of which he attributes to Soulié de Morant (1879–1955). Schnorrenberger translates qi as "vital strength or breath" and notes that qi "is certainly not equivalent to the Western term 'energy'." In addition to meaning air, atmosphere, and weather conditions, the character qi can mean a person's outward expression or countenance, and is also applied to mean function or functional activity (Figure 2.1). Substituting meridians for distribution and collateral vessels, or *jingluo* (经络), and energy for vital air, or qi, has kept Chinese medicine on the fringes of conventional care since the 1930s and 1940s.

One of the truly unique discoveries of the Chinese was their recognition that those neurovascular nodes (acupoints) located on the body (soma), associated with superficial vessel branching and related nerves, could reflect disease conditions in the internal organs (viscera). Body-organ, or somatovisceral, relationships were established by the Chinese through correlating the location of body pain with observed problems in particular organs (Chapter 3). The Chinese further realized that nodes distributed along the body surface could be physically stimulated to relieve pain and treat internal organ problems. This is the essence of needling, heating, and physically stimulating superficial locations, now generally categorized under the umbrella of acupuncture. It was not until the early 1890s that William Head discovered organ-referred pain in the West (Head: 1893). Research since the 1980s is providing insight into autonomic and somatic neural reflexes associated with needling stimulation, and the somatovisceral relationships described by the ancient Chinese (Chapter 14).

From the fifteenth century onward, almost all areas of Chinese thought were influenced and revised by Western views and mistranslation, including areas of philosophy and religion. Through the process of redaction, these incorrect terms were adopted by the Chinese to represent the accepted Western terms for the original Chinese. Adherents of the Western idea of energy-meridians truly believed the concept to be an accurate interpretation—however, those familiar with the Chinese classics apparently knew differently. Unfortunately, they thought the new concepts were additions promoted by the Chinese after Western contact. As a consequence, the Chinese were criticized for distorting their own original theories, as typified by the comments of Jurgen Thorwald (1962) in his book, *Science and Secrets of Early Medicine*:

> It struck Western critics as partly "a grandiose intellectual construct" and partly "absolute nonsense." The core of truly original ideas and sound data is overlaid with later additions. This is characteristic of all the medical works of China and makes it difficult to distinguish genuine early conceptions from the highly imaginative speculations of later ages.

Early Western Exposure

Prior to the thirteenth century, exposure to Chinese medicine was limited to China's nearest neighbors, including Japan, Korea, Thailand, Malaysia, Indonesia, Brunei, Singapore, and the Philippines (Huard and Wong: 1968; Chen: 1996). Both Japan and Korea hold the ancient Chinese texts in high regard, and developed their own rich heritage in Oriental medical and acupuncture practice that is similar to the Chinese approach. Knowledge of Chinese medicine, including herbs, moxibustion, and acupuncture, reached the Middle East, Eastern Europe, and India in ancient times along the Silk Route. Chinese medicine was known in Persia and Greece, and in what is now known as Lebanon (Huard and Wong: 1968). Moxibustion using carded cotton was adopted and practiced to some extent by the Egyptians (ca. 1500). Chinese anatomical drawings were in great demand along the ancient trade routes. Although the artistic style is quite primitive by today's standards, the drawings nevertheless were sensational for their time.

Information concerning the Chinese art of pulse diagnosis was introduced as well, with a translation of the *Pulse Classic* of Wang Shu He (ca. 280) into Persian during the fourteenth century (Ma, K.: 1983). Because the extent of these early contacts is not accurately known, it is difficult to say if early Greek, Persian, and Indian medicine influenced the Chinese, or if the Chinese influenced the medical systems of these other countries. It is also possible, because of geographical and language barriers, that the mutual interchange of information between China and other cultures was limited. It is known, however, that certain herbs from India and Persia found their way into Chinese medicine, and some Chinese herbs were adopted by those countries (Kong and Chen: 1996). Important food items were also traded. Many rumors abound that acupuncture originated in India or even in Tibet. However, Heinrich Laufer (1900) notes that the Tibetan historical classics, written ca. 630, record the derivation of Tibetan medicine as being from China (Cowdry: 1921a). Archaeological and historical data confirm that the theories of Chinese medicine and acupuncture are truly the product of China.

European Exposure

One of the first known Europeans to witness Chinese medical practice was Marco Polo from Venice, Italy. He resided in China from 1275 to 1292, and may have brought the first reports to Europe. However, the subject of Chinese medicine was not included in his *Travels*. The Venetian archives contained a now-lost letter that Marco Polo wrote to the Doge of Venice mentioning "needles that cure." Jesuit missionaries who visited China in the fifteenth century were the first to introduce Chinese medicine to Europe. They made use of needling therapy and moxibustion, and taught it to others. A century later the first European work on the subject was published, more than one hundred years before ten Rhijne, by Girolamo Cardano (1508–1576), a physician and medical teacher in Milan (Roccia: 1974). His information was based on reports by travelers who had been treated with needling therapy and moxibustion in Asia. By 1549, a Jesuit mission was already established in Japan where the missionaries were knowledgeable about needling therapy, moxibustion, and Chinese and Japanese terms of anatomy, physiology, and pulse diagnosis (Michel 1993).

More information was obtained after European trade was established with China and Japan during the late sixteenth and seventeenth centuries. One early mention was provided by Jakob de Bondt (1598–1631), the surgeon general to the Dutch East India Company, who observed acupuncture and moxibustion being used in Java. A paragraph in his book, *Historia Naturalis et Medica Indiae Orientalis* (Bondt: 1769), was devoted to acupuncture as practiced in Japan. Some forty years later, Herman Buschof, a Dutch minister and friend of ten Rhijne, wrote an early account of moxibustion in the treatment of gout and arthritis in his book, *Het Podagra*, published in 1674. Englebert Kaempfer (1651–1716), a German physician who worked at Dejima, Nagasaki Bay, for the United East India Company, wrote the most comprehensive Western account of moxibustion, with essays on acupuncture, in 1712 (Bowers: 1966; Bowers and Carrubba: 1970). Scattered reports on Chinese medicine continued from the time of these early introductions until relatively recently. Few Western physicians actually practiced Chinese medicine during this time frame, so intervals of twenty, thirty, or more years lapsed between periods of interest in its use.

Chinese pulse diagnosis—which had been introduced to Japan as early as the seventh century—was now given much attention. A Jesuit missionary working in Guangzhou, China, provided the initial Western translation of the Chinese *Pulse Classic* in 1671. This report was followed by the efforts of Andreas Cleyer, a German physician, who served with ten Rhijne in Java. He wrote on acupuncture and the pulse in his book, *Specimen Medicinae Sinicae, sive Opuscula Medica ad mentem Sinesium*, published in 1682. Cleyer attributed several parts of his book to the work of a Jesuit missionary, possibly the one from Guangzhou noted above. Still another translation of the Chinese *Pulse Classic* was provided by Michael Boym (1612–1659), a Polish Jesuit missionary, entitled *Clavis Medica ad Chinarum Doctrinam de Pulsibus*, published in 1686. A study of Cleyer's work inspired Sir John Floyer (1649–1734) to invent a mechanical clock device to measure pulses, and to write *The Physician's Pulse-Watch* in London in 1707. He included a paraphrased version of Cleyer's translation of the Chinese *Pulse Classic*.

By the start of the nineteenth century, early reports on acupuncture were just a historical curiosity for European physicians. It was considered that no further investigation on this topic was warranted, and the practice of needling therapy was in a state of ridicule. Ten Rhijne's report on acupuncture had little or no impact until Louis Berlioz (1776–1848) of France, father of the famous composer, used it to start experimenting with acupuncture in 1810 (Roccia: 1974; Agren: 1977). Berlioz is considered a pioneer in acupuncture, and perhaps the first physician in France to actually practice the art. Berlioz published an article in 1816 on the efficacy of acupuncture in treating digestive and nervous disorders (Agren: 1977; Tailleux: 1986). Another important contributor was Sarlandiere le Chevalier (1825), who practiced in Paris, and in 1815 reported on curing a cataleptic. In 1825 he was the first to use an electrical device attached to inserted needles. This was the first known application of percutaneous electrical nerve stimulation (PENS, or electroacupuncture).

Shortly after the efforts of Berlioz in 1816, numerous French articles appeared in medical journals attesting to the utility of acupuncture. The use of acupuncture continued in Italy, along with the publication of articles and books on the subject (Roccia: 1974). Electrical stimulation applied to inserted needles was also reported by da Camino of Venice (1834, 1837). Renewed interest was stimulated in other European countries—Germany in particular, and several authors quoted favorable results in Sweden in the *Annals of the Medical Association* in 1825 and 1826. A summary of acupuncture practice in Europe during this time is contained in the academic thesis of Gustaf Landgren (1805–1857), for his degree of Medicinae Doctor at Uppsala University, May 16, 1829 (Agren: 1977). Landgren also treated some cases with acupuncture but apparently made no lasting contribution. By the year 1900, electroanalgesia promoted by Sarlandiere le Chevalier was already in disrepute (Stillings: 1975).

Report by Willem ten Rhijne

The fullest early account of Chinese medicine was provided by Willem ten Rhijne in 1683. He served as a physician to the Dutch East India Company in Java, Indonesia, before being sent to Japan. Here, he spent two years at the small Dutch trading post on the artificial island of Dejima in Nagasaki Bay (Bowers: 1966). He traded information on Western medicine of the time for an explanation of the four Chinese diagrams he had acquired. He learned that Chinese medicine was based on circulation of blood and vital air (qi), and that the Chinese spoke of arteries, veins, and nerves being involved. He noted that the Chinese focus was on blood circulation, and the structure and function of the vessels. He discussed the Chinese idea of vessels dividing into smaller and smaller branches, and seems to indicate that this information was unknown in Europe. Ten Rhijne also noted that needles are never inserted into the internal organs. His findings were published in 1683 under the title *Dissertatio de Arthritide; Mantissa Schematica; de Acupunctura* (Carrubba and Bowers: 1974). Clinical success is reported in treating a wide range of disorders of the internal organs, pain, emotional complaints, and infectious diseases that were prevalent at the time. After the concept of energy flowing through meridians gained a foothold in Europe during the 1940s and 1950s, ten Rhijne's report on Chinese medicine being based on vessels, nerves, and blood circulation was discredited as erroneous.

A Chinese physician taught ten Rhijne the names, pathways, and length of the twelve main distribution vessels, and four of the eight singular vessels (Chapter 10). This information corresponds accurately with data from the *Yellow Emperor's Internal Classic* (*Huangdi Neijing*) (ca. 300 BCE) (Yu: 1983). Ten Rhijne used the principles of the "wetness (humidum) radical" and "innate heat" of Galen and Aristotle, respectively, for the Chinese concept of yin and yang, as used in the name of the vessels.

Learning that Chinese medicine involved the circulation of blood and air (qi), and that disease is caused by "winds" (*feng*, 风) invading the body, ten Rhijne interpreted this as being the same as the "winds" of Hippocrates, and Galen's "circulation of humors," which were both in disfavor during his time. Once this label was applied to Chinese medicine, it persisted through the years. Even Cowdry (1921a) considered the Chinese of his era to be "still saturated with the doctrine of circulating 'humors,' and in this respect, still primitive people." After characterizing the Chinese views on anatomy, physiology, and medicine as identical to that of the ancient Greeks, the physical basis of Chinese medicine was not given serious consideration until the 1980s and 1990s. Ten Rhijne wrongly supposed that the Chinese and Japanese practitioners needled, or heated by moxibustion, to disperse entrapped air to cure ailments. He likened the process of needling to sticking a fork in a sausage, swollen during frying, to release the built up airs before it explodes.

From Europe to America

A few doctors in the United States tried their hand at needle therapy as early as 1822 (Cassedy: 1974). These early pioneers expressed concern that acupuncture might go the way of other radical therapies or pseudomedical innovations introduced from Europe, including mesmerism, homeopathy, phrenology, hydrology, and others. Ten Rhijne's dissertation was first translated into English in 1826, and published in the *North American Medical and Surgical Journal* (1826; 1: 198–204), which coincided with the American interest in needling at that time (Rosenburg, D. B.: 1979). One of the most notable practitioners was the Canadian physician, Sir William Osler (1848–1924). He practiced a variant form of acupuncture, and recommended its use for the treatment of lumbago and sciatica. This is noted in his classic textbook, *The Principles and Practice of Medicine* (Osler: 1912):

> For lumbago acupuncture is, in acute cases, the most efficient treatment. Needles of from 3 to 4 inches in length (ordinary bonnet-needles, sterilized, will do) are thrust into the lumbar muscles at the seat of pain, and withdrawn after five to ten minutes. In many instances the relief is immediate, and I can corroborate fully the statements of Ringer, who taught me this practice, as to its extraordinary and prompt efficacy in many instances.

Introduction of the Energy-Meridian Theory

As a young man, Georges Soulié de Morant went to China in 1901 employed by the Banque Lehideux. He remained there until 1917, once serving as French Consul of Shanghai. During his long stay he became interested in the study of Chinese medicine, which was to become his lifelong dedication. After returning to Paris he popularized acupuncture in France through clinical practice and published papers, and also wrote articles on Chinese art, music, history, and literature. Soulié de Morant taught acupuncture to physicians, and translated qi (vital air) as energy, supposedly "for lack of a better word" (Zmiewski: 1994). Substituting energy for vital air brings into question whether either the etymology or usage of the Chinese character qi was given any serious study. Soulié de Morant also translated the character jing, in jingluo, as meridian, since jing can also refer to the straight lines used in laying out agricultural fields. Jing is further used as the first character in the Chinese terms *jingxian* (经线) and *jingdu* (经度), which respectively mean meridian and longitude. Because of this, jingluo was incorrectly translated as meridian, even though the terms jing and luo both refer to blood vessels. Unfortunately, this error has been widely promoted in the West, as noted by Unschuld (1998): "Soulié de Morant coined the term 'meridian,' which despite its lack of faithfulness to the underlying Chinese concepts, has been retained by nearly all authors writing for a Western public."

Soulié de Morant considered that the intake of air, food, and water; emotional components; celestial rhythms; and atmospheric forces were all essential to the maintenance of his energy concept. He also included in his idea of energy most of the physiological processes of the body, such as needling reaction, propagated sensation, organ functional activity, and vital substances. He thought that modern medical science would someday verify the existence of meridians and his energy model, which is often referred to as French energetics. Soulié de Morant produced three texts entitled: *l'Energie* (Energy) (1939); *le Maniement de l'Energie* (Management of Energy) (1941); and *Physiologie de l'Energy* (Physiology of Energy) (1955). After his death in 1955, these three volumes were published as a single volume (Soulié de Morant: 1957). Later, two additional volumes, *les Meridiens, les Points, et leur Symptoms,* and *les Maladies et leur Traitements,* were published in 1972 by Soulié de Morant's lifelong physician collaborator, Dr. Thérèse Martiny. Because of his lengthy stay in Asia, Soulié de Morant was well known to the Chinese and Japanese experts of his day—a fact which may have influenced the Chinese to accept his explanation of energy flow through meridians as the correct European translation for Chinese theories.

Despite the misconceptions, Soulié de Morant's work was nevertheless a useful contribution. His efforts helped spread the clinical application of acupuncture in France and the rest of Europe. Practitioners studied his texts, and by the time of opening communications with mainland China in the early 1970s, acupuncture was already established in France. As a result of Soulié de Morant's efforts in the past, new books were published in English and German. The English books, based on the energy model, served as some of the early source material for an understanding of acupuncture as it made its way to America (Mann: 1962, 1964; Palos: 1963). Information was later obtained directly from China, which opened up a whole new world of understanding about the physical basis of Chinese medicine.

Chinese books published in English typically use the term meridian, along with the pinyin term qi, without referring to it as meaning energy, but inadvertently refer on occasion to vessels, and do describe other genuine physiological features. In bilingual books in both English and Chinese, the Chinese is true to the vascular system and circulation of nutrients, while the English refers to qi and meridians. To this day many Chinese experts understand their theories involve vascular circulation and the nervous system, but use the terms qi and meridian when writing in English, or when addressing Westerners. However, there are many Chinese practitioners who embrace the energy-meridian view, sometimes promoting the mystical aspects of Chinese thought. In addition, many English versions of Chinese textbooks reduce the original concepts of nutrients (*ying*, 营), defensive substances (*wei*, 卫), organ vitality substances (*shenjing*, 神精), and vital air (qi) to a single word, qi, without providing a translation for this concept. This practice makes it almost impossible to comprehend the original ideas. Writers of these books have expanded the meaning of qi to include everything in the physical world, elevating it to a cosmic level.

Authenticity of Chinese Medicine

Physicians in ancient China developed a total medical system that has survived virtually unchanged to present times. Further, Chinese medicine is complete within itself in that there is consistency between physiological concepts, etiology, methods of diagnosis, and principles of treatment. Disease-causing factors include environmental conditions, dietary habits, emotions, and stress (Chapters 6 and 7). Either poor nutrition, including overeating, or excess in any of the other three factors disturbs physiological balance, resulting in illness (Chapter 13). Chinese herbs, needling therapy, and other treatment approaches are used to promote particular effects to restore critical physiological balance (Chapter 15), called *zheng* (正) in Chinese (Figures 2.3 and 13.1). Claude Bernard (1813–1878), the renowned French physiologist who is universally recognized as one of the great scientists of all time, had a concept similar to that of zheng. He believed that health is the result of maintaining the constancy of the body's internal environment, what he called the *milieu interieur* (Bernard: 1865). Walter Cannon (1871–1945), an American physiologist, was the first to define these same ideas in modern biological terms as homeostasis (Cannon: 1914, 1932; Fleming: 1984).

Chinese medicine is best characterized as physiological medicine, which depends on maintaining the internal functional balance, which in turn relies on the vascular circulation of blood, vital air (qi), and vital substances. This concept makes Chinese medicine unique compared with other primitive medical practices that existed at about the same ancient period, such as those in India, Egypt, and Greece. Medicine in these regions was empirical in nature, an example being the medicine of Hippocrates (460–351 BCE). In his book, *An Introduction to the Study of Experimental Medicine* (1865), Claude Bernard stated that medicine has to be physiologically rooted and subject to scientific principles. The scientific standards he established are: (1) medicine must have an experimental base derived from anatomical and physiological studies; (2) disease must be described in terms of physiological mechanisms and manifestations; and (3) medicine must have a clinical practice essential to restoring or normalizing physiological function.

Physiological Base

Chinese medicine meets Bernard's criteria, having been firmly established on a keen understanding of anatomy and physiology. Early Chinese studies may be viewed as crude by modern standards, but nonetheless, they were scientific in the truest sense. Most of the physiological information cited in this present text was translated from the *Yellow Emperor's Internal Classic* (*Huangdi Neijing*) (ca. 300 BCE), often referred to in this book as the *Internal Classic* or *Neijing*. Careful study of this ancient book reveals most of the important Chinese discoveries. As the story unfolds it becomes clear that the physiology of Chinese medicine is essentially the same as that of Western medicine. However, the Chinese emphasis on physiology is subtly different from that of the West, particularly with regard to concepts of vitality (*shen*, 神) (Chapter 7), how the body systems dynamically interact, and how external and internal factors cause disease. Perhaps most crucial to the Chinese view is the highly integrated nature of the body, involving neurovascular systems, the internal organs, and the external body, which includes the musculoskeletal system. These major aspects of the body give rise to viscerosomatic (internal organ–to-body), somatovisceral (body-to–internal organ), and somatosomatic (body-to-body) relationships important in health, disease, and clinical practice.

It is imperative to ascertain a true and correct understanding of Chinese physiology in order to establish a baseline for clinical practice, and also to provide a starting point from which more study can take place. Western science has developed an excellent comprehension of human physiology that is recognized by the world medical community, with the understanding that continuing studies are pursued to keep improving the physiological database. Conventional medical practice is firmly based on Western physiology and its latest findings. The ancient Chinese physicians had the same concept in mind, and developed treatment approaches consistent with their understanding of physiology. There can be a diversity in how clinical methods are applied, with different means applied to treat one disease, or a single treatment approach may be applied to treat different disorders. However, it was considered critical that all practitioners were well versed in the same basic understanding of human physiology. The *Neijing* was written to standardize the Chinese physiological concepts and clinical strategies. The Western-generated energy-meridian model, which gained prominence in the 1940s and 1950s, introduced impossible, or at best, incomprehensible, physiological ideas, resulting in an erroneous view of Chinese medicine as being metaphysically based.

Chinese medicine, with its own unique view of physiological organization, must play a role in the process of understanding human physiology, if to accomplish nothing more than to determine whether the postulated theories of Chinese medicine are correct or not. An integral part of this task is to explain the Chinese theories using universally accepted anatomical and physiological terms. Fortunately, research in neurophysiology over the past two decades is providing sufficient insight to help explain the Chinese theories. This includes explaining how the insertion of fine needles can bring about profound restorative reactions in the human body (Chapter 14). If Chinese medicine is truly a physiologically based system, then it can be studied by accepted scientific means. The Chinese view of physiology offers a unique insight into bodily function and organization that would be of interest to Western medical practitioners as well.

Organization and Branching of Vascular System

The ancient Chinese distinguished the arterial and venous circulation routes, and identified all major blood vessels (*mai*, 脉) in the body (Chapters 9 and 11). Critical junctures or nodes (jie) are formed where finer branches (arterioles, venules, and capillaries), and related nerves, of collateral vessels (luo) of specific longitudinal distribution blood vessels (jing) supply the superficial regions of the body (Figure 9.3). For this reason the ancient Chinese placed great emphasis on the distribution and collateral vessels. The four diagrams of ten Rhijne, and other so-called acupuncture charts, are a depiction of the nodes located on a particular vascular route, represented by the distribution and related collateral vessels that supply a particular region of the body (Chapter 11).

The Chinese used one set of diagrams to show the distribution vessel routes, and another diagram to indicate the nodal (acupoint) pathway, without connecting the nodes with a line (Veith: 1949). Since Westerners understood neither what the diagrams represented, nor the Chinese concept of vascular branching, the diagrams could not be reconciled with known vessel pathways. Also, given the fact that needling-induced sensations (propagated sensations or PS) could propagate along the nodal pathways, the idea of imaginary pathways may have been reinforced. To some, Soulié de Morant's substitution of meridian for distribution and collateral vessels perhaps seemed a reasonable choice. However, Lu and Needham (1980) point out that using the word meridian to describe a nodal pathway is misleading and inappropriate. Unfortunately, they too were in error—they interpret the distribution vessels as longitudinal pathways, and the collateral vessels as horizontal pathways, such as north–south and east–west city streets laid out in a grid. Lu and Needham interpret vital air (qi) as being similar to the Greek concept of pneuma.

The notion of invisible pathways may have partly resulted from incorrectly understanding the discussion in *NJLS 10* (*Distribution Vessels*), which states that distribution (jing) vessels (arteries and veins) lie hidden within the striated muscles, and consequently are not visible to the naked eye. Visible vessels consist of superficial collateral (luo) vessels, such as the veins on the back of the hand (Chapter 9). These are clearly descriptions of blood vessels, and are easily identified as such. Because the vessels on the back of the hand are veins, both Veith (1949) and Wang (1926) incorrectly translated luo as vein and jing as artery. The energy-meridian school created more confusion by extending the idea of imaginary pathways when they also replaced the Chinese character mai, which strictly means vessel (Figure 9.2), with the word meridian. Navigational meridians are invented, and do not physically exist, just as the idea of meridians has never existed in Chinese medicine concepts.

Blood Circulation of Nutrients

The Chinese undoubtedly discovered the continuous circulation of blood, given their detailed description of both the vascular system (Chapters 9 and 11) and blood circulation (Chapter 10). The precise time in primitive history when this discovery was made is not known. To the Chinese, blood circulation was the most important physiological feature. Impaired blood flow in any region of the body, including internal organs, can result in pain and dysfunction (Xiu: 1988). External environmental factors, emotions, and stress can have adverse effects on blood flow. One complication in trying to comprehend the details of blood circulation as explained in Chinese medicine is the emphasis on the circulation of nutrients in the distribution vessels. Because external factors are thought to penetrate the body initially by means of the superficial vessels, emphasis was placed on circulation through the linear pathways of all distribution vessels that serve the superficial regions. In the West, blood circulation is usually viewed in terms of the turnover rate of total blood volume circulation.

William Harvey's explanation of blood circulation in 1628 cannot be ignored or undervalued by the Chinese discovery. Harvey's verification of blood circulation is considered the greatest single event in Western medicine. His work was a brilliant experimental proof, which led to a new scientific exploration of medicine, and the consequent rejection of the flawed ideas of Hippocrates and Galen. When Chinese medicine was equated with the Greek ideas that Europe abandoned in light of Harvey's work, it is understandable that there was no rush to embrace what was seen as yet another "inscrutable and backward" medical approach. It is not clear that anyone in Europe either knew about or comprehended the significance of the Chinese blood circulation model before or even after Harvey's efforts.

The energy-meridian theory refers to blood and energy-qi flowing through the meridians in a particular circulation order. However, the context of the Chinese classic *NJLS 16* (*Nutrients*) only refers to the circulation of nutrients (ying) through the distribution vessels (Figure 10.2). The Chinese were aware that blood and vital air (qi) are circulated only in the vascular system. It is not physically possible to distribute blood and vital air (qi) via imaginary or invisible pathways in the body. To rationalize how blood circulates through invisible pathways, the energy-meridian theory makes the contention that Chinese blood is a dense material form of qi, and hence not real blood. But the blood of the ancient Chinese is the same as all blood in the twenty-first century (Figure 2.2). According to the Chinese, the vessels are connected to the heart, forming a continuous loop for blood circulation, like a ring without end, and the motive force of the heart circulates blood, nutrients, and vital air (qi). No one has explained what force circulates blood and energy in the imaginary meridians. If it involves the heart, then the vessels have to be involved.

The role of the heart in circulating blood is confirmed by the palpation of body pulses, which is used to diagnose ailments. According to the Chinese, pulses are only detected in arteries (Chapter 10). The pulse is the result of a pressure wave—created by contractions of the left ventricle of the heart—transmitting through the arterial blood vessels. Pulses can be palpated at certain superficial locations on vessels assigned to specific internal organs and nodal pathways. For example, pulses at the wrist are palpated at three locations, represented by nodes (acupoints) on the lung distribution vessel, which happens to be the radial artery. The node Renying (ST 9),[6] located on the stomach distribution vessel, is the site for palpating the carotid pulse. There are nine further areas on the body where pulses are palpated, and all of these involve arteries (Table 10.1). Many of the pulses are located on the so-called meridian pathways, which indicates that it is actually blood vessels that are involved.

Toward Understanding

Despite characterizing Chinese medicine as unexplained energy flow in meridians, practitioners can still be taught its effective application. However, meridians do not exist in any physical sense, and hence cannot be described by any known facts. Without facts, there is no possible way to evaluate the idea in terms of medical science. Void of a credible foundation, some practitioners have difficulty in achieving repeatable clinical results. Researchers are having trouble formulating protocols that demonstrate conclusively that acupuncture is any more effective than a placebo (Ceniceros and Brown: 1998; Ernst: 1998). Given this situation, it is partly understandable why the energy-meridian theory can be confused with metaphysical ideas. To some this leaves the impression that Chinese medicine and acupuncture represent a belief system, such as a religion (Breivik: 1998). Others have suggested that most United States acupuncturists "practice metaphysically explained 'meridian theory' acupuncture using needles to supposedly remove blockages of a hypothesized substance Qi" (Ulett, Han and Han: 1998).

Why does anyone care whether Chinese anatomy and physiology are explained as energy flowing through meridians, or by the circulation of blood, nutrients, other vital substances, and vital air (qi) through the vascular system? The answer to that lies in the moral obligation of every practitioner to provide each patient with the latest medical understanding available. The need to continually search for the truth is the most fundamental principle of science and medicine. If the functioning of the human body cannot be understood under normal physiological conditions, then there is little hope of knowing how to treat it when disease conditions exist. Research so far shows that the true concepts of Chinese medicine operate under known physiological principles, involving the complex organization of the neural, vascular, endocrine, visceral, and somatic systems, sustained by the circulation of nutrients, vital substances, and oxygen from vital air.

Inherent Problems with Energy Circulation

There is no question that people can subjectively feel energetic, or can experience a lack of vitality or energy; however, the idea of energy circulating in the body is clearly inaccurate. The word energy, meaning "in work," is an abstract concept, which per se cannot be circulated in anything. Some active process or work must take place for it to be expended. Propagated sensation induced along a nodal pathway may have been thought by some as being energy circulation, but this phenomenon is the result of neural activation. However, nutrients (ying) that supply the basic fuel for energetic processes of the body do have potential energy, and are considered by the Chinese to be the most critical of the substances circulated in the vessels. Other material substances that can be ignited to release heat have potential energy as well. Light can be radiated in the form of photons streaming from the sun to warm the earth, or heat can be radiated from a fire, but both of these examples are the result of energy being released due to some physical process. Sunlight is produced by nuclear fusion processes expending energy in the sun. Radiant heat from a fire is produced by burning a fuel in the presence of oxygen. Gasoline is another example of potential energy that needs to be pumped (circulated) to the automobile engine, mixed with air, then ignited with an electric spark to produce the explosive release of energy that makes the engine work. Electric power transmission lines, with electrons flowing back and forth, do not deliver electrical energy, although they do provide power in terms of potential energy. Energy is dissipated in the end-use appliance, such as in an electric motor, electric light, television, or computer connected to the electric potential supplied by the power line.

The bioenergetics of life on earth is one of the more subtle but profound processes that directly supports most life, especially that of plants, animals, and humans (Figure 6.5). For animals and humans this involves adenosine diphosphate (ADP) being converted to adenosine triphosphate (ATP) by the combustion of glucose derived from nutrients (ying), and oxygen from vital air (qi) in cellular mitochondria, with the consequent formation of water and release of carbon dioxide (CO_2). Characteristics of the energy-rich phosphate ATP fit the description of the Chinese concept of *zhen* (真), or true function (Chapter 8). ATP serves as a carrier of potential energy in all living organisms from bacteria, fungi, and plants to animals and humans. While fueling all energetic processes that support growth and function, including muscle, neural, and visceral activities in humans and animals, ATP reverts back to ADP, with the release of CO_2 and water. Meanwhile, plants and other organisms, that will later be consumed by animals and humans, utilize CO_2 and water through sunlight-induced photosynthesis to form the ATP that is needed to supply energy for growth and the formation of complex organic compounds, with the subsequent release of oxygen into the atmosphere. All human bioenergetic processes take place within individual cells of the body; energy is not circulated. Nutrients (ying), other vital substances, and oxygen from vital air (qi) circulating in the blood represent the potential energy needed to fuel the formation of ATP, which in turn serves as the cell's energy currency.

Improving Clinical Effectiveness

Crucial to any medical system is a rational explanation of health and disease, and a reliable clinical approach that is consistent with its physiological basis. This is true of the Western biomedical model where there is a consistency between disease and its treatment, explained in terms of modern pathophysiology, providing the etiology of the ailment is understood. Chinese physiological medicine, presented in subsequent chapters of this text, meets the standards of consistency between physiological theory and clinical practice. However, the Western energy-meridian explanation of Chinese medicine permeates most acupuncture training programs, and is fundamentally at odds with the physiological basis of both Chinese and Western medicine. Through a misunderstanding of the true basis of Chinese medical theories, it has been difficult to obtain consistent clinical and research results. Although acupuncture has been determined a safe and effective alternative medical therapy, researchers contend that this treatment modality requires more controlled research to understand its full range of clinical application (Ceniceros and Brown: 1998; Ernst 1998). Even though clinical practice produces excellent results, thirty years of active research using the energy-meridian model has failed to demonstrate unequivocally the effectiveness of acupuncture (Moroz: 1999). Many clinical studies of acupuncture have apparent methodological flaws (Zaslawski et. al.: 1997). Additional problems arise in trying to use "sham acupuncture" when its so-called energetic and biomedical effects are unknown (Ryan: 1999).

Reinventing Chinese Medicine and Acupuncture

Some practitioners of Chinese medicine and acupuncture become frustrated in their attempt to rationally comprehend terms such as acupoints, meridians, energies, qi, and yin-yang, which they think represent Chinese medical concepts (Fraust: 1998). A number of practitioners want to make a complete break with Chinese medical ideas and create a new and simplified approach that Fraust calls contemporary acupuncture. Others use the term medical acupuncture, to distinguish it from Chinese medicine (Helms: 1998; Filshie and White: 1998), although acupuncture is an obvious medical procedure. This is all well and good, except that the theories involving energy-meridians do not represent the original theories of Chinese medicine. Dr. Felix Mann, a pioneer in acupuncture and its scientific explanation, and a prolific writer, now realizes that after years of popularizing meridians, they in fact do not exist. He, too, is promoting the idea of reinventing acupuncture (Mann: 1992, 1998). Unquestionably, humans have a great capacity for reinventing; the only problem is that the valid theories of Chinese medicine first have to be understood. Reinventing acupuncture will eventually lead back to rediscovering the truth about what the ancient Chinese had previously discovered. This is the time to consider the advice of George Santayana (1863–1952), from his book *The Life of Reason* (five volumes, 1905–6): "Progress, far from consisting in change, depends on retentiveness. Those who cannot remember the past are condemned to repeat it."

Trying to summarize the principles of Chinese medicine before they are completely understood was a problem faced by ancient physicians as well. An example is provided in *NJLS 48* (*Obeying the Taboos*), where a physician named Leigong struggled to condense his medical knowledge acquired during training into useful treatment principles. The Yellow Emperor advises Leigong:

> Reducing medical information to basic principles is like collecting items in a bag. When the bag is full but not bound, the information spills out and is lost. When the study of medical materials is completed, but not summarized into principles, it cannot be applied to obtain marvelous results.
>
> Those who summarize medical knowledge before their bags are full, may think they are skilled physicians, but they cannot be considered teachers of anyone.

Variant forms of needling therapy, termed neural therapy, were considered in the 1920s in Germany by the brothers Ferdinand and Walter Huneke (1928). This approach involves the injection of local anesthetics into various locations on the body, and is still practiced with books illustrating the needling locations for treating various problems (Dosch: 1985). This therapy is used to treat chronic pain and illness by injecting anesthetics into scars, peripheral nerves, autonomic ganglia, trigger points, glands, and other tissues (Frank: 1999). Similar to acupuncture, treatments are based on normalizing dysfunction in the autonomic nervous system. The term trigger point was coined by Travell and Simons (1983) to describe sensitive points that spontaneously develop in relation to pain and musculoskeletal problems. The ancient Chinese called these sensitive areas *ahshi* (阿是), which literally means "oh yes!," the typical patient response when one of the sites is pressed. Travell and Simons also pioneered the injection of anesthetics and other methods, including stretching and spraying the skin with an evaporative coolant. Another form of trigger point therapy uses dry needles (acupuncture needles) and ischemic pressure, instead of injecting anesthetics (Baldry: 1989, 1993).

Understanding the Mechanisms of Action

Given the confusion that exists about acupuncture, there is clearly a need for understanding how it works in order to better discern its possible utility (Langevin and Villancourt: 1999). Needling therapy activates complex defensive mechanisms in the body, involving the immune system, tissue reactions, blood vessels, sensory nerves, somatovisceral pathways, autonomic nervous system (ANS), central nervous system (CNS), brain, and endocrine glands. These mechanisms involve the entire body, and cannot be demonstrated by any one single experiment. The same is true of the Western biomedical model, which is verified by the body of work that constitutes Western medical research. Consequently, any model depends on numerous experiments that deal with only one aspect of the overall scheme. This is also true with explaining the scientific mechanisms of action due to needling.

The process is complicated by the fact that inserting a needle almost anywhere in the body will produce some response. One of the areas of interest is to determine if there is anything unique about the nodes (acupoints) associated with the distribution vessels. The nature of the needling response depends on the method and strength of stimulating a node to bring about a desired effect. Eventually, descending control processes of the CNS mediate pain relief, relaxation of muscles, restoration of blood flow, and visceral normalization. This model is presented in Chapter 14, along with the latest research on specific elements of the model.

Genuine Theories of Chinese Medicine

The accomplishments of the ancient Chinese have not previously been examined in sufficient objective detail to validate the importance of their discoveries. Many of the problems relate to unintended gross mistranslation and misinterpretation. Translations of the ancient texts were typically very superficial, vague, and incomplete. But, a major part of the problem also involved the background of the early translators. Some were historians and religious people, while others were diplomats with no training in anatomy, physiology, or medicine. The *Internal Classic* or *Neijing* is basically a medical book. The *Lingshu* volume, which is one half of the total *Neijing,* contains most of the anatomical and physiological information. This material cannot be reliably translated without a good understanding of the human body. Also, it is important to understand the general concepts of Chinese medicine. Therefore, an iterative process is involved in trying to understand Chinese medicine while trying to correctly translate the material.

This book provides a fresh look at the ancient theories of Chinese medicine, and describes them using consistent and understandable terms in the English language. The primary goal is to present the true way (dao)[7] of Chinese medicine, and its important anatomical and physiological findings, along with its consistency with respect to the cause and treatment of disease. For those students and practitioners who were trained in the energy-meridian school, this book provides a physiological view that is consistent with what they have learned with respect to diagnosis and clinical applications. Their knowledge and experience base is still applicable. The information presented here will provide a greater understanding and appreciation of the ancient healing art of Chinese medicine.

The Chinese consider the *Neijing* the ultimate source book on the foundation of Chinese medicine—this classic is referenced throughout the text to clarify the fundamental theories and discoveries. Some 200 citations to 80 treatises of the *Neijing* provide detailed discussion of each important idea, thus freeing the reader from having to read the classic themselves. On the other hand, the citations do allow the reader to research a specific treatise if they are interested in studying the *Neijing* directly. Hopefully, sufficient information is provided that permits Chinese medicine to be examined in the same light as any other rational medical approach. This will provide an accurate basis for investigating and applying this ancient healing art to serve the needs of the public at large. No new theories are created or introduced. Where additional information is presented to provide understanding of the Chinese ideas, it is so noted.

2

Ancient Beginnings

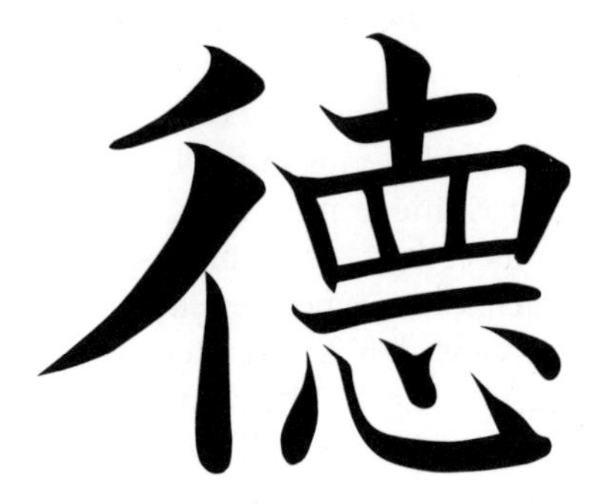

De: Virtue

> I have heard that the ancient teachers acquired precious knowledge that is not yet written down in books. I wish to hear about such theories and take them as current criteria by which to govern the people and to control the human body, and apply them to prevent disease for the common people, promote harmony among the classes, and spread the beneficence of virtue, so that our children and grandchildren are worry free, and pass on this knowledge to later generations without end.
>
> Yellow Emperor, *NJLS 29 (Knowledge Passed Down by the Masters)*

What is known as Chinese culture evolved along the Huang (Yellow) and Chang (Yangzi) River basins of central and south-central China. As the Stone Age Chinese people progressed they eventually developed agriculture, a written language, and a medical system to serve the needs of a civilized community. The first remnants of their recorded history date to around 3000 BCE. Important information was passed down by oral tradition, knotted cords similar to the Peruvian *quipos*, notched sticks, and primitive writing. The Chinese maintained a memory of their much earlier times, long before the founding period (3000–2200 BCE), when life was uncomplicated. The people then lived in harmony with nature (the dao). They were relatively free of disease, or at least disease could apparently be resolved by simple meditative techniques. As civilization began to develop it brought with it additional strains on life. A highly evolved society emerged by the end of founding period, bringing with it the full measure of physical and emotional stresses still apparent in the world today. Henceforth, it was necessary to understand details of human physiology, and how the body is adversely affected by internal and external forces, in order to effectively diagnose and treat the diseases of civilized people.

Out of the Stone Age

During the 2,700 years or so from the founding period to the end of the Zhou dynasty (221 BCE), China made incredible progress. The early founding period started with some groups still living in caves. By the end of the Zhou dynasty, China was a very sophisticated society, with an attendant evolution in medical ideas. Early beliefs involved the idea of evil spirits as the cause of disease, which was later replaced by accurate concepts consistent with a physiological basis of disease. The primitive Chinese expelled disease-causing spirits by pricking the skin with stone points to release blood. This practice was eventually substituted by a well-organized system of needling therapy using metal needles. Medical theories were passed down through the centuries by oral tradition and primitive writing. Written medical texts started appearing around 1300–800 BCE. The single most important text to be compiled in this period was the *Yellow Emperor's Internal Classic*, which may have been written during the later phases of the Zhou dynasty, and which established the entire framework of Chinese medicine (see Yellow Emperor's Internal Classic, page 25).

Need for a Written Language

As Chinese society became more complex, the development of a written language became increasingly necessary. This was especially true for recording medial theories, classifying diseases, and the diagnosis of ailments. Fu Xi (ca. 2953 BCE), first ruler of the founding period, and Huangdi (ca. 2697 BCE), or the Yellow Emperor, the third original ruler, along with the statesman Cang Jie (ca. 2700 BCE) are credited with developing the "tadpole figure" and "chicken tract" forms of pictographic writing. Primitive writing continued through the Xia dynasty (2100–1600 BCE), and character writing as presently recognized appeared during the Shang period (1751–1128 BCE). The Shang people inscribed characters on beautiful bronze castings to commemorate events or to dedicate a particular work to a specific person.

True character writing also appears on Shang oracle bones dating from 1300–1100 BCE. These writings consist of identifiable characters etched on tortoise shells and animal bones. Many of the pictographs and ideographs represent disease names and symptoms. Other characters indicate early classification of diseases by their location on the body. The use of characters in this way indicates that early Chinese writing may have derived from the need to diagnose ailments. The process involved etching characters on tortoise shells and bones to represent the disease symptoms of the patient. The bones and shells were then heated to produce cracks. Analysis of the cracks allowed the shaman to diagnose and treat the disease (Yu: 1983).

Underlying Principles

Certain fundamental principles of the universe were recognized long before the founding period of Chinese culture. These ideas became ingrained in Chinese thought. Thus, it is no surprise that these same concepts were later incorporated into the basic foundations of Chinese medicine: two significant ideas include the Zhou concept of virtue (*de*, 德),[1] and their view of vitality or spirit (*shen*, 神) (Chapter 7). However, three elementary concepts date back even further in history: the way (dao), qualities of opposition (yin and yang), and phases (*xing*, 行).

Dao, the way or the path, represents the laws of nature. These are basic principles which all phenomena, including human behavior, follow. The way is the principal feature of Daoist philosophy. The quality of opposing but interdependent forces of nature is described by the two Chinese adjectives, yin and yang (Chapter 4). The relative position of one item to another can also be described by these terms. Using the concept of oppositions to describe relationships permits a dynamic, rather than static, view of the world. This is extremely useful in describing the nature of certain diseases or even physiological processes. The phases (xing) represent sequential time-dependent relationships that are apparent in many processes (Chapter 6), such as annual climatic periods or growing seasons. Trees and plants also exhibit predictable phases or changes in their annual cycles. Living species experience logical phases of conception, birth, growth, maturing, reproducing, aging, and finally death. The idea of phases is a general concept that governs everything in the universe.

The early Chinese cultivated rice in the Chang (Yangzi) River basin and millet in the Huang (Yellow) River basin. Success in agriculture depended on a detailed knowledge of growing seasons. Thus, like other primitive societies, the people developed complex systems for predicting seasonal changes based on five climatic phases[2] and six dominant weather conditions[3] for each year. Five-phase relationships are applied to explaining other correspondences. Associations between things in specific categories, such as internal organs, body tissues, vitalities or spirits, emotions, and the flavors of foods and herbs, are typically viewed in terms of phases. Hence, examination of the five-phase relationships of diverse items, including disease-causing factors, transformation of diseases, and physiology, is fundamental to Chinese medical thought.

Emergence of the Zhou Dynasty

Several major tribes coexisted in central China during the founding period, with Fu Xi being the first of the five legendary rulers. Each tribe held sway over particular areas and each waged war on and captured slaves from the others. In 2100 BCE the Xia people established a ruling dynasty that lasted 500 years, following which the Shang tribe took over the leadership role. The Shang subsequently dominated central China for the next 600 years. The Zhou tribe, who had existed as far back as the founding period, overthrew the Shang in 1128 BCE. This was to be the most significant event in the early period: China entered its true golden age during the reign of the Zhou, during which time China evolved from a slave society to a feudal society. The Zhou dynasty is often viewed in terms of the Western Zhou (1128–770 BCE), Spring and Autumn (770–476 BCE), and the Warring States (475–221 BCE) periods.

Virtue of the Zhou

The Zhou believed that man's mortal and immortal destiny is dependent upon an individual's virtue (de), moral deeds, and personal effort. Destiny is neither dependent upon the idea of a soul before birth or after death, nor at the pleasure of some whimsical spiritual or mysterious force. Zhou leaders replaced Shang superstitions with the idea that the sky or heaven (*tian*, 天) represented the ultimate spiritual reality. The personal power of the rulers was considered to be the direct result of their human virtue and effort. The Shang had considered that their ancestors were directly associated with God, and therefore could be used as mediators to ask for favors from God. The Zhou had a very different view, respecting their ancestors based on their moral deeds and accomplishments while alive. Virtue is one of the main principles of the Daoist book, the *Dao De Jing* (*Classic on the Way and Virtue*), attributed to Laozi (ca. sixth century BCE).[4] Both virtue (de) and the way (dao) are important in the theories of Chinese medicine.

Golden Age of China

The Zhou concept of virtue freed their people from the superstitious dogma of the past, allowing individuals to be judged on their merits. Virtue provided the spark that resulted in the greatest developmental period in China's history. This effort rivaled, and in many ways exceeded, the accomplishments of the Greek golden age that occurred later. It was this philosophical transformation that gave rise to early scientific and medical developments. These ancient scientific efforts established the rational basis of Chinese medicine. Expanded thinking under the Zhou eventually led to their own downfall by enabling strong individual states to develop under the new philosophy.

Chinese culture experienced the greatest development during the Zhou period. Outstanding achievements occurred in astronomy, mathematics, engineering, science, and medicine. Important philosophical ideas were formalized during this time: two significant schools of thought included the Confucian doctrines of Kong Fuzi (551–479 BCE), and the Daoist principles of Laozi on the way and virtue. These philosophies continue to have a great influence on China. Daoist ideas are incorporated into the fundamental concepts of Chinese medicine.

The dominance of the Zhou declined during the waning years of their dynasty. Many powerful states, allowed to develop under the Zhou kings, struggled for control during the Warring States period. The state of Qin, under the leadership of Qin Shi Huang, conquered the other warring factions in 221 BCE, uniting them into a single country. The short-lived Qin dynasty collapsed in 207 BCE, some three years after the death of Qin Shi Huang, but the idea of a united country remained. The new country was named after the state of Qin, from which the name China is derived. Remnants of the Zhou dynasty disappeared and China never saw another period of such extraordinary development. Perhaps the greatest treasure of the Zhou dynasty was their medical system, which has been passed down through the centuries virtually unchanged.

Early Medical Concepts

Ancient people understood that food, water, and air were needed to sustain life. They also understood the critical importance of blood for humans and animals alike. Hence, air breathed in from the atmosphere, along with the absorbed essence of food and water that circulated in the blood, were appropriately regarded as fundamental to life and the maintenance of physiological balance. The gift of the ancient Chinese was to recognize that even a slight impairment in blood flow restricts the distribution of nutrients, defensive substances, vitality substances, and vital air. If not corrected this eventually results in pain, dysfunction, and disease.

Vital Substances from Food and Water

Food and water, usually referred to as water (*shui*, 水) and grains (*gu*, 谷), supply the raw material from which absorbed nutrients (*ying*, 营) and defensive substances (*wei*, 卫) are derived. Nutrients are needed for growth and to sustain the body, while defensive substances perform a protective and warming function (Chapter 8). These ideas are consistent with Western concepts. The liver, heart, spleen, lungs, and kidneys are thought to store refined substances of the spirit or vitality (*shenjing*, 神精) that circulate in the bloodstream. Organ vitality substances affect behavior and emotions, and are biologically active substances associated with each organ, which are now known to include hormones produced in the endocrine glands (Chapter 7) and other biologically active substances.

Vital Air from the Atmosphere

The Chinese character for air, *qi* (气), is pronounced "chee," as in the word cheetah. Originally the character was a pictograph showing heat waves rising from the ground or a heated surface (Figure 2.1). Later the character also indicated exhaled breath that can be seen on a cold day; thus the character qi became the breath radical, and is still used today as a written component for words associated with breath. Sometimes, qi is thought of as vital air, since it is now understood to include oxygen from atmospheric air. The ancient Chinese appreciated that vital air inhaled from the atmosphere was necessary to sustain life and for the utilization of nutrients, as noted in *NJSW 9* (*The Six Junctures and Manifestations of the Viscera*):

> The sky is the source of air [qi] for sustaining life. The earth is the source of the five flavors [herbs and food] for nourishing human life. The five airs are breathed in through the nose and stored in the lungs and heart. The flavors and vital air [qi] are distributed above [in the vessels] to reflect five colors [on the face] to provide a bright complexion. The fact that air is responsible for producing the sound of the voice is evident.

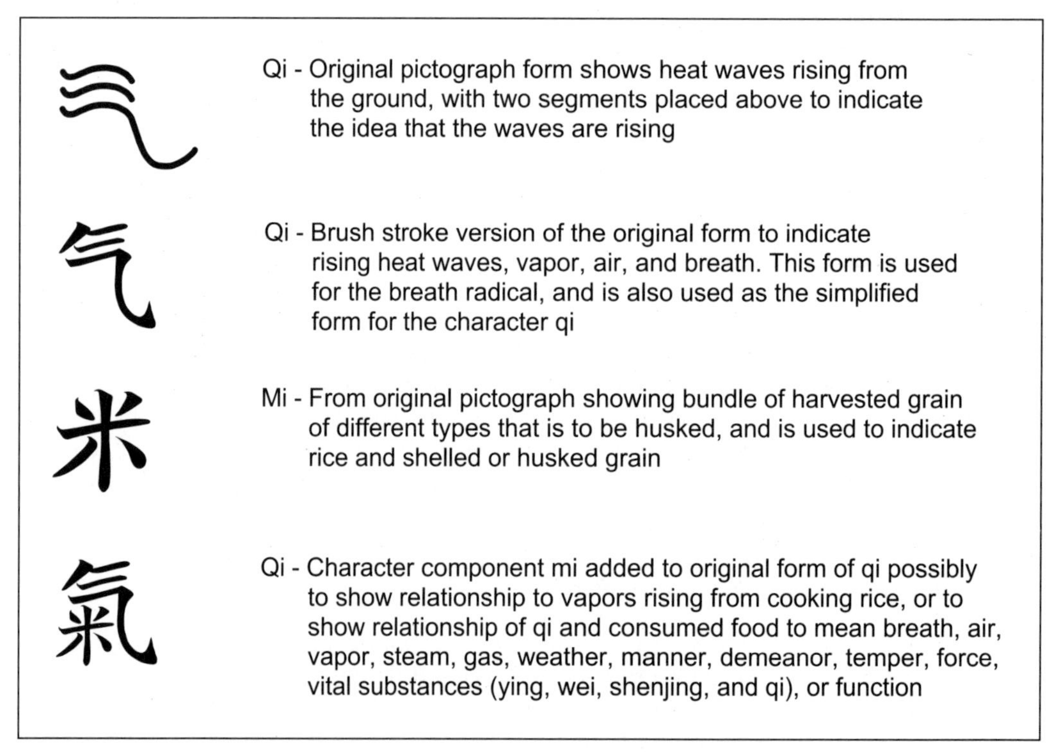

Figure 2.1 Derivation of the Chinese character *qi* used in Chinese medicine to denote air, vital air, and functional activity; also to refer collectively to nutrients (*ying*), defensive substances (*wei*), substances of vitality (*shenjing*), and vital air.

The earth's atmosphere is called *daqi* (大气), or big air. The ancient Chinese thought the atmosphere held up the earth. Weather or atmospheric conditions are also known as qi, and are called *tianqi* (天气), which means sky-airs. Air in automobile and bicycle tires is also called qi: the single character qi written on large signboards in China indicates where to get air to fill tires. Circulating nutrients, defensive substances, vitality substances, and vital air, collectively, are sometimes referred to as qi. A person's countenance or outward expression of vitality is also referred to as a reflection of one's qi, while functional activity, including organ function, can be referred to as qi as well.

The Role of Blood

Just as in other primitive cultures, the early Chinese performed blood sacrifices, or bloodletting of animals, and applied bloodletting in the treatment of humans. Interest in the effects of bloodletting led to detailed anatomical studies of the vascular system (Chapter 9). From this, the Chinese improved their understanding of the role of blood in circulating nutrients, immune substances, vitality substances, and vital air (Chapter 10). These efforts led to remarkable discoveries in physiology and of the mechanisms of human disease. Evidence for bloodletting is provided by the character *xue* (血), for blood (Figure 2.2). The original pictographic representation shows a small, wide-lipped, three-legged vessel used for collecting blood, containing a substance. In this case a horizontal line is used to denote blood in the container. The modern brushstroke form of xue still conveys this idea. These wide-lipped sacrificial vessels were originally made of clay, suggesting that the practice of bloodletting goes back to the earliest periods. During the Shang period these vessels were crafted in bronze.

Concepts of Excess and Deficiency

One of the more subtle but critically important Chinese ideas was the recognition that external environmental forces are always present, and have a potential adverse effect when excessive.

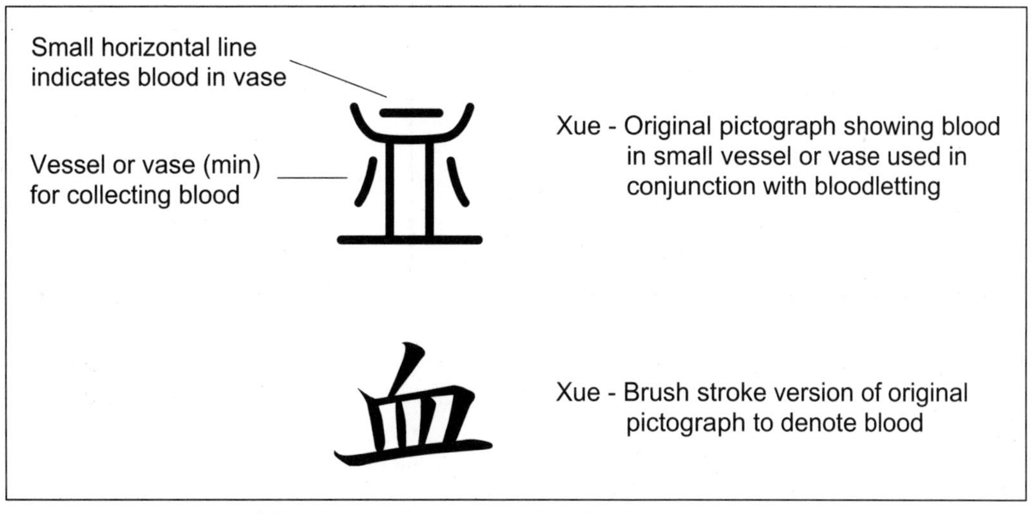

Figure 2.2 Derivation of the Chinese character *xue* for blood.

A state of health exists when physiological balance (*zheng*, 正), or internal homeostatic function, is near its optimum and the external environment (*xie*, 邪) is within a range that permits normal response without inducing ailments (Figure 2.3A). When external forces are excessive, as may occur with exposure to extreme cold or other agents that result in a fever or ailment, the body will mount a defensive reaction. Internal homeostasis in this situation is normal, and a strong antipathogenic response is provoked to defend against the external assault. This is defined as a solid (*shi*, 实) or excess condition (Figure 2.3B). When internal homeostasis is below its optimum level, either due to long-term external exposure or internal conditions, including emotional factors, a situation can result known as a hollow (*xu*, 虚) condition or deficiency, even though the external exposure is within normal range (Figure 2.3C). Internal problems are often the result of impaired blood flow, resulting in a deficient distribution of nutrients, immune substances, vital air, or biologically active substances of vitality.

Medicine as a Rational System

By the time writing evolved, Chinese medicine seems to have already attained a high level of refinement and its use was widespread. This is illustrated by a biography of a famous fifth century BCE physician, contained in the *Records of the Historian*, by Si Ma Qian (145–86 BCE), written in 100 BCE The physician was named Bian Que, and he specialized in herbs and acupuncture. Among many of his achievements is credit for reviving a provincial governor's

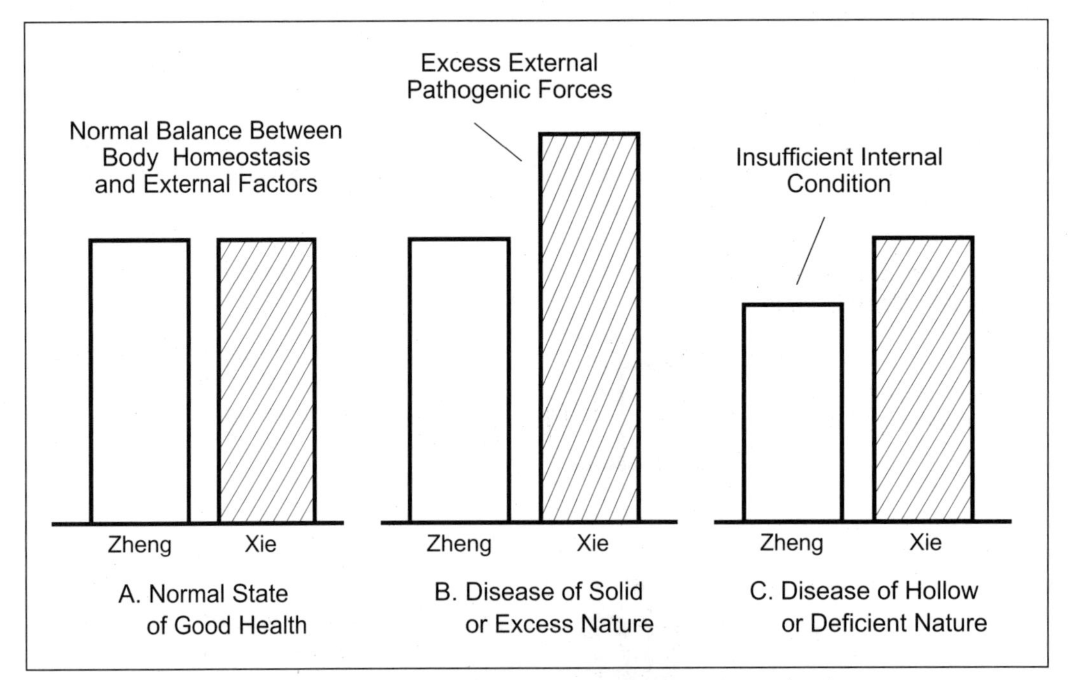

Figure 2.3 Fundamental Chinese concept of disease involving the relationship between physiological balance (homeostasis or *zheng*) and the external environment (*xie*), illustrating: A, normal health; B, excess disorder; and C, deficiency disorder.

son who had apparently died suddenly. Bian Que heard about the boy's death while traveling through the state of Guo. He came upon a group of people standing outside a palace weeping, crying, and making sacrifices. After asking about the circumstances of the death he sought permission to examine the boy, including palpation of the body and pulse diagnosis. He decided that the boy was possibly in a coma and announced that the "death" might be reversible. He proceeded to revive the young man with the application of acupuncture. After the use of moxibustion the boy could sit up, and he fully recovered after being treated with herbal medicines for the next twenty days. Bian Que's fame was so great that after his death he was known as the God of Medicine. Stone monuments and a temple were built in his honor near his hometown (Chuang: 1978). Several physicians over the next following centuries also used the name Bian Que, perhaps for fame or recognition.

Healing Herbs and Arrows as Medicine

Herbalism and needling therapy are an intrinsic part of Chinese medicine. Even the ancient character *yi* (医), meaning medicine or cure, is an ideograph illustrating both ideas. The top half of the primitive form depicts a quiver full of arrows (Figure 2.4). Next to that, another component indicates the right hand, above which is a representation of a bird's wing to denote the idea of the hand making a quick action. Such would be the case in pulling back a bowstring and releasing an arrow. This conveys the notion of shooting arrows to release the harmful influences that cause disease (Wieger: 1965).

The lower half of the character shows a vessel or amphora for the decoction and storage of an herbal remedy. Combining these two components results in the complete ideograph for

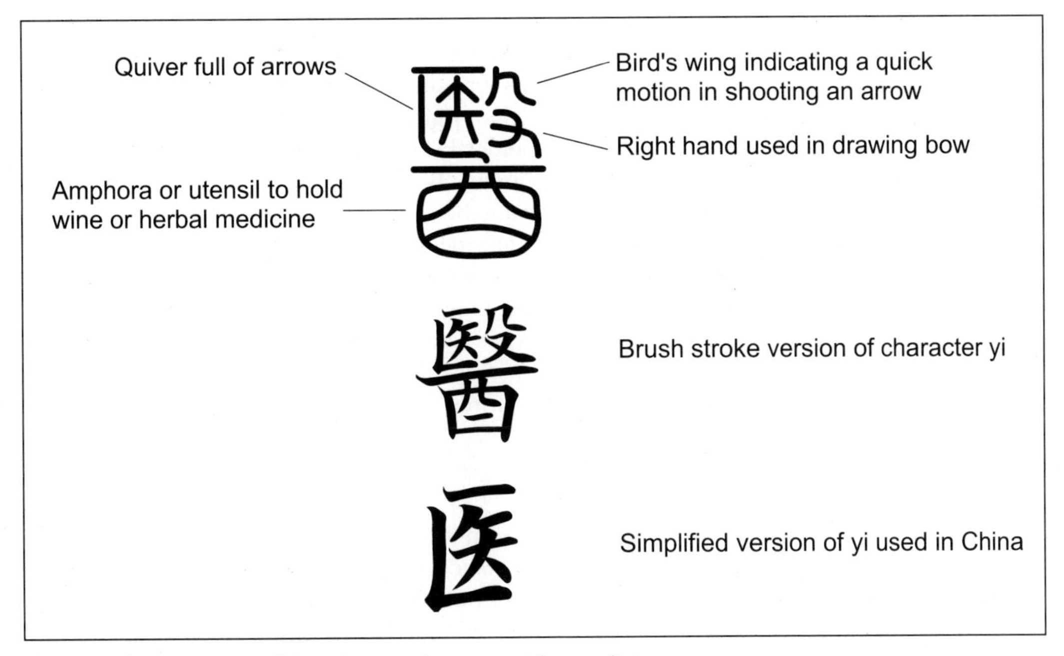

Figure 2.4 Derivation of the Chinese character *yi* for medicine or cure.

medicine or cure. The character conveys the idea of treating illness by using herbs to strengthen the body and needling therapy to restore balance. The lower component of yi is the character currently used to denote wine (*jiu*, 酒). This may be consistent with the onetime practice of the ancient Chinese, especially the Shang people, of using wine as medicine (Chapter 5). Wine is still used today as an important means of preparing some herbal remedies.

With the invention of the writing brush, the character for yi took on its modern form, which is consistent with the original form. However, Mainland China has simplified the character yi to show only the original quiver containing the modern character for arrow.

First to be Needled

No one really knows how far back in prehistory it was first noticed that pain or disease could be relieved by pricking superficial body regions. One could speculate that needling therapy derived as a result of accidental encounters with thorns or barbs. After such an event, someone may have felt relief from a previously painful condition. Also, it is possible that primitive people, out of the sheer frustration of dealing with pain, may have intentionally jabbed themselves with sharp objects. The Stone Age Chinese were hunters and warring tribes who had considerable awareness of injuries, wounds, and bleeding, especially due to encounters with sharp, pointed projectiles.

These early observations led to the concept that piercing the body with small sharp objects, to liberate a few drops of blood, was beneficial. Releasing a small amount of blood dispersed the pain and disease-causing bad spirits or adverse environmental influences. This was a common belief among many primitive cultures, even to present times. But it was the Stone Age Chinese who developed the practice of pricking and puncturing the skin into a useful medical approach. Node locations (acupoints) are stimulated to bring about reactions that are directed to specific superficial or internal areas of the body (Chapters 14 and 15). This is the physiological basis of utilizing certain locations to treat different ailments or pain conditions.

Smaller versions of the sharp projectile points for hunting were fashioned by the Chinese. These stone points, or *bian* (砭), were used as the original devices for therapeutic bleeding. Bian stones could only be used to prick the superficial skin. They were too large and crude to be inserted into the body without significant injury. Bian points were also used to reduce abscesses and boils, and to massage areas between the muscles. The true practice of inserting needles into the body did not actually occur until metal needles appeared. This happened perhaps as early as 800 BCE. Few clues exist as to why the practice of bleeding points was mostly replaced by the insertion of fine needles. One comment is provided in *NJLS 1* (*Nine Needles and Twelve Sources*) on possible concerns over the safety of stone projectiles. It is also noted that better control over restoring blood distribution is achieved by the practice of inserting fine metal needles than by using bian stones.

Treatment Approaches

All diseases known to affect the human population are classed in terms of solid or hollow conditions. Thus, the main principle of treatment is to either drain off (*xie*, 泻), or reduce an excess, or to mend (*bu*, 补), or strengthen a deficiency. On the surface this may seem oversimplified—however, the challenge to the skilled practitioner of Chinese medicine lies in the complexities of determining the cause of the problem: which internal organ is affected;

the possible impairment of blood, nutrients, immune substances, vital air, or biologically active substances; or whether the problem is due to impaired functional activity.

Herbs and needling are employed to drain off or clear excess heat, and can be employed to reduce an excess functional condition. Herbs, needling, and heat (either moxibustion or heat packs) are used to warm a cold condition. The three principal treatment approaches—herbs, needling, and heat—are used to mend blood, promote circulation, strengthen vital substances, or restore functional balance. Dietary approaches are also employed to address internal organ problems, excess conditions, and deficiency disorders. Food is also used to strengthen the body and to counteract the effects of overconsumption of certain flavors (Chapter 6).

Celebrated Texts

Most of what forms the present understanding of Chinese medicine comes from ancient Chinese texts, many of which were compiled between 600 and 300 BCE, when ancient Chinese science reached its developmental epoch. Unfortunately, many early books have been lost over the centuries. The most devastating loss occurred immediately after the Zhou dynasty, during the reign of Qin Shi Huang, the first major ruler in history to systematically burn books on a massive scale. Happily, a few surviving copies of the key texts have provided sufficient detail to preserve the basic source material.

During the Zhou dynasty, the court housed a major library containing many books. At one time, Laozi himself, who is thought to have written the Daoist classic, was in charge of these great archives. Many books were written on bamboo slips and bound together with leather strips; some were written on silk. Four major encyclopedic works were compiled by a number of individuals, although they were jointly attributed to the Yellow Emperor, known respectively as the *Upper Classic* (*Shangjing*), *Lower Classic* (*Xiajing*), *External Classic* (*Waijing*), and *Internal Classic* (*Neijing*) *of the Yellow Emperor.* These classic volumes contained a collection of the latest cumulative information of their time. One or two copies of the *Internal Classic,* which deals with Chinese medicine, have survived. The *Upper* and *Lower Classics* are now lost. In 1973, a Han-dynasty tomb located in Mawangdui, China, dated to April 4, 168 BCE, yielded one copy of the *External Classic.* This book has yet to be translated into English. Many other books are known to have existed during the Zhou period, since reference is made to them in surviving books.

Yellow Emperor's Internal Classic

The most outstanding of the surviving ancient medical works is the *Yellow Emperor's Internal Classic* (*Huangdi Neijing*), compiled sometime between 600 and 300 BCE. This classic is commonly referred to simply as the *Neijing,* the pinyin transliteration of its name in Chinese. Most of the basic ideas of physiology and medicine are contained in this incredible text: it provides surprisingly accurate and detailed information on the human body, with some of the ideas clearly equivalent to those of modern Western physiology. It is written in a condensed and archaic style of dialogues between the Yellow Emperor and his physicians, the main one being his chief physician and teacher, Qibo. The *Neijing* is divided into two volumes: the *Suwen* (*Common Conversations*), and the *Zhenjing* (*Classic on Needling*). Later, in 762, this second volume was renamed the *Lingshu.*

The *Neijing* is based on the Daoist philosophy of virtue (de) and the natural way (dao). The underlying theme for maintaining health is to live a balanced life consistent with the virtues of humankind and the laws of nature. The main concern is to live in accordance with the changes in seasons and subsequent environmental and climatic conditions. A balanced lifestyle, in terms of dietary intake and habits, as well as minimizing emotional stress and strain, is also viewed as essential.

The first historic reference to the *Neijing* was provided in the *Annals of the Former Han Dynasty* (206 BCE–25 CE), where it was noted to contain eighteen scrolls. Zhang Zhongjing (150–219) mentions the *Neijing* in his classic book on treatment of diseases due to cold (see Treatise on Diseases due to Cold, page 29). During the Jin dynasty (265–419), Huang Fumi refers to the *Neijing* in his own classic on Chinese medicine, *Jia Yi Jing*. At that time the *Neijing* was still acknowledged to consist of eighteen scrolls, equally divided into the *Suwen* and the *Zhenjing*. The *Annals of the Sui Dynasty* (581–618) lists the *Neijing Suwen* as containing only eight scrolls. Then in 762, during the Tang dynasty, an individual named Wang Ping was presented with a nearly intact copy of the complete *Neijing*.

Wang Ping set about restoring parts of the *Neijing* using material from other surviving texts at the time. He also deleted obvious duplications and added some characters to improve the text. In addition, Wang Ping and others that followed wrote comments, separate from the *Neijing* text, to help clarify some of the seemingly vague passages. Unfortunately, many of the comments do little to help explain some of the characters in the original texts. Wang Ping renamed the *Zhenjing* volume the *Lingshu*, which is often translated as miraculous pivot. However, Wang Ping's intended meaning in using the characters *Lingshu* may have been to classify this volume as the comprehensive treatise on physiology and needling. The characters (*ling*, 灵 and *shu*, 枢) are more appropriately translated as center of knowledge, or hub of brightness. Wang Ping also divided both volumes into eighty-one treatises or sections. Two of these from the *Suwen* could not be restored and are considered permanently lost. These are *NJSW 72* and *NJSW 73*, respectively entitled *On the Method of Needle Insertion* and *On the Origin of Diseases*. Fortunately most of the information from the lost chapters is repeated in the *Lingshu* volume.

Wang Ping's annotated version is the most common edition currently available. Concern has been expressed that he and others altered the *Neijing* over the years to bring it more in line with contemporary thinking. The consistency of the theories, however, indicates that the original concepts are intact. These cannot be measurably altered without destroying the integrity of the whole text. It seems that Wang Ping's contribution was truly to restore the original copy and to clarify the text by appending interpretations in the Chinese of that period. (For more details of Wang Ping's efforts, see Veith: 1949, Introduction: *Analysis of the Huang Ti Nei Ching Su Wen*, plus Appendices I, II, and III to that chapter.)

Possibly by the time of the Tang dynasty (618–907), it had already been forgotten that Chinese medicine had a rational physiological basis. Knowledge gained through postmortem examinations during the Zhou period may not have been fully understood. One of the problems contributing to the lack of continuity with earlier times is the *Neijing* itself, which was written as the final authority on Chinese medicine. Thus, further or continued research was no longer considered necessary, since the fundamental tasks were already completed. After a period of time, the classics took on a certain reverence, and the idea of altering the content or adding new information was out of the question. To understand this way of thinking one only has to imagine the problems that would be involved in adding more information to the *Dao De Jing* of Laozi. Even today, many devotees of Chinese medicine consider every word in the *Neijing* to be absolutely correct.

The *Neijing* covers anatomy, physiology, pathology, medicine, diagnostic techniques (including pulse diagnosis), treatment modalities, herbal medicine, and needling therapy. For this reason it is sometimes called the *Classic on Internal Medicine.* The *Neijing* also contains the first-known herbal formulas. This key text presents a complete medical system based on the theory of main distribution vessels and their collateral branches for the continuous circulation of blood, nutrients, defensive substances, vital air, and refined substances of vitality.

References to other classics on needling and pulse diagnosis are cited in the *Neijing,* giving a hint that once there were even older documents. The *Upper* and *Lower Classics* are mentioned as well. The discovery of silk manuscripts in 1973 dealing with needling, moxibustion, and pulse diagnosis confirms that other medical writings did exist. These may have actually preceded the *Neijing,* or at least existed during the same period (see Mawangdui Texts, page 28).

The *Neijing* is written in a very condensed, concise manner typical of the literary style of ancient times. The writing style may be thought of as a form of shorthand, and for this reason, some consider it next to impossible to accurately translate into English. Another point to note is that throughout the *Neijing,* one or two specific characters are used to add a certain balance or rhythm to some of the sentences, suggesting that it was originally composed in verse, which would have made it easier to commit to memory. The use of verse was indispensable in ancient times when information was handed down orally from one generation to the next before formal texts were compiled. A similar tradition was involved with the ancient Greek classics, including Homer's *Iliad,* where stories were memorized as verse and passed down from the time of the Trojan war until the Greeks invented their system of writing.

Ten Rhijne (1683) mentioned Chinese and Japanese practitioners who possessed copies of the *Neijing,* which they guarded jealously and which they did not allow him to examine. Other early Europeans exposed to Chinese medicine may not have been aware of the *Neijing.* No serious attempt was made to translate it into English until Ilza Veith undertook the task in 1949. Her excellent effort, eventually published by the University of California Press (Veith: 1949), only covered the first thirty-four treatises of the *Suwen.* Unfortunately, this left forty-seven remaining in the *Suwen,* along with the entire *Lingshu* volume, containing another eighty-one treatises, to be translated. The *Lingshu* is the more technical of the two volumes, and contains most of the anatomical and physiological information.

Veith's translation nevertheless correctly identified qi as referring to air that is circulated with blood in the vascular system. She uses the term vessel, and never mentions the word meridian nor energy. Since the character for vessel (*mai,* 脉) is also used to mean pulse, she does incorrectly identify some named vessels as pulses. Veith also incorrectly assumes that all collateral vessels are veins.

To illustrate how many Western translators have failed to accord the *Neijing* its proper weight in the understanding of Chinese medicine, one translator of the *Suwen* concluded that *NJSW 19* (*Inscriptions on the Jade Astronomical Instrument and True Visceral Function*) alone was sufficient to explain all the main ideas of Chinese medicine (Dawson: 1925).

Classic on the Difficulties

The *Classic on the Difficulties* (*Nanjing*) is thought to have been written later than the *Neijing*, perhaps between 403 and 221 BCE. Some scholars, however, think that it first appeared around 100 CE, or even later. The *Nanjing* is a companion volume to the *Neijing*, providing further clarification of the principal features or difficult topics contained in the *Neijing*. Its authorship is unknown, but it is often attributed to several people, including Qin Yue Ren, who lived around 255 BCE. This person also used the name Bian Que—perhaps in a laudatory sense. Not surprisingly, the *Nanjing* provides elucidation on eighty-one specific topics or questions. The inclusion of precisely eighty-one numbered difficulties may indicate that the writing of this text occurred much later than thought, or that it was revised and numbered later.

Mawangdui Texts

An incredible treasure of ancient silk manuscripts and some text on bamboo slips was recovered in 1973 from a Han-dynasty tomb, dating to 168 BCE, in Mawangdui in a suburb of Changsha, Hunan Province, China. The find comprises some fifty different medical books. Included are four books entitled: *Zu Bi Shi Yi Mai Jiu Jing* (*Eleven Vessels for Moxibustion of the Arms and Legs*); *Yin Yang Shi Yi Mai Jiu Jing* (*The Yin-Yang System of Moxibustion for the Eleven Vessels*); *Mai Fa* (*Methods of Taking the Pulse*); and *Yin Yang Zheng Hou* (*Symptoms of Yin and Yang Pulse Patterns*). The content of these books suggest that they might be forerunners of the *Neijing*. One possible clue to their antiquity is that they describe only eleven main distribution vessels, whereas the *Neijing* contains the complete system of twelve vessels. The early manuscripts from Mawangdui indicate the initial use of naming vessels by their appropriate area of the body in the yin-yang classification system (Chapter 4).

Some forty-four pieces of silk, annotated and illustrated with drawings of male and female human figures, were also recovered in this tomb. These are instructions for *daoyin* (导引) or guided stretching exercises involving breathing techniques (*qigong*, 气功). Qigong (*qi*, 气, meaning breath, and *gong*, 功, exercise) is a Daoist therapeutic breathing practice. Some of the daoyin exercises show the *wuqinxi* (五禽戏) movements, or five animals at play, representing the tiger, bird, monkey, deer, and bear.

Two copies of the *Dao De Jing*, the primary Daoist classic attributed to Laozi, were also recovered from the same tomb. Indications are that one copy of this book was made prior to the reign of Emperor Liu Pang (206–194 BCE), and the other copied during his reign (Hendricks: 1989). Perhaps noteworthy is that neither text is divided into eighty-one verses as presently found in later copies. Furthermore the virtue (de) half of the book precedes the chapters on the way (dao), in contrast to the organization of later copies.

Early Herbal Texts

Key books were also written about Chinese herbal medicine during the time that needling therapy progressed through its great developmental phase. Early texts other than the *Neijing* mention the use of natural remedies derived from vegetable, animal, and mineral sources. These texts include the *Shi Jing* (*Book of Odes*) (ca. fifth century BCE) and the *Shan Hai Jing* (*Classic of Mountains and Rivers*) (ca. 400–250 BCE), which contained a total of 120 herbal remedies (Hsu and Peacher: 1981; Cai: 1983). The first true Chinese materia medica appeared during the second century BCE, entitled *Shen Nong Ben Cao Jing* (*Materia Medica of Shen Nong*), which deals with 365 different medical remedies.

Treatise on Diseases due to Cold

One of the more important early medical books attributed to a specific author was written by Zhang Zhongjing (150–219), originally known as the *Treatise on Febrile Diseases Caused by Cold and Miscellaneous Diseases.* It was later reedited during the Western Jin (265–316) and the Song (960–1279) dynasties into two separate books: the *Treatise on Febrile Diseases Caused by Cold* (*Shang Han Lun*) (Hsu and Peacher: 1981; Luo and Shi: 1986), and the *Synopsis of Prescriptions of the Golden Chamber* (*Jin Gui Yao Lue Fang Lun*) (Luo: 1987). Zhang's original work contained more than 300 detailed medical prescriptions carefully organized for specific diseases. These herbal formulas are the forerunners of subsequent prescriptions. Zhang formalized diagnostic techniques used in the *Neijing* and used the "four methods": examination, auscultation, inquiry, and pulse feeling. He also developed the rudimentary concept of applying the "eight keys" of the *Neijing* to analyzing the nature of disease, namely yin and yang qualities, internal and external factors, heat or cold, and deficiency or excess (Chapter 13). These are called the eight conditions, or eight principles.

3

Early Understanding of Physiology

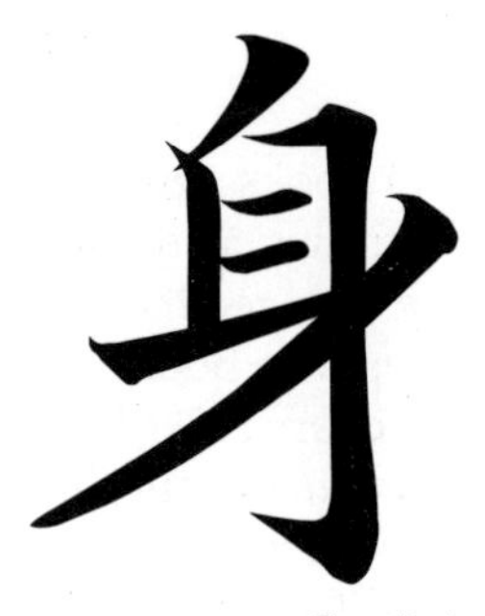

Shen: Body

> I have heard that the sages of ancient times understood the logic of the human body and classified and differentiated the viscera and bowels. They also understood the principles of collateral and distribution vessels.
>
> Yellow Emperor,
> *NJSW 5 (Great Treatise on the Proper Representation of Yin and Yang)*

Early medical concepts and superstitions of the founding and Shang periods gave way to rational studies by the middle of the Zhou dynasty. These efforts distinguished fine details of anatomy, physiology, and disease processes. All the main internal organs were correctly identified, and organ pathology was viewed on a physiological, rather than empirical, basis. Another significant observation of the ancient Chinese involved the organization of the body. When viewing a standing subject it is obvious that, for the most part, major vessels, muscles, peripheral nerves, and propagated sensation (PS) pathways are distributed up and down the body longitudinally. From this the specifics of somatovisceral relationships, referred pain, and sensitive locations were determined. Recognizing the importance of this physiological feature is the true genius of the early Chinese physicians. Chinese treatment approaches incorporate this longitudinal organization. This results in a systematic treatment approach to stimulating the superficial body to bring about a highly directed and controlled restorative response (Chapters 14 and 15). It is now understood that longitudinal functional relationships, noted by the Chinese, are related to how the spinal cord is organized in terms of spinal afferent processes.

Many early books were lost after the fall of the Zhou dynasty, so the full extent of ancient Chinese medical knowledge is unknown. The Mawangdui texts (Chapter 2) may provide additional insight into Chinese anatomical knowledge, but these documents have yet to be examined in detail. Consequently, the *Neijing*, and to a lesser extent the *Nanjing*, are the main sources of information on Chinese medical concepts. Key features of this anatomical and physiological information are presented in this and subsequent chapters. Ancient Chinese physicians recorded measurements of the body, skeleton, viscera, and gastrointestinal tract. They identified the protective tissue membrane that surrounds the heart (pericardium), and also the internal membrane system (*sanjiao*, 三焦) that surrounds and protects the other internal organs. Given the methods and techniques of measurement that were employed, it may seem surprising that the data is essentially consistent with twenty-first century findings.

Anatomical drawings date back to the Han dynasty (206 BCE–220 CE), and show the detailed arrangement of the internal organs within the body cavities (Cowdry: 1921a, 1921b; Veith: 1949). Drawings of individual internal organs and bowels are clearly identifiable (Figure 3.1). Other drawings illustrate the body's distribution vessel pathways, nodal (acupoint) pathways, and site locations for the application of moxibustion. It has been suggested by some that these drawings somehow found their way to China from the West, but the character and style of the drawings are typically Chinese. There are Chinese records that indicate anatomical dissection studies were performed, and the results were recorded by means of sketches and illustrations.

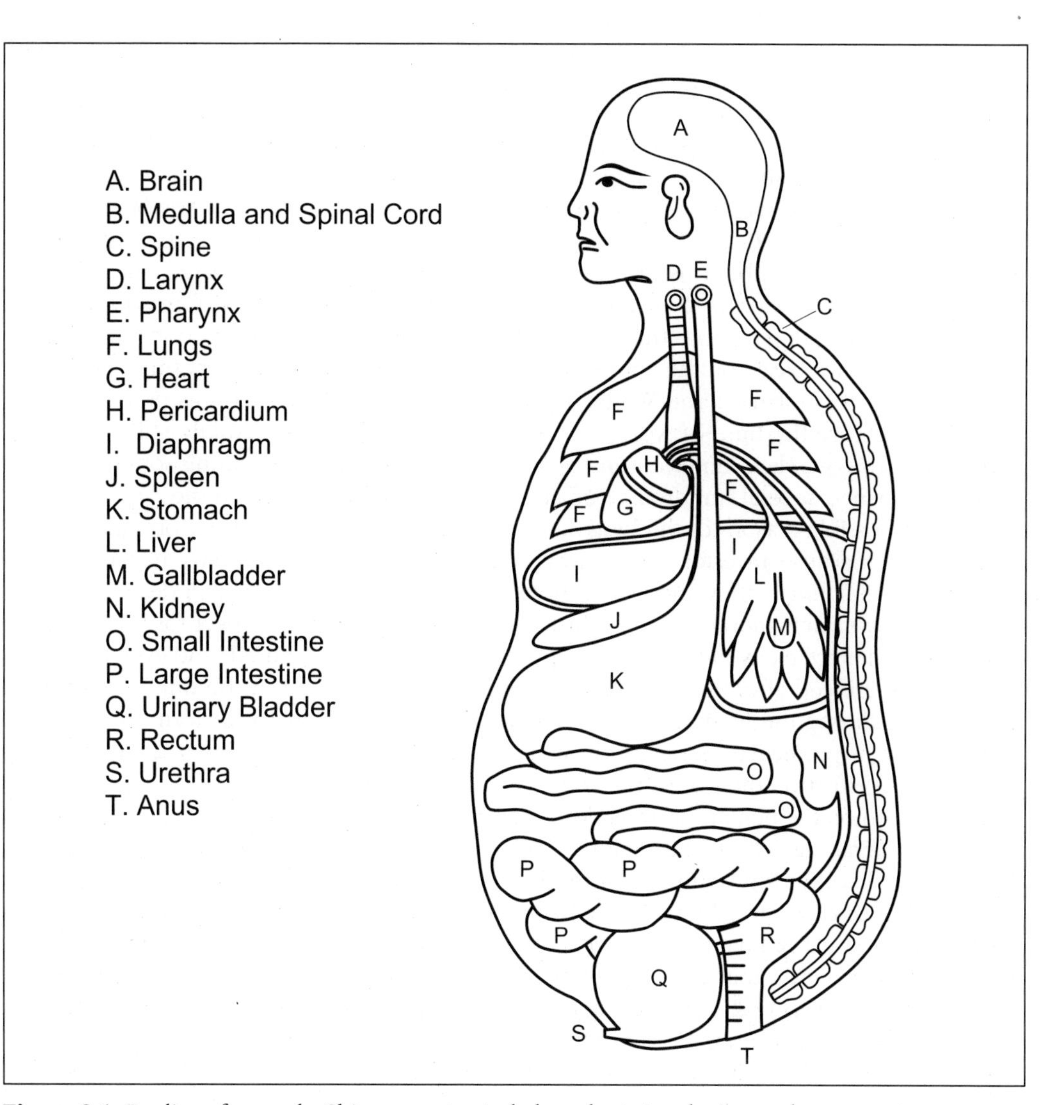

Figure 3.1 Replica of an early Chinese anatomical chart depicting the internal organs.

Postmortem Studies

An understanding of human body morphology can only be obtained by postmortem examination. In this effort, the ancient Egyptians were early innovators. Preparing the deceased for the afterlife by removing the internal organs and mummifying the body was prevalent in Egypt for many centuries. This practice may have led to a profound comprehension of the body and development of a sophisticated medical system. According to the Egyptian priest-historian Manetho (ca. 300 BCE), the third king of the first dynasty, Djer (Athothis or Teta) (ca. 3000 BCE), practiced medicine and compiled a papyrus on anatomy. No evidence of this work presently exists; the important extant papyri on ancient Egyptian medicine date from about 1800 to 1200 BCE (Nunn: 1996). This information suggests that the Egyptians were slightly ahead of the Chinese, and perhaps a thousand years ahead of the ancient Greeks. One of the main differences between the ancient Chinese and Egyptians is that the Chinese undertook postmortem examinations specifically as a means of understanding the cause of death and to gather information about the human body, while the Egyptians perhaps only inadvertently acquired anatomical information through the embalming and mummification process.

The Egyptian contribution to anatomical science and medicine is partially acknowledged by medical historians, while the efforts of the ancient Greeks, especially Aristotle (384–322 BCE) and Galen (ca. 130–200 CE), are considered paramount. However, the anatomical investigations and contributions of the ancient Chinese have basically been ignored; some Western medical historians have even contended that the Chinese never performed anatomical studies. It is interesting to note that this fact is still doubted by some experts, an incorrect assumption perhaps based on the impression that Confucian beliefs did not permit postmortem autopsy (Veith: 1949; Huard and Wong: 1968). However, it is likely that this practice was in vogue long before the time of Kong Fuzi (551–479 BCE), and was actually still in practice during his lifetime. In later times autopsies may have been prohibited during some dynasties, but this happened several hundred years after the initial studies noted in the *Neijing*.

Another possible reason for thinking that the ancient Chinese did not perform autopsies is the belief that, because ancestor worship was common, the Chinese must have had a particular reverence for the human body and would therefore not violate its integrity after death. However, even a cursory examination of Chinese history reveals no particular respect for human life in ancient times. In fact, many of the feudal emperors frequently had hundreds and even thousands of subjects sacrificed after building their secret burial chambers or at the time of their own deaths. Also, during the many internal wars, a common tactic was to stack up the enemies' bodies to use as protective barriers from which to carry on the battle. This had a devastating psychological effect on the opposing side.

Information on the human body as described in the *Neijing* can only be obtained by direct observation. Tracing out all the major blood vessels in the body, for example, including vessels to and within the brain, including nerves and vessels supplying the eyes (*NJLS 21: Cold and Hot Diseases*, and *NJLS 80: On Major Puzzlements*), cannot be accomplished by any intellectual construct or imaginative speculation. Descriptions of the internal organs, including their weight, size, and capacity, along with their functions, likewise cannot be ascertained by observing the external body. Describing the arteries separately from the veins, and indicating which vessels contain more blood than air, or vice versa, is only feasible if the body is dissected. Given all this, it is not surprising that the *Neijing* itself contains details on postmortem dissection and even refers to standard procedures for its accomplishment.

Standard Procedure for Autopsy

Postmortem dissection was described in 2697 BCE (Wang: 1926), and procedures for conducting such a study is referenced in *NJLS 12* (*The Distribution Rivers*):

> With regards to a person, even eight-Chinese-feet tall,[1] they can be examined by a trained practitioner providing that the skin and flesh are still intact. Externally the body can be completely measured in accordance with established standards. In case of death, a dissection study can be performed to examine the condition of the internal organs to determine the firmness or fragility of the viscera, and the size of the bowels and contents of the digestive system. The length of the vessels can be measured, and whether the blood is either clear or deep and thick. The total air content of the body can be determined, as well as the ratio of blood to air in the twelve longitudinal distribution vessels. It can also be determined if the body contains considerable blood and air, or if there is a lesser amount of both. Quantitative measurements can be derived for all of these parameters.

During the Han dynasty, Emperor Wang Mang (ca. 6–24) ordered his physicians to dissect the body of a captured revolutionary. Measurements were made of his internal organs, and the length and route of the vessels were measured by the insertion of fine bamboo rods. According to Wang Chi Min (1926), many such records are described in the ancient literature. One study was conducted in 1045 with drawings made to illustrate the anatomical details (Miyakawa: 1996). These studies were later augmented by the efforts of Yang Jei, between 1102 and 1106. After the Japanese were exposed to Western medicine by the Dutch physician ten Rhijne, some Japanese practitioners wanted to learn more about the human body. Additional anatomical information was also obtained from the Portuguese and Spanish. In 1754, Yamawaki Toyo conducted the first Japanese dissection study (Yeo and Hwang: 1994). Twenty years later (1774), Sukita Kenpaku translated a Western anatomy book into classical Chinese.

Anatomical Understanding from Earlier Times

Many anatomical details are provided throughout the *Neijing*, with one reference indicating that a comprehensive knowledge of anatomy possibly existed before the *Neijing* was written. This clue is provided in *NJSW 5* (*Great Treatise on the Proper Representation of Yin and Yang*):

> I have heard that the sages of ancient times understood the logic of the human body and classified and differentiated the viscera and bowels. They also understood the principles of collateral and distribution vessels and noted the six confluences between deep and superficial vessels. They discovered and named the sites for needling, determined the distribution of muscles and their attachments to the bones, as well as the origins of these muscles, and also identified the skin zones. They understood the upstream [venous] and downstream [arterial] flow in the vessels and their proper order of circulation. They appreciated the relationship of the four seasons and their yin and yang characteristics, and how to manage their extremes. They understood the agreement of the external environment and the internal body and all the superficial and deep [somatovisceral] relationships.

Skeletal and Body Measurements

The ancient Chinese attempted to standardize body measurements, and also devised an anatomical orientation reference using the Chinese adjectives yin and yang to describe the external and internal body regions (Chapter 4). During the Zhou period, the Chinese value for an inch (*cun*, 寸)[1] was taken as the width of the thumb, and the character for cun is a pictographic representation of the thumb. The English inch is also taken as the width of the thumb, or the length of three barely corns placed end to end. The difference between the two values is about 10 percent, with 1 cun equal to 0.902 inches (2.30 centimeters). A Chinese foot (*chi*, 尺) is made up of 10 cun, and 10 Chinese feet amounts to one measure called a *zhang* (丈). In setting the standard for human measurement, the average height was taken as 75 cun (or 5 feet 6 inches in U.S. equivalent). However, a significant number of people are either taller or shorter than this average value. An individual's height could be measured in absolute terms, and consequently could be more or less than 75 cun tall. Thus, in order to derive a standard, the Chinese developed a system whereby measurements of the body were derived from relative measurements for each particular person.

System of Body Measurements

As the size and shape of every human body is different, locations, lengths, and spacing are measured in proportional terms. The use of relative measurements is essential to locating nodal sites. Nodes are referenced to recognizable anatomical features in each individual. Sites exist at unique locations mainly due to the arrangement of bones and muscles, and the distribution of blood vessels and nerves.

Features related to node locations are relatively consistent between individuals, with only rare exceptions. The only differences have to do with size. A tall person, for example, will have longer leg and arm bones than a small or short individual. But the number of nodes located on the extremities is the same for each person, although there will be a variation in the relative spacing of these sites. By using a relative inch measurement, based on some anatomical feature in each individual, then distances and lengths have standard values. Thus, the standard length of the arm, measured from the elbow to the wrist crease, is 12 cun (relative value), regardless of the actual measurement compared to a fixed standard.

Measurements are calculated by determining the length of the Chinese body inch (cun) for an individual, and then using this value to locate critical features and nodes. The body cun is taken as either the width of the individual's thumb, or the length of the second phalanx of their index finger. The width of a person's four fingers, on one hand, provides a standard measurement of 3 cun. Certain features on the body, such as bone lengths or spacing between joints or regions, are assigned fixed relative values. For example, the distance between the nipples on the chest is considered to be 8 cun, and the distance from the top of the pubic bone to the navel is fixed at 5 cun. Other relative measurement values were established for all the major anatomical features (Table 3.1).

Table 3.1 Detailed measurements of the human skeleton, from *NJLS 14* (*Bone Measurements*).

Body Measurement	*Cun*	*Inches*[4]
Girth of head	26	23.5
Girth of chest	45	40.6
Girth of waist	42	37.9
Anterior to posterior hairline (over top of head)	12	10.8
Anterior hairline to lower edge of jaw	10	9
Posterior hairline to lower edge of jaw	22	19.8
Between two mastoid processes	9	8.1
Between two regions in front of tragus, Tinggong (SI 19)	13	11.7
Distance between zygomas	7	6.3
Laryngeal prominence to line connecting Quepen (ST 12)	4	3.6
From line connecting Quepen (ST 12) to xiphoid process	9[1]	8.1
Distance between two nipples	9.5	8.6
Xiphoid process to umbilicus	8[2]	7.2
Umbilicus to pubic symphysis	6.5[3]	5.9
Distance between two sides of pubic bone	6.5	5.9
Upper edge of pubis symphysis to medial condyle of femur	18	16.2
Medial condyle of femur to below medial condyle of tibia	3.5	3.2
Lower edge medial condyle of tibia to medial malleolus	13	11.7
Medial malleolus to ground	3	2.7
Midpoint of popliteal fossa and upper edge of heel tuberosity	16	14.4
Upper edge of heel tuberosity to ground	3	2.7
Frontal eminence of forehead to atlas (cervical vertebrae, C1)	10	9
C1 to head of axilla transverse crease (which is hidden)	4	3.6
Axilla to hypochondrium	12	10.8
Hypochondrium to greater trochanter	6	5.4
Trochanter to lateral midpoint of patella	19	17.1
Medial edge of thigh to front of thigh	6.5	5.9
Lateral midpoint of patella to lateral malleolus	16	14.4
Lateral malleolus to tuberosity of fifth metatarsal	3	2.7
Tuberosity of fifth metatarsal to ground	1	0.9
Posterior edge of heel to tip of second toe	12	10.8

1. If shorter, then lungs are smaller; if greater, lungs are bigger.
2. If longer, then stomach is larger; if shorter, then stomach is smaller.
3. If longer, the ileum (Chinese) is wider and longer; if shorter, then ileum is narrower and shorter.
4. Approximate value using 1 cun = 0.902 inches, or 2.30 centimeters.

Skeletal Measurements

Detailed measurements and relative spacing of all bones (*gu*, 骨) in the body are provided in *NJLS 14* (*Bone Measurements*) (Table 3.1). These measurements are also based on a person being 75 cun tall. The accurate measurement of bones could have been obtained from old skeletal remains, and not necessarily from dissection studies. However, the other anatomical information involving organs, vessels, body tissues, and fluids noted in the *Neijing* could only have been obtained by observation of fresh cadavers.

Function and Classification of Internal Organs

All the major organs were identified by the early Chinese. The principal viscera, including the heart, lungs, liver, kidneys, and spleen, are critical for the distribution and dispersion of nutrients, whereas the bowels and intestines perform the important role of digestion and elimination. Internal organs in Chinese medicine are grouped into five discrete functional systems. Each viscus is assigned certain physical, physiological, and emotional attributes, and each is matched with a particular bowel (Table 3.2). The paired viscera and bowels are also thought to relate in terms of interior and exterior relationships. In this case, interior refers to the internal organs, including the brain, while exterior refers to the body (soma), including all the muscles and superficial regions. In modern nomenclature, interior and exterior associations are termed viscerosomatic relationships. Interior and exterior relationships are important to mechanisms of disease, as well as to treatment approaches.

Chinese physiology also views interactions between the organ systems with respect to the five-phase geophysical model (Figure 3.2). Some of the relationships that involve one organ's ability to either act upon (victorious mode) or counteract (insulting mode) another organ are

Table 3.2 Assignment of internal organ concordances with respect to the five earth phases.

Viscera (Zang)	*Liver*	*Heart*	*Spleen*	*Lungs*	*Kidneys*
Bowel (*Fu*)	Gallbladder	Small Intestine	Stomach	Large Intestine	Bladder
Internal Membrane		*Sanjiao*[1] and Pericardium[2]			
Tissue	Muscles[3]	Vessels	Flesh	Skin and Hair	Bones
Body Fluid	Tears	Sweat	Saliva	Mucus	Urine
Offensive Odor	Perspiration or Odor of Urine	Burnt	Sweet Smelling	Fishy	Putrid
Orifice	Eye	Ear	Mouth	Nose	Anus and Urethra
Sense Organ	Eye	Tongue	Mouth	Nose	Ear
Sense	Sight	Speech	Taste	Smell	Hearing
Vitality	Mood	Overall Vitality	Intent	Vigor	Drive
Emotion	Anger	Joy	Pensiveness	Grief and Worry	Fear and Fright
Endocrine Gland[4]	Pineal	Pituitary	Pancreas	Thyroid	Adrenal
Earth Phase	Wood	Fire	Soil	Metal	Water

1. *Sanjiao* refers to the internal membrane system surrounding the organs in the thoracic, abdominal, and lower abdominal cavities, excluding the pericardium.
2. Protective membrane surrounding the heart.
3. The Chinese character *jin*, for muscle, has typically and incorrectly been translated as tendon.
4. Inferred assignment based on the functional characteristics, vitalities, and emotions attributed to each organ system.

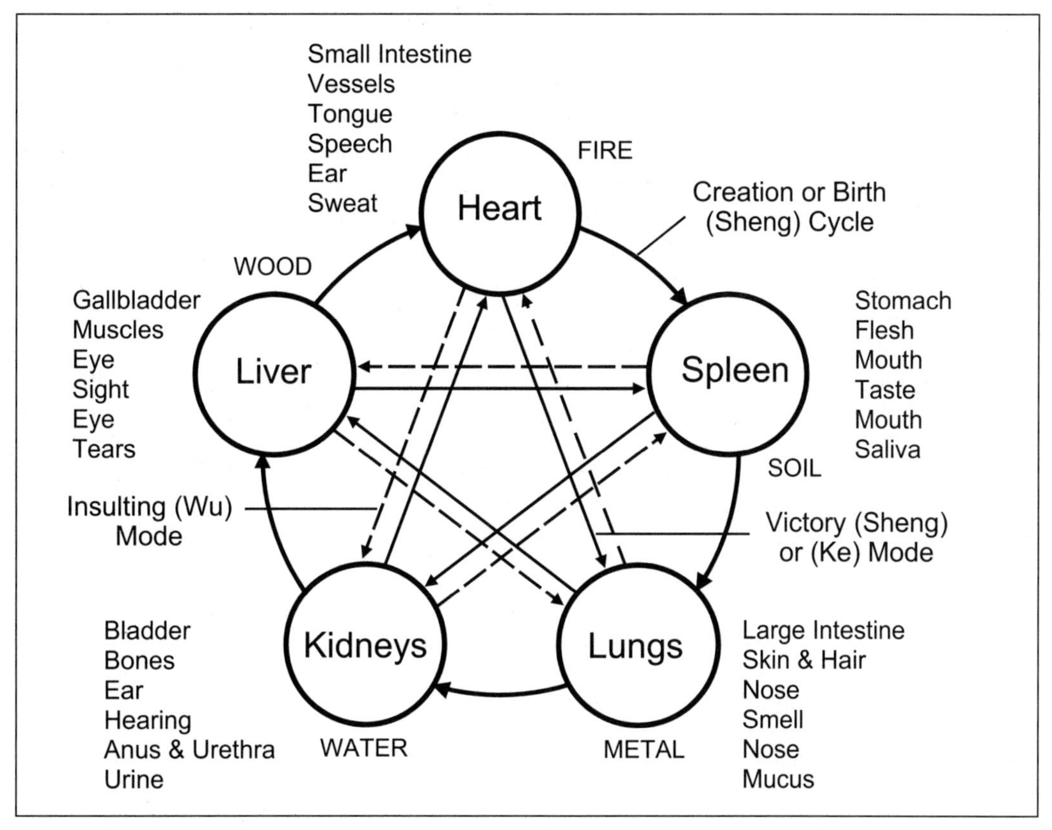

Figure 3.2 Five-phase relationships between the internal organs, indicating the nourishing (*sheng*), victorious/controlling (*sheng/ke*), and insulting (*wu*) modes, with each related bowel, dominant tissue, sense organ, sense, body orifice, and body fluid.

a matter of common sense (Chapter 6). This is true with respect to overconsumption of certain flavored foods and herbs, organ vitalities, and emotions. However, relationships involving the creation or mother-son cycle, where one organ is thought to influence the next organ, are not so apparent. Each viscera is thought to be preferentially nourished by one of the five flavors during fetal development, which gives rise to the initial creation cycle, as summarized in *NJSW 67* (*Motion of the Five Phases*):

> The sour flavor gives birth to the liver, which in turn creates muscles, and muscles then create the heart... Bitter flavor gives birth to the heart, which in turn creates blood, and blood then creates the spleen... Sweet flavor gives birth to the spleen, which in turn creates flesh, and flesh creates the lungs... Pungent flavor gives birth to the lungs, which in turn creates skin and hair, and skin and hair give birth to the kidneys... Salty flavor gives birth to the kidneys, which in turn create bones, and bones gives birth to the liver.

While the ancient understanding of the internal organs is similar to modern understanding, there are important differences involving assigned functional responsibilities for each organ

(Table 3.3). Viewing the internal organs in terms of physiological features provides a consistent model for describing organ and body functions and pathology. A summary of the main visceral functions follows: the heart provides the motive force for blood circulation; lungs breathe in air from the atmosphere and exhale respiratory gases; the liver is responsible for metabolic processing and dispersing nutrients; kidneys filter metabolic waste products from the blood through the formation of urine; and the spleen is responsible for lymphatic, immune, and blood coagulation functions. In addition, the stomach, spleen, and bowels break down food, absorb nutrients, and eliminate waste products. Organ functional activity is also expressed in terms of visceral qi, which is further described by yin and yang attributes.

Except for the spleen, the classification of these functions is consistent with Western physiology. No spleen-related metabolic functions are recognized in the Western view of spleen physiology; however, the Chinese assigned role of the spleen in processing nutrients does correlate well with pancreatic function. Functional activities attributed to the spleen, with respect to the immune and lymphatic systems, are consistent with Western understanding. The Chinese also consider the spleen responsible for keeping blood circulating within the vessels, which is now known to be mediated by a vast array of complex plasma proteins involved in controlling the blood coagulation system.

Table 3.3 Functional responsibilities assigned to each internal organ in Chinese medicine.

Internal Organ	*Traditional Responsibilities*
Lungs	Controls vital air and respiration, dominates the pores, manifests in the skin and body hair, promotes circulation of vital air, regulates the passage of water (due to their relationship with the kidneys), and opens into the nose.
Large Intestine	Reception and elimination of waste material, and absorbtion of fluids from it.
Spleen/Pancreas	Governs digestion, keeps blood in circulation, dominates muscle tissue, is the prime organ of immune function, opens into the mouth, and manifests on the lips and corners of the mouth.
Stomach	Reception and breakdown of food.
Heart	Controls blood circulation, dominates all other organs, manifests on the face, houses the mind, is the seat of overall vitality, and opens into the tongue.
Small Intestine	Reception and digestion of food, and nutrient absorption.
Kidneys	Dominates development and reproduction, stores refined substances, controls water metabolism, assists in receiving vital air, dominates bones and teeth, manifests in hair on the head, opens into the ears, and dominates lower body orifices.
Bladder	Temporarily stores urine.
Liver	Disperses nutrients, stores blood, maintains functional activity, dominates muscles (including tendons and fascia), manifests in the nails, and opens into the eyes.
Gallbladder	Stores and excretes bile as an aid to digestion.

Pairing of Viscera and Bowels

Correlating human physiology with the five earth phase geophysical model constrained the grouping of the internal organs into five discrete functional systems. Pairing each viscus with a related bowel was based on examination of the internal organs. A close anatomical and physiological relationship is obvious between the liver and gallbladder. An anatomical and functional relationship between the kidneys and the urinary bladder is also noted. Hence, the liver was paired with the gallbladder, and the kidneys were paired with the urinary bladder. Matching the remaining viscera and bowels is not as obvious.

The early Chinese understood the stomach's role in the initial process of breaking down ingested food. The spleen lies against the left lateral posterior aspect of the stomach, while the pancreas lies between the stomach and the spleen, and shares certain blood vessels with the spleen. The pancreas also connects with the intestinal tract at the output of the stomach. Because of the intimate anatomical association of the spleen, stomach, and pancreas, the spleen and stomach were paired. Pancreatic functions were included in the spleen-stomach organ system, without clearly identifying the pancreas on an anatomical basis. Pairing the spleen with the stomach results in the spleen having both metabolic and immune system functions. Recognizing that the pancreas is included with the spleen is crucially important, since it provides a clue to what was known about the other endocrine glands.

The digestive role of the small intestine was understood by the early Chinese, who correctly identified the veins of the small intestine as the means of absorbing nutrients into the bloodstream. One major difference from the Western view is that the Chinese only included the duodenum and jejunum in their description of the small intestine. The heart is responsible for circulating blood, and the greatest number of arterial vessels supply the small intestine (heart distribution vessels). Hence, the heart was paired with the small intestine.

All the bowels are considered exterior organs since they are part of the alimentary canal that communicates with the exterior via the mouth and anus. The only exception is the bladder, which communicates directly to the outside by means of the urethra. The viscera are considered to be interior organs since they do not communicate with the outside world, except for the lungs, which communicate via the nostrils. Skin is considered dominated by the lungs. The large intestine also communicates with the skin at the anus. This results in the lungs being paired with the large intestine. It is interesting to note that the anus is called the door of vigor and is responsible for passing on the incoming flavors as flatulence. Vigor (*po*, 魄) belongs to the lungs. Perhaps the passing of gas by the large intestine during physical exertion or exercise, which is commonly observed in many animals, was viewed by the ancient Chinese as a corollary to lung function.

Classification of Viscera and Bowels

The heart, lungs, liver, kidneys, and spleen are classified as solid organs. Each is capable of maintaining a store of specific refined substances of vitality (*shenjing*, 神精) unique to each organ. Because of this long-term storage capability, the viscera are named *zang* (藏), which means to hide, conceal, or hoard, and also means storehouse. The main function of the solid organs is to process and distribute blood.

The Chinese designated the bowels by the character *fu* (府), which means treasury or storehouse. But, here the concept is short-term storage, since the items normally found in the storehouse or treasury are constantly moving in and out. The six treasures of ancient times consisted of wood, fire, metal, water, soil, and grain. Thus, the stomach and the intestines are also considered the storehouse or treasury of water and grains. Bowels associated with each viscus are hollow organs incapable of storage for long periods, and because of this short-term storage capability are called fu organs. Bowels include the stomach, small intestine, large intestine, internal membrane system[2] (sanjiao), and bladder. The gallbladder stores bile for long periods and therefore is considered to be an extraordinary[3] or singular fu organ. The fu organs mostly function by breaking down food and eliminating waste products. The nature of fu and special fu organs is described in *NJSW 11* (*On the Differentiation of the Five Viscera*):

> The brain, medulla and spinal cord, bones, vessels, gallbladder, and uterus are six organs generated by the earth's environment. Similar to the earth, they all store substances and have the capacity for storing and not draining off. They are called extraordinary persevering storehouses.
>
> With respect to the stomach, large intestine, small intestine, internal membrane system [sanjiao], and urinary bladder, these five organs are generated from atmospheric forces. Their function is similar to the sky in that they drain off and do not store. They gather the foul odor of the five viscera, and are called the transmitting and transforming [digestive] bowels. Their contents do not remain for long and are transported to be drained off. The anus [door of vigor] is employed by the five viscera so that water and grains [food] do not remain in storage for long.
>
> The five viscera store refined substances but do not drain off, therefore they can be full but not oversupplied. The six bowels are for transmitting and transforming things without storing, therefore, they can be oversupplied but not filled to capacity.

The bowels, including the visceral peritoneum (sanjiao), also have a critical role in maintaining blood volume and body fluids. The following is noted in *NJLS 47* (*Root of the Viscera*):

> The six bowels are the organs that transform water and grains into useful nutrients, and facilitate the flow of body fluids.

The sanjiao refers to the internal membrane system of the body, including the pleura, as well as the parietal and visceral peritoneum of the abdominal cavities. Because the visceral peritoneum surrounds the intestines and other organs, it is thought of as a bowel and is referred to as a fu organ. The sanjiao relates to the internal organ membrane system of the thorax and abdominal and lower abdominal cavities. The membrane that acts as a yin counterpart to the sanjiao (classed as a yang fu organ) is the pericardium that surrounds the heart, which is itself not considered to be a true organ. Both the pericardium and the internal membrane system (sanjiao) are similar in that they both consist of membrane tissue. Since the pericardium is associated with the heart, and the largest part of the visceral peritoneum (middle *jiao*) is associated with the small intestine, they are both assigned to fire in the five earth phase arrangement. The five viscera, six bowels, and the pericardium make up the twelve main internal organs and are collectively referred to as the *zangfu* (脏腑) (Table 3.2).

Nutrient Absorption by Small Intestine Vessels

Surprisingly detailed information is provided in *NJLS 81* (*Carbuncle*) describing the branching of small intestine vessels, starting with the capillaries, as the means of absorbing nutrients into the venous bloodstream:

> The intestines and stomach receive food, and the organs of the thoracic cavity [lungs and heart] distribute vital substances [nutrients, *ying* (营); defensive substances, *wei* (卫); vital air, *qi* (气)] to warm up the striated muscles, nourish the bones and joints, and facilitate function of the pores. Organs of the abdominal cavity [spleen, stomach, small intestines] distribute nutrients that are like distilled fluids that flow above into the rivers of deep valleys, oozing and seeping into the small intestine capillaries and venules [*sunmai*, 孙脉]. When the thin and thick fluids are harmoniously mixed, they are changed and transformed to make the blood red. The harmonious blood first overflows to fill the capillaries and venules, and then flows into the collateral veins, which all overflow into the distribution vessel [portal vein].

Differentiation of the Intestines

Strong evidence is provided that the Chinese performed detailed examination of the intestines and their associated collateral vessels. This is born out by the way they differentiated between the small and large intestines. By considering the vessel patterns that supply these organs they were able to discern the functional roles of the intestines. The small intestine was believed to comprise only the duodenum and the jejunum, while the large intestine included the ileum and what the Chinese called the wide intestine. The Chinese definition of the ileum consists of the same small intestine region as in Western anatomy, but also includes part of the large intestine. This resulted in the Chinese assigning the cecum, ascending colon, and the right half of the transverse colon to the ileum. The wide intestine is identified to include the left half of the transverse colon, descending colon, sigmoid colon, rectum, and anus. The reason for this seemingly strange classification of the intestines becomes clear when viewing the network patterns of the distribution vessels supplying the gut.

The jejunum is provided with a dense supply of collateral vessels (jejunals) from the superior mesenteric artery. The ileum, cecum, ascending colon, and right half of the transverse colon, which together constitute the ileum as defined by the Chinese, are also supplied by the superior mesenteric artery. However, the collateral vessels (ileals, ileocolic, right colic, and middle colic) supplying the Chinese ileum are much fewer. The Chinese wide intestine is supplied by collaterals of the inferior mesenteric artery.

The ileum absorbs nutrients, water, and other substances, and the wide intestine principally absorbs water. Because of these unique anatomical and physiological features, the Chinese considered the small intestine to dominate digestion, liquids, and juices, and the large intestine (Chinese ileum and wide intestine) to dominate body fluids.

All descriptions of the small and large intestines in the *Neijing* consist of the small intestine, ileum, and wide intestine. When referring to the large intestine, it is assumed that it includes the ileum and wide intestine. Early drawings of the large intestine show it with its sixteen bends and curves, incorporating the Chinese ileum and the wide intestine as described in the *Neijing*. The transition between the jejunum and the ileum is not distinguishable by any anatomical features of the intestine itself, except for differences in the density of blood vessel supply patterns. Nevertheless, the Chinese identified a specific location for this region, naming it the pass-door (*guanmen*, 关门). Drawings of the large intestine show it to begin with the guanmen and end with the anus. One bilateral nodal site (ST 22) located on the abdomen, 3 cun above the navel and 2 cun on each side of the centerline, is named after the guanmen transition region. This location is used to treat conditions such as abdominal distension, anorexia, diarrhea, and edema.

Reality of the Sanjiao

The pleural and peritoneal membrane tissues (*jiao*, 焦) are viewed in terms of the three (*san*, 三) divisions of the body cavities (Figure 3.3). These include the thoracic (upper jiao), abdominal (middle jiao), and lower abdominal (lower jiao) regions, collectively called sanjiao in Chinese. Major portions of this system are the serous membranes that enfold the lungs in the thorax and invest the organs in the abdominal cavity, separately from the pericardium. Peritoneum membranes form mesenteries with the abdominal organs that hold and support the numerous vessels and nerves supplying these organs, and are important to water transport and the function of digestive organs. When viewing the interconnected alimentary organs the visceral peritoneum forms a protective tube surrounding the esophagus, stomach, small intestine, and large intestine. This tube-like arrangement was identified by the early Chinese as an external hollow organ, responsible for water transport and influencing the digestive process. Reference to these ideas is made in *NJLS 2* (*Origin of Communication Sites*) and in the *Nanjing* (*Difficulty 38: Regarding the Five Viscera and the Six Bowels*), respectively:

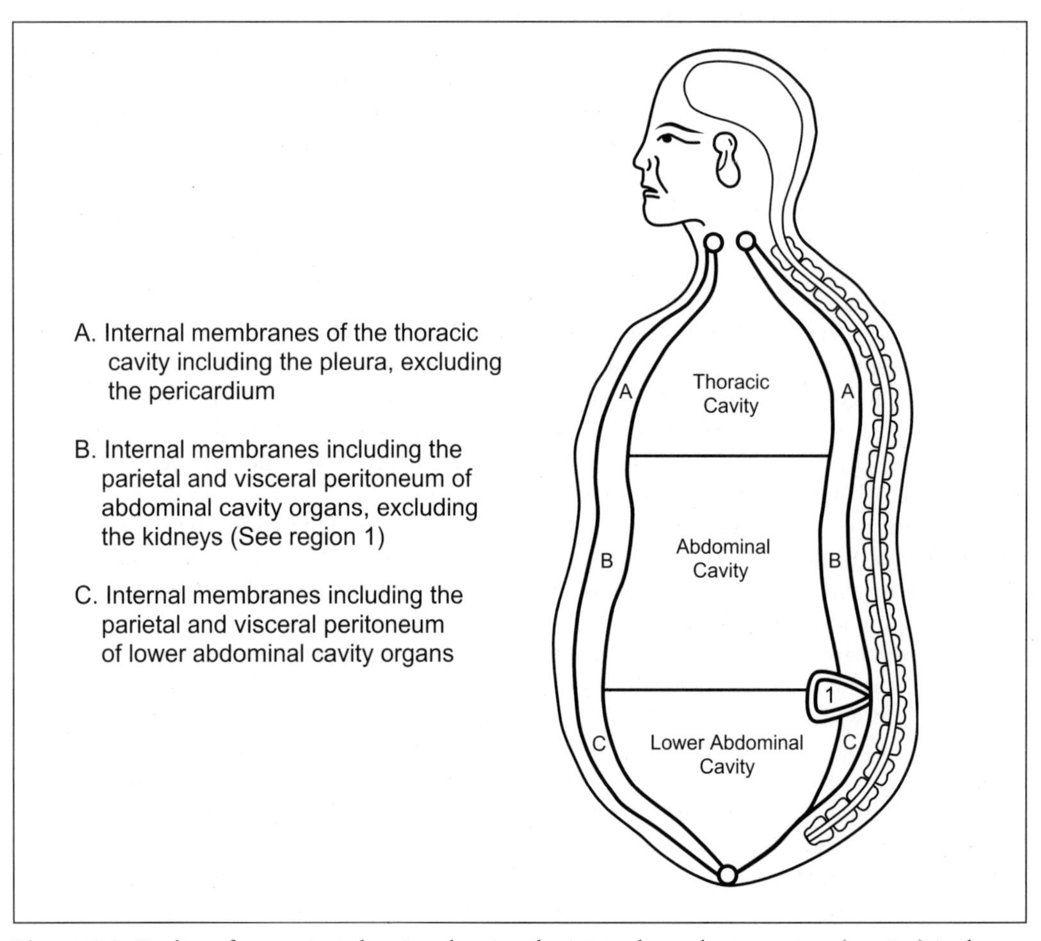

Figure 3.3 Replica of an ancient drawing showing the internal membrane system (*sanjiao*) in the thoracic, abdominal, and lower abdominal cavities (*shangjiao*, *zhongjiao*, and *xiajiao*).

> The kidneys are in control of the bladder and the internal membrane [sanjiao]. The visceral peritoneum is a bowel functioning as a middle waterway through which water runs, and it belongs to the bladder. The visceral peritoneum is a solitary bowel with no corresponding viscera.
>
> The internal membrane system is an external bowel.

Other similar references are noted in *NJLS 8 (Origin of the Spirit)*, and the *Nanjing (Difficulty 31: The Location and Function of the Internal Membrane [Sanjiao])*, respectively:

> The internal membrane system [sanjiao] is like the irrigation official who determines the course of the waterways.
>
> The internal membrane system [sanjiao] is involved in the passage of water and grains through the body, and therefore is involved in vital substance production along the alimentary tract from beginning to end.

The *NJLS 18 (The Meeting and Interaction of Nutrients and Defensive Substances)* notes that nutrients (ying) are derived from the tissue membranes of the abdominal cavity (middle jiao), which originate at the stomach, and defensive substances (wei) are derived from the lower abdominal tissue membranes (lower jiao), which originate at the ileum. In the Chinese view, the abdominal cavity tissue membranes invest the stomach, duodenum, and the jejunum portion of the small intestine, while the lower abdominal tissue membranes invest the ileum portion of the small intestines and the large intestine (see Differentiation of the Intestines, page 41). Because of the anatomical relationship between the internal membrane and the organs it covers, the middle tissue membranes are considered to have a role in the digestion and absorption of nutrients, while the lower tissue membranes have a role in the absorption of defensive substances (in the deep lymphatics) and in passing on the dregs to the large intestine.

From *NJLS 18*, the upper tissue membranes (upper jiao) originate at the upper opening of the stomach (cardiac orifice), travel up the esophagus, cut across the diaphragm, spread inside the thoracic cavity, move through the axilla, travel with the divisions (lobes) of the lungs, and finally return to the stomach. Above the thoracic cavity they travel up to the tongue and below to the stomach.

The interpretation of the ancient idea of the internal membrane system (sanjiao) has been confused from the time of initial Western exposure. One reason for this may lie in the fact that the internal membrane system is not viewed as an organ in the West, and that the character jiao was misunderstood from the start. The ancient pictograph for jiao shows a bird being roasted over a fire. Since the sanjiao is described as having influence on metabolic functions, the character jiao has been commonly translated as heater. However, the present and historical use of the character means something that is burnt, shriveled, or dried, as a bird roasted over a fire. During dissection studies (or when slaughtering animals) it is necessary to remove the protective membrane tissue, including the visceral peritoneum, to gain access to the internal organs. This thin membrane feels moist at first; however, after exposure to the atmosphere it becomes dried and brittle, taking on a wrinkled and shriveled appearance. Therefore, the character jiao actually describes the nature of the membrane after it is exposed to the air.

Organ Pathology

All the viscera reflect disease conditions that are either related to functional disorders or are the result of pathogenic factors. Due to the physiological attributes of the organs, they exhibit a basic set of clinical manifestations that appear in many disorders (Table 3.4). There are additional patterns of organ pathology indicating physiological dysfunction or attack by a pathogenic factor, details of which are beyond the scope of this text (O'Connor and Bensky: 1981; Cheng: 1987). These conditions can be characterized as deficiency syndromes, involving a deficiency in functional activity (visceral qi) affecting the lungs, spleen, heart, or kidneys; deficiency in yang function affecting the spleen or kidneys; and deficiencies in yin substance affecting the lungs or kidneys. There can also be blood deficiencies affecting the heart or liver. Pathogenic wind conditions, such as wind heat, phlegm heat, and phlegm damp, can affect the lungs. The spleen is particularly affected by cold damp. The liver is affected by stagnation that impairs its dispersing function, by liver fire, and by liver vessel cold. Each organ displays particular tendencies and acute symptoms (Table 6.6). Heat and fire conditions usually refer to some type of infection caused by a pathogenic agent, except in the case of deficient heat due to a yin substance deficiency. Some of the above conditions can be complicated by involving another organ, and there are also syndromes associated with the bowels.

Anatomical Information on Internal Organs

The size and weight of all the internal organs were measured and recorded by the early Chinese physicians. The capacity of the hollow organs, such as the stomach, intestines, bladder, and gallbladder, were also noted, as was the internal volume of the heart. Measurement standards have fluctuated over the past centuries, so it is not possible to accurately correlate some of the parameters, especially volumetric measurements. Using the Han-dynasty value of the cun results in an accurate correlation of linear anatomical measurements noted in the *Neijing* and the *Nanjing*. For volume standards, the Chinese equated 10 *ge* (合) with 1 *sheng* (升); 10 sheng with 1 *tou* (头); and 10 tou with 1 *shi* (石). Modern standards set 1 sheng at 1 liter,[4] which appears to be significantly greater than the value used during the Zhou period.

Similar problems exist with correlating ancient weight measurements. Here, modern usage equates 10 *qian* (钱) with 1 *liang* (两), and 10 liang with 1 *jin* (斤).[5] The current value of 1 jin is 1.1023 pounds, or 500 grams, resulting in 1 qian being equal to 5 grams. During the Zhou dynasty 1 jin may have contained 16 liang, and if its value was the same as the present jin (500 grams), 1 liang would be equal to 31.5 grams (approximately 1 ounce), and 1 qian would equal 3 grams. These latter values are applied to weights used in measuring herbs contained in formulas (Bensky and Gamble: 1986). Although an accurate comparison of modern volume and weight measurements with those of the Zhou is not possible in an absolute sense, the relative measurements between values in the ancient texts do compare well (Tables 3.5 and 3.6).

Measurement of Viscera, Stomach, and Intestines

Several chapters of the *Neijing*, especially in the *Lingshu* volume and the *Nanjing* (*Difficulty 42*: *The Human Anatomy of the Viscera and Bowels*) provide detailed anatomical measurements. The size, weight, and capacity of the viscera (Table 3.5) and the bowels (Table 3.6), and related structures, are accurately depicted. These anatomical features, especially the weight,

Table 3.4 Basic profile of visceral pathology due to environmental extremes, from *NJSW 22* (*On Visceral Function and Seasonal Rules*).

	Indications	*Treatment*
Liver Disease	Pain below both sides of ribs (hypochondriac pain) with stretching sensation down to lower abdomen, and patient easily given to fits of rage or anger.	Select liver and gallbladder distribution vessels.
Deficiency	Blurred vision, vertigo with impaired perception, impaired hearing, patient can experience fear of being grabbed, as in being arrested.	
Inverse Function[1]	Headache, deafness, inability to hear, and swelling of cheeks.	Bleed above distribution vessels.
Heart Disease	Pain in center of chest, fullness in branches of ribs, pain between region of pectoralis major (breast), back, and scapula, and pain along the medial (inside) aspect of both arms.	Select heart and small intestine distribution vessels.
Deficiency	Fullness or swelling in chest and abdomen, and pain below ribs and in the loins mutually affecting each other.	Bleed vessels on underside of tongue.
Spleen Disease	Heavy sensations in body, weak muscles with difficulty in walking, twitching of hands and feet, and pain in underside of feet.	Select spleen and stomach distribution vessels.
Deficiency	Abdominal fullness and intestinal rumbling, diarrhea with undigested food.	Bleed kidney vessels for pain in bottom of feet.
Lung Disease	Gasping for breath (asthma), cough, congested chest,[1] pain in scapula and back, perspiration, and pain along the hip, medial thigh, thigh bone, knee, tibia, and foot.	Select lung and bladder distribution vessels superficially.
Deficiency	Shortness of breath with impaired breathing, deafness and dry throat.	Bleed liver vessel for deeper conditions.
Kidney Disease	Abdominal distension, swelling of tibial region, gasping for breath (asthma) and cough, heavy sensations in body, night sweats, and hatred of wind.	Select kidney and bladder distribution vessels for bloodletting.
Deficiency	Pain in chest, pain in upper and lower abdomen, cold extremities, and unhappy thoughts.	

1. Counteracting activity.

Table 3.5 Size of the solid organs in terms of their width and length, along with their weight and capacity, as noted in the *Neijing* and *Nanjing*.

Viscera	*Width*	*Length*	*Features*	*Capacity*	*Weight*
Tongue	2.5 cun[1]	7 cun			10 liang
Heart			Seven holes, three hairs	3 ge[2]	12 liang
Spleen	3 cun	5 cun	Contains additional 0.5 jin of tissue spreading around it		2 jin,[3] 3 liang[4]
Larynx	2 cun	12 cun	Contains nine segments		12 liang
Lungs			Six lobes, two ears		3 jin, 3 liang
Liver			Seven lobes		2 jin, 4 liang
Kidneys					1 jin, 1 liang

1. Approximate value using 1 cun = 0.902 inches, or 2.30 centimeters.
2. 10 ge make 1 sheng, which is equivalent to 1 modern liter. This value seems to be significantly larger than that used during the Zhou dynasty.
3. 1 jin is 1.1023 pounds, or 500 grams.
4. 1 liang is 50 grams, or one-tenth of a jin. However, during the Zhou dynasty 1 jin contained 16 liang, each liang equivalent to 1 ounce, or 31.5 grams.

Table 3.6 Size of the hollow organs in terms of their width or circumference, diameter, and length, along with their weight and capacity, mainly from *NJLS 31 (Intestines and Stomach), NJLS 32 (Fasting of a Healthy Person),* and *Difficulty 42 (The Human Anatomy of the Viscera and Bowels).*

Bowel	*Width/ Circumference*	*Diameter*	*Length*	*Capacity*	*Weight*
Esophagus	2½ cun[1]	1½ cun	16 cun		12 liang
Stomach	15 cun	5 cun	26 cun (23.5")	20 sheng[3]—grains 15 sheng—water	2 jin,[4] 3 liang[5]
Small Intestine (Duodenum and Jejunum)	2½ cun	8⅓ fen[2]	320 cun (24')	24 sheng—grains 6 sheng, 3⅔ ge[3]—water	2 jin, 14 liang
Ileum	4 cun	1½ cun	210 cun (15.8')	10 sheng—grains 7½ sheng—water	2 jin, 12 liang
Wide Intestine	8 cun	2½ cun	28 cun (2.1')	9 sheng—grains 3⅓ ge—water	12 liang
Bladder			9 cun	9 sheng, 9 ge	9 1/12 liang
Gallbladder				3 ge	3⅛ liang

1. Approximate value using 1 cun = 0.902 inches, or 2.30 centimeters.
2. 1 fen is equal to one-tenth of a cun.
3. 10 ge make 1 sheng, which is equivalent to 1 modern liter. This value seems to be significantly larger than that used during the Zhou dynasty.
4. 1 jin is 1.1023 pounds, or 500 grams.
5. 1 liang is 50 grams, or one-tenth of a jin. However, during the Zhou dynasty 1 jin contained 16 liang, each liang equivalent to 1 ounce, or 31.5 grams.

size, and capacity can only be derived by postmortem examination. At first glance it seems the intestines and bowels are too long. The difference between these and modern values arises from the methods employed by the Chinese in taking their measurements. In a live person, the length of the bowels is approximately half of that in a cadaver because of the intestinal smooth muscle tone, which is lost after death when the bowels become relaxed and elongate to about 18 to 20 feet. The Chinese made their measurements of the stomach and intestines in this postmortem relaxed and elongated state, and while stretching the organs out in a straight line. Stretching the intestines may have resulted in an abnormal length measurement.

The *NJLS 31* (*Intestines and Stomach*) provides additional anatomical details on the intestines and stomach in order to determine their capacity to receive grains and water. The length and pathway of every section of the digestive tract, including major bends and features from the pharynx to the rectum, including the diameter of the small intestine and colon, are provided. Thirty-two bends or curves are recorded: sixteen associated with the duodenum and jejunum, sixteen with the ileum and large intestine. The overall stretched-out length from the mouth to the anus is given, and the capacity of the stomach and its size, both in its normal configuration and when stretched out, is also described. The size of the mouth, tongue, and pharynx is also given, in addition to the weight of the tongue and larynx (Table 3.5).

Effects of Fasting

One interesting study, reported in *NJLS 32* (*Fasting of a Healthy Person*), involved measuring the size and volumetric capacities of the gastrointestinal system organs (Table 3.6). This anatomical data was used to estimate how long a person could survive without food and water. It was known that even a healthy person could possibly die by not eating and drinking for several days. When the stomach was full the intestines were thought to be empty. As food traveled down through the gut, the stomach was then empty. Based on the measured capacities of the gastrointestinal organs, it was assumed that the intestines and stomach normally contained a total of 35 sheng of grain and water at the time an individual started fasting. Assuming a person had two bowel movements each day, for a total daily elimination of 5 sheng of dregs, the food supply would be exhausted in seven days and the person would be at risk of dying.

Physiological Relationships

In addition to the functional activity of the internal organs, key physiological relationships are integral to the theory and practice of Chinese medicine. One of these is associating human physiology with the five earth phase dynamic relationships. This results in a unique and highly practical way of viewing bodily processes in terms of health, disease, and treatment strategies. The Chinese also considered the internal organs to have chronobiological[6] relationships, whereby each organ is assigned a dominant two-hour period each day (Table 4.4), as well as having dominance during specific seasons (Figure 6.3). Organ pathology may therefore predominate or lessen during certain times of the day and in different seasons, and treatment approaches take into consideration the time of optimum recovery potential. Other important relationships include the internal-external relationship of the bowels and viscera, as represented by matched venous and arterial collateral vessels (*luo*, 络) paired in the extremities.

Dynamic Interplay between the Internal Organs

Physiological interrelationships between the internal organs are viewed in terms of the five earth phases (Figure 3.2). The resulting five-phase physiological model is used to explain how the major visceral systems function in relationship to each other. These affiliations might seem overly simple at the beginning of the twenty-first century, however they are still useful. This is particularly true when viewing the dynamic effects of one viscus on another, especially when it affects an organ's functional activity. The five-phase schema is also essential in understanding various aspects of treatment plans. Here, five-phase nodes (acupoints) related to each earth phase can be used to restore functional balance between the organ systems. Specific nodes are employed to produce functional changes consistent with the five-phase arrangement with respect to the mother-son relationships (Chapter 15).

Internal-External Relationships

The twelve internal organs (zangfu) have internal and external relationships. First, the viscera are referred to as interior, while the bowels are thought of as exterior. The reason for this classification is that the bowels make up the alimentary tract and are connected to the outside in the upper regions by the mouth and esophagus, and in the lower region by the anus. A major portion of the visceral peritoneum (sanjiao) surrounds the gastrointestinal tract. For this reason the sanjiao is also considered to communicate externally.

The second consideration involves the correspondence between the vessels in the interior and exterior regions. Internally each viscus is connected to its corresponding bowel through related distribution and collateral vessels. The matched internal-external organ pairs are supplied by the specific arteries and veins that distribute to those organs. In the exterior areas of the body the distribution vessels of the internal-external pairs also communicate by distributing to the same superficial anatomical regions (Chapter 9). These matched organ pair vessels involve specific arteries and return-flow veins that supply the same general area.

Body-Organ Relationships

The Chinese found that blood vessels are distributed to the superficial body (soma) and to the organs (viscera) like a "ring without end." Based on critical observations, they theorized that these pathways create communication links between the internal and external body. This means that a specific location on the superficial body corresponds with a specific internal organ. Sorting out which vessel distributions relate to which organ was deduced by analyzing the locations on the superficial body that involved pain referred from a known diseased organ. How the ancient Chinese stumbled on the idea that organ pathology can be reflected in the superficial body regions is not known. They were certainly aware that conditions such as appendicitis cause protective muscle contractions over the inflamed area, and that certain menstrual problems will result in cramps as well. In the case of heart disease, involving pectoris angina, the correlation is straightforward. This condition was recognized as being associated with chest pains reflected in the shoulder, down the arm (usually the left arm), and onward to the little finger. The distribution vessel traveling along this pain pathway was discovered to be associated with the heart. Other correlations between referred pain and diseased internal organs may have been just as easily determined. Viscerosomatic communication was not observed in the West until William Head described organ-referred pain in 1893.

The correlation between referred pain in the superficial body and internal organ pathology confirms the existence of viscerosomatic relationships. This phenomenon can only occur if there is a convergence of the afferent visceral nerve fibers and corresponding inputs from some specific part of the body. These relationships are all part of the same complex protective system mediated by the propriospinal system of the spinal cord. Modern neurological studies (Cervero: 1986; Foreman, Hammond and Willis: 1981) have confirmed that the integration of afferent somatic and visceral information, along with the propriospinal system, is fundamental to how the body is organized.

Correlation between Internal Organs and Distribution Vessel Pathways

With the limited materials and procedures available to the ancient Chinese it may seem surprising that they determined which distribution vessel pathways were related to specific internal organs. Originally the Chinese named the vessels for the region to which they distributed, but later renamed them after the internal organs they represent in the yin-yang orientation system (Chapter 4). Correlating vessels with specific organs was accomplished by observing pain referred to the superficial body due to organ pathology. Postmortem correlation with a noted pain area then gave clues to the vascular organization of the body. Meaningful references that verify this supposition include *NJLS 66* (*Origins of All Disease*):

> The areas of pain should be carefully examined in order to determine which organ is involved. The conditions may be either excess or deficient. In case of deficiency, it should be regulated by mending; in case of excess, it should be regulated by draining off.

Another reference, *NJLS 73* (*Official Abilities*), provides direct evidence that referred pain was used to determine which distribution vessel was involved:

> With respect to the five viscera and six bowels, careful examination of their referred pain, both on the left and right sides, and the upper and lower portions of the body, permits understanding of whether it is a cold or warm condition, and which distribution vessel is involved. The skin can be further examined to determine if it is either cold or warm, or smooth or uneven to determine the nature of the painful condition. The area above and below the diaphragm should be examined when locating the disease.

Inference of Endocrine Gland Involvement

One major absence in the Chinese information is a clear description of the endocrine glands. Except for the ovaries and testes, these structures were never anatomically described. Some Chinese scholars contend that endocrine glands were possibly identified along with the fatty tissues associated with specific organs, a plausible suggestion, especially for the spleen-pancreas and kidney-adrenal associations. This idea is partly borne out by the fact that the Chinese included the tissue between the spleen and the stomach as part of the spleen (Table 3.5). If this is the correct interpretation, then the pancreas could easily be included in the description of the spleen. A similar correlation applies to the adrenal glands, which sit on top of each kidney. These glands are not discussed; however, the activities of the adrenal glands are grouped with responsibilities attributed to the kidneys.

Certain physiological activities for each specific organ system can only be explained by including a particular endocrine gland. The correlation is accurate and helps to explain the vitality characteristics (organ spirits) assigned to each viscus. Organ vitalities are noted as being mediated by physical substances that circulate in the blood system, which may be different from other vital substances maintained by the viscera, as previously noted in *NJSW 11* (see Classification of Viscera and Bowels, page 39). Vitality substances appear to describe biologically active agents, possibly including hormones (see Chapter 7 for a discussion of organ vitalities and endocrine glands).

Four Seas of the Human Body

The Chinese also viewed anatomical and physiological features by considering certain areas of the body as similar to the four seas of ancient China, a continuation of the idea of describing the function of each distribution vessel in reference to one of the twelve main rivers of China. Fundamental to the Chinese physiological model is the need for nutrients, vital air (containing oxygen), blood, and nervous system function. Any abnormality in these four components, including deficiencies or excesses, is thought to result in either disease or dysfunction (Table 3.7). Certain nodal sites were noted to have special communication with a particular sea, and thus could be employed in treatment to bring about normalization. Details of the four seas is provided in *NJLS 33* (*On the Seas*):

> Yellow Emperor: I have heard considerable information about the techniques of needling where you specifically state that these methods are dependent on nutrients [ying], defensive substances [wei], blood [*xue*, 血], and vital air [qi]. The twelve distribution vessels internally

Table 3.7 Clinical manifestations as a result of either surplus or deficiency in the four seas of the human body.

Four Seas	*Surplus*	*Deficiency*
Sea of Vital Air (Air-Qi)	Air fills the thoracic cavity, causing difficult respiration and a red complexion (hyperventilation).	Lesser amount of air affects the ability to speak.
Sea of Blood	Causes a feeling that the body is larger than normal, producing a flushed sensation with no awareness of disease location.	Causes an impression that the body is smaller than normal, with a shrunken feeling and no awareness of disease location.
Sea of Grains and Water	Abdominal fullness.	Hunger sensation due to not receiving food.
Sea of Neural Tissue (including Brain and Spinal Cord)	Causes sensation of lightness with great strength, with the individual being able to exceed their normal limits.	Causes a turning or whirling sensation in the brain, ringing in the ears, weakness and aching in the limbs, dizziness, blurred vision, sluggishness, and a desire to sleep.

are connected to the bowels [fu] and viscera [zang], externally they have major branches that distribute to the extremities and joints. Can you tell me how [the distribution vessels] are united with the four seas?

Qibo replies: The human body has four seas and also twelve distribution vessels that are similar to the twelve rivers. The twelve distribution-like rivers [on earth] all flow into the sea, and the seas are located in the east, west, south, and north, and this is why they are called the four seas.

The Yellow Emperor asks: How do they agree with respect to the human body?

Qibo replies: The human body has a sea of neural tissue [*sui*, 髓], a sea of blood, a sea of vital air [qi], and a sea of nutrients [food, i.e. water and grains]. These are commonly referred to as the four seas... The stomach is the sea of grain and water [food], with communication nodes above at the street of vitality [Quepen, ST 12], and below down to Sanli [Zusanli, ST 36]. The thoroughfare vessel [*chong* 冲 aorta] serves as the sea [of blood] for the twelve distribution vessels, with an important communication site in the upper region at Dazhu [BL 11], and in the lower regions at the upper and lower Juxu locations [Shangjuxu, ST 37, and Xiajuxu, ST 39]. The center of the chest serves as the sea of vital air [qi], with communication sites in the upper region of the spinal column above [Yamen, DU 15] and below [Dazhui, DU 14], and in the frontal area at Renying [ST 9]. The brain[7] is the sea of neural tissue [including the medulla and spinal cord], with one communication site in the upper region at the vertex [Baihui, DU 20], and one in the lower area at Fengfu [DU 16].

Nerves in Ancient Times

Considerable effort was made by the Chinese to identify all the vessels in the body, but little detail was applied to mapping out the nerves. The Chinese noted that something equivalent to nerve function is involved in nodes (acupoints), and they made reference to certain areas of critical neural connections, along with corresponding blood vessels. This includes specific areas, such as the networks supplying the heart and nerves to the eyes. It is now known that the most important neural involvement includes the autonomic nerves, which provide motor signals to control the blood vessels and organs, and the afferent fibers that transmit somatic and visceral sensory signals back to the central nervous system (CNS). Qibo's description of the brain, including the spinal cord, as the sea of neural tissue indicates that the Chinese were aware of the function of the nerves (see *NJLS 33*, in Four Seas of the Human Body, above).

Nerve signals or functions are described in terms of spirit or vitality (*shen*, 神), and it was recognized that nerves have afferent and efferent properties. This means nerves can conduct signals to cause something to happen (efferent signals), such as a motor signal to contract a muscle, as well as conducting sensory information (afferent signals), such as sensations of pain and temperature. In modern China nerve signals are still called spirit or vitality signals (*shenqi*, 神气). References to afferent and efferent nerve functions, especially related to nodes, are noted in *NJLS 1* (*Nine Needles and Twelve Sources*). Here a distinction is made between nerve function and other tissue, such as skin, flesh, tendons and muscles, and bone:

> That which we call critical junctures or nodes are the places where vitality signals [shenqi] transmit inward and outward [afferent and efferent nerve signals], and are not just skin, flesh, tendons and muscles, and bones.

The Greeks provide a rudimentary description of nerves slightly later. Herophilus (ca. 300 BCE) and Erasistratus (ca. 290 BCE) described vessels that conveyed vital, natural, and animal spirits. The idea that nerves as vessels conveyed vital, natural, and animal spirits persisted in the West until the eighteenth or nineteenth centuries. The description is basically the same as that of the ancient Chinese, except that in the *Neijing* the peripheral nerves are not clearly identified as independent structures. Nevertheless, the function of the nerves is included in the physiological processes described by the Chinese. This is particularly true in explaining the function of nodes, control of blood vessels, and connections to the internal organs. Neural processes are also basic to explaining the function of muscle distributions.

Spirit and Sensory Function

The relationship of spirit to nerves and refined substances of vitality helps explain sensory functions and capabilities, including vision, taste, smell, hearing, speech, and propagated needle sensation (PS). Collateral vessels supplying the sensory structures are assigned to specific viscera. These vessels in turn supply refined substances to the sensory organs. Thus, each of the main organs is responsible for one of the sensory functions. While discussing the pathway and length of the distribution vessels in *NJLS 17* (*Length of the Vessels*), Qibo notes the relationship of the senses to the organs:

> Internally, the five viscera constantly communicate with the seven orifices in the upper regions [two eyes, two ears, two nostrils, one mouth]. Therefore, the refined substances of the lungs communicate with the nose. When the lungs are in normal condition [harmony], the nose is able to smell odors and fragrances. Refined substances of the heart communicate with the tongue. When heart function is normal, the tongue is able to taste the five flavors. Refined substances of the liver communicate with the eyes. When liver function is normal, the eyes are able to distinguish the five colors. Refined substances of the spleen communicate with the mouth. When spleen function is normal [harmony], the mouth can savor the five grains. Refined substances of the kidneys communicate with the ears. When kidney function is normal, the ears are able to hear the five sounds. If the five viscera are not functioning properly [not in harmony], there is impaired communication with the seven orifices.

Propagated Needle Sensation

Clues to the unique organization of the body were provided when the ancient Chinese first observed a propagated sensation as a result of needling. Directing PS to specific body areas was found to be therapeutically useful. The ancient Chinese may have understood that this involved the CNS. One explanation is provided in *NJLS 75* (*Needling Nodes for True Function and Pathogenic Forces*), where the Yellow Emperor inquires about the treatment of a disorder that may include vertigo, loss of hearing, and ringing in the ears. He asks:

> I do not know the meaning of the needling technique said to treat an attack of confusion. With respect to attack of confusion, the ears are not able to hear and the eyes are not able to see, and you said to needle the communication locations of the bowels to resolve diseases of the bowels. What communication nodes are used to bring about such effects? I wish to hear the reasons for this.

> Qibo replies: What a wonderful question. This technique is the utmost point of needling therapy. It is understood by the spirit and the mind, while neither the spoken nor written word is able to reach this level of explanation. The attack of confusion I talk about is the acute or urgent attack of confusion... For this condition needling must be applied at midday by stimulating Tinggong [SI 19] until the sensation propagates [PS] to the pupils and a sound is heard inside the ear... After needle insertion, the patients should use their fingers to firmly press the two nostrils and temporarily hold their breath, and a sound can be heard inside the ear when the needle is manipulated.
>
> The Yellow Emperor replies: Excellent. This discussion is about something invisible that the eye cannot see, but is like seeing the sensations propagated [PS] by needling. These phenomena involve the mutual participation of the spirit and the mind [possible reference to the nervous system].

An example of enhancing the therapeutic effect by stimulating PS is noted in *NJLS 26* (*Internal Diseases*) in treating pain in the area of the heart:

> For pain in the region of the heart, select the site below the ninth thoracic spinous process [Jinsuo, DU 8] for needling, and massage this area before and after needling. There will be immediate relief of the pain. If the pain is not immediately relieved, stimulate sites on the upper and lower extremities; when a radiating sensation [PS] is produced, the pain will be immediately relieved.

Speech

Speech is a result of complex processes involving brain function to control the voice box and tongue. One's overall vitality or spirit and mental state are reflected in one's voice, which is thought to be dominated by the heart. Important vessels supplying the tongue and the brain belong to the heart distribution vessels. The *Neijing* notes that the sound of the voice is the result of air passing through the voice box, and it was understood that the brain controlled the process of speech. Chinese physicians considered that cerebral vascular accident (stroke) can result in brain damage and subsequent paralysis. They noted that the patient would be likely to recover if the function of speech was not impaired. This observation is presently supported by clinical findings in the West.

The function of speech is further discussed in *NJLS 69* (*Loss of Voice due to Grief and Rage*), where Shao Shi, another physician-teacher, notes that the tongue is the engine of the voice:

> The pharynx is the passageway for water and food. The larynx provides for the in and out passage of vital air [inhaled air moving down into the body; exhaled breath moving up and out]. The epiglottis is the door of the voice. The tongue is the engine of the voice. The uvula is the gate of the voice. The upper part of the throat [nasal pharynx] communicates with the nose where the incoming air and outgoing breath are separated and discharged. The hyoid bone enables the spirits [possible reference to nerve signals] to control the tongue.

Arteries supplying the tongue are collateral vessels assigned to the heart. Thus collateral vessels and nerves of the tongue are related to the heart.

Sight

Vision was understood to be the most complex sensory function that depends on refined substances contributed by the five organs, as well as nerves and blood vessels. Of the viscera, the liver has the greatest influence on vision because the veins that supply the eyes are collateral branches of the liver distribution vessels, and because of the liver's role in dispersing refined substances. It was understood that vision involved nerves, which belong to the brain. The area of the brain responsible for vision (visual cortex) was understood to be located in the occipital region.

The following dialogue from the *Neijing* serves to illustrate the detailed level of understanding when explaining the complexities of sensory function. Here Qibo explains to the Yellow Emperor the process of bewilderment or temporary dizziness. This discussion is noted in *NJLS 80*, where the Yellow Emperor asks:

> Whenever I climb up to the clear cool terrace, midway up the stairs I turn and look around, and then I creep and crawl ahead due to the bewilderment it causes. I personally feel different and internally strange and I close my eyes. When I open my eyes, it takes a while to calm my mind and not feel disrupted. When I reach the top I am still dizzy. I unroll my hair and kneel, bowing my head and looking down, after which my feelings do not change for some time. Then suddenly my feelings become normal. What vital functions are involved in this?
>
> Qibo replies: The refined substances of the five viscera and six bowels flow up to be the refined substances of the eyes. Refined substances of the bones [kidneys] serve the pupil of the eyes, refined substances of the muscles and tendons [liver] serve the iris [dark of the eye] of the eyes, refined substances of the blood [heart] serve the collateral vessels of the eyes, refined substances of vital air [lungs] serve the white of the eyes, and the refined substances of the flesh [spleen] serve the eyelids.
>
> The collected refined substances of the tendons and muscles, bones, blood, and lungs merge in the vessels that serve the eye connections [optic nerve and related vessels]. In the upper regions these belong to the brain and externally relate to the posterior surface of the nape of the neck [surface overlying the visual cortex]. Thus, when pathogenic environmental forces attack the nape of the neck, when the body is in deficiency, the effects penetrate deeply to follow along to the eye connections [optic nerve and vessels] in the brain. After pathogenic factors enter, there is a turning sensation generated in the brain. This turning sensation in the brain causes an acute tightening of the eye connections. This acute condition results in eye-related dizziness with a whirling sensation [vertigo]. An internal pathogenic assault on refined substances results in disruption of their mutual coordination, causing their dispersion. Dispersion of refined substances causes double vision [diplopia], seeing one thing as two.
>
> With respect to the eyes, the refined substances of the five viscera and six bowels, including nutrients and defensive substances, mood [*hun*, 魂], and vigor [*po*, 魄], are regularly supplied to generate spirit vitality or function. Thus, when the spirit is fatigued, mood and vigor are dispersed, and drive [*zhi*, 志] and intent [*yi*, 意] are confused. Since the iris and pupil of the eyes are ruled by the yin viscera [kidneys and liver], and the white of the eyes and the red vessels are governed by the yang viscera [lungs and heart], therefore coordination of yin and yang conveys good vision.

The eyes are the messengers of the heart, and the heart is the humble abode of the spirit or vitality. Therefore, disorders related to refined substances of the spirit cause an inability to turn with sudden and extraordinary visual effects, along with dispersion and subsequent loss of mutual coordination of refined substances, vitality or spirit, mood, and vigor. This is called bewilderment.

4

Qualities of Opposition

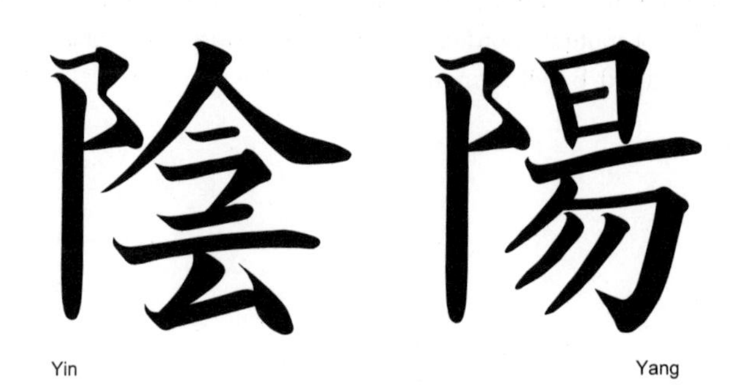

> Yin and yang are the way of sky and earth, are fundamental to all things, are the parents of change and transformation, the origin and beginning of birth and destruction, the palace of gods, and are necessarily considered in understanding the basis of treating disease.
>
> Yellow Emperor,
> *NJSW 5 (Great Treatise on the Proper Representation of Yin and Yang)*

In ancient China the world was viewed as the interplay of opposites. These opposite qualities, called yin and yang, can apply to materials, processes, reactions, or behaviors. Just as the world can be divided into yin and yang attributes, these classifications can be further subdivided into yin and yang. Grammatically, yin and yang are mostly used as adjectives to describe the dominant nature or quality of something, or applied in reference to a fixed or relative position. Characteristics may change with respect to time, thus altering a classification: day (yang) giving way to night (yin) as the hours of each day pass is one example. Daily cycles of the sun (great yang) and the moon (great yin) provided the fundamental basis from which the ancient Chinese developed their principles of yin and yang.

As day and night wax and wane, a small amount of light shines in the skies before the sun actually rises. Hence, there is yang within the last phase of the night (yin). Similarly, the effects of night coming on are apparent at dusk, so there is yin within the last phase of daylight (yang). The nature of these daily variations of yin and yang is also applied to the human situation and to the body. This results in the classification of external and internal anatomical features, physiological function, and disease and treatment processes in terms of yin and yang. Part of the story is provided in *NJSW 4* (*On the Virtuous Word of the Golden Cupboard*) where Qibo says:

> It is said, there is yin within yin, and there is yang within yang. Yang [sun] is in the sky from dawn to noon, and there is yang within yang. Yang is in the sky from noon until dusk, and there is yin within yang. Yin [moon] is in the sky from dusk until the cocks crow, and there is yin within yin. Yin is in the sky from the crowing of the cock until dawn, and there is yang within yin. The human being likewise complies with

yin and yang [classifications]. With respect to the human and yin and yang, the exterior belongs to yang and the interior belongs to yin. When yin and yang are applied to the body, the back is yang while the abdomen is yin. When yin and yang are applied to the viscera [*zang*, 藏] and the bowels [*fu*, 府], the viscera belong to yin and the bowels belong to yang. The liver, heart, spleen, lungs, and kidneys are the five viscera that belong to yin. The gallbladder, stomach, large intestine, small intestine, bladder, and the internal membrane [*sanjiao*, 三焦] are the six bowels that belong to yang.

Why is it necessary to understand yin within yin, and yang within yang? Because, disease attacks yin in winter, disease attacks yang in summer, disease attacks yin in spring, disease attacks yang in autumn, and needling treatment is applied according to the affected region. Furthermore, the back belongs to yang, and the heart is yang within yang. The back belongs to yang, and the lungs are yin within yang. The abdomen belongs to yin, and the kidneys are yin within yin. The abdomen belongs to yin, and the liver is yang within yin. The abdomen belongs to yin, and the spleen is extreme yin within yin. This all describes the reciprocal compliance of yin and yang with respect to superficial and deep, interior and exterior, and to female and male [of all species], and wherefore yin and yang comply with the heavens.

Further explanation of yin and yang concepts is detailed in this chapter. There are certain advantages and disadvantages with using the generalized terms yin and yang. It is useful to classify processes, functions, and substances in terms of a balance between mutually opposing properties. However, problems result in using yin and yang as nouns. The most common mistake is to view yin and yang as representing people, places, or things, rather than the quality or nature of these things. An incorrect use of yin and yang can be confusing to those first exposed to these concepts.

Classification of All Things

Interacting forces and substances are viewed in light of their yin and yang properties. The designation of appropriate categories is applied at all levels to describe the characteristics of diverse subjects. This includes describing interactions of environmental forces, anatomical features, physiological mechanisms, and pathological conditions. A general list of yin-yang oppositions is given in Table 4.1, while a yin-yang comparison with some Western physiological items is provided in Table 4.2.

Inappropriate use of yin and yang can result in the oversimplification of complex processes. On the other hand, there is an advantage in using specific terms to categorize things or to classify consistent sets of related items. This benefit is apparent when relating physiological processes, or in grouping diagnostic and other data related to pathogenic factors, disease, or dysfunction under yin and yang. When these manifestations are viewed in terms of yin and yang qualities, it greatly improves the understanding of the clinical problem being observed. All physiological and pathological processes can be examined with respect to yin and yang classifications. Treatment approaches are also considered in terms of yin or yang. This type of information is critical in determining the cause of the ailment and the likely course of action in formulating a treatment plan.

Table 4.1 Comparison of yin and yang classifications for general items.

Yin	*Yang*
Earth, Water	Sky, Air
Moon, Planets	Sun, Stars
Cold, Damp, Cloudy	Hot, Dry, Clear
Down, Under, Lower, Bottom	Up, Above, Upper, Top
Internal, Hidden, Deep	External, Exposed, Superficial
Front	Back
Night, Dark, Shady	Day, Light, Sunny
Black	White
Slow	Fast
Heavy	Light
Even Numbers	Odd Numbers

Table 4.2 Comparison of yin and yang classifications with physiological items or processes.

Yin	*Yang*
Meditation	Stress
Parasympathetic Outflow	Sympathetic Outflow
Bradycardia	Tachycardia
Diastole	Systole
Asleep, Rest, Relaxation	Awake, Motion, Exercise
Blood	Vital Air
Nutrients	Metabolic Processes
Anti-inflammatory	Inflammatory
Neurotransmitters	Nerve Function
Hormones, Biologically Active Substances	Visceral Function
Inhibition	Stimulation
Coagulation	Anticoagulation
Tissue Repair	Tissue Damage
Hypotension	Hypertension
Hypofunction	Hyperfunction

Fixed and Dynamic Relationships

In the Chinese system of cosmology, objects and processes are given fixed yin and yang classifications. These do not change with respect to time or spatial relationships. The sun is yang and will always remain so. Likewise the earth is yin and this will not change. Fire is always yang and water yin. A subject is categorized as yin or yang, based on physical qualities, position, or time affiliations. Many items, especially those involving physiological processes, have a dynamic interplay with opposite reactions. In these cases it is necessary to evaluate the relative balance between the two interacting entities in order to classify the overall nature as either yin or yang. What may appear to be an excess of yang qualities could in fact be a deficiency of yin.

Symbols of Yin and Yang

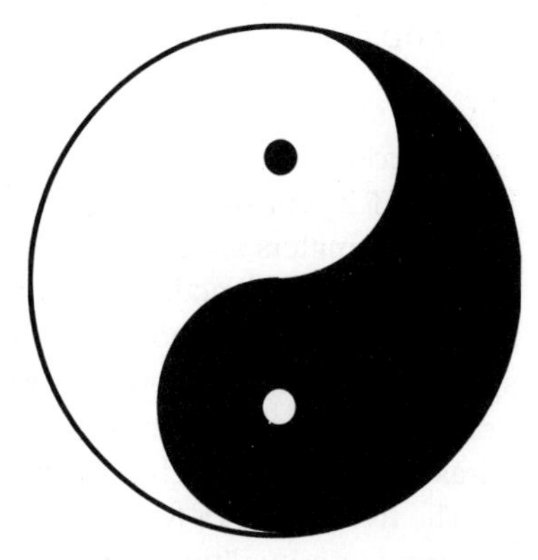

Figure 4.1 The *taiji* symbol used to denote the dual nature and interdependence of yin and yang, with the white portion representing yang and the black, yin.

The most famous graphic symbol used to illustrate the dual nature and interdependence of yin and yang is the *taiji* (太极) figure, which first appeared in the *Yijing* (*The Simple Classic*) around 600 BCE (Figure 4.1). The taiji graphic shows a black comma-shaped region that takes up one half of the area of a circle, while a similarly shaped, but opposite, white region fills in the rest. Black represents yin qualities while white represents yang. A small white circle is contained in the black region and a small black circle is contained in the white area. These smaller circles convey the idea that there is always a certain amount of yin quality within yang, and conversely there is always some yang quality within yin. The taiji graphic is commonly referred to as the "yin-yang symbol."

Material substances, such as water, wood, and blood, are characterized as yin in nature. Nonmaterial substances such as air, flames, and sunlight are considered to be yang. The natural world can be viewed in terms of its yin and yang qualities. The importance of this concept lies in recognizing the dual aspects of most dynamic relationships and allows us to view processes in terms of interplay and balance. When applied to humans, these ideas provide a great insight into understanding bodily function and disease.

Something classified as yin is usually a physical or material substance, while a yang classification could represent something that is nonmaterial or insubstantial. Water and fire, respectively, embody the characteristics of yin and yang, and these were adopted as the metaphorical symbols for yin and yang. Reference to these symbols is noted in *NJSW 5* (*Great Treatise on the Proper Representation of Yin and Yang*)—"Water represents yin qualities while fire represents yang qualities"; and *NJSW 67* (*Motion of the Five Phases*)—"Water and fire are the symbols of yin and yang."

Ancient Pictographs

The qualities of yin and yang were originally derived from the idea that shady and cloudy conditions represent yin, while sunny and bright conditions represent yang. Ancient pictographs depicted the nature of yin and yang as cloudy and sunny, respectively. Traditional brushstroke characters still convey this original idea. The yang character shows a picture of the sun above the horizon with its rays streaming down. The character for yin is more complicated because it uses the ideograph *jin* (今) and the pictograph *yun* (云): jin conveys the idea of actuality, presence, or the actual moment; yun shows warm vapors rising into the sky to condense into clouds.

Later the *fu* (阜) radical was added to both yin and yang to denote steps, or earthwork on the side of a hill or cliff. Yang became known as the sun shining on a hillside, or the sunny side of the hill; yin became known as the shady side of a hill. More recently, China further simplified the characters to show only the present fu radical with the sun pictograph (*ri*, 日) for yang, and with the moon character (*yue*, 月) for yin. This simplification is understandable because the sun is referred to as the great yang (*taiyang*, 太阳) and the moon is known as the great yin (*taiyin*, 太阴).

Yin Substance

Physical substances are considered as yin and serve as the material basis for yang function, or can be converted to something with yang properties. Wood is classified as yin; however if it is ignited it will burn and produce flames, which are yang in nature. Neurochemicals or neurotransmitters are also classified as yin, and are critical in the production of neural activity, which is a yang function. Although neurotransmitters are classified as yin, these are further segregated into yin and yang types. Nerve function is typically classified as yang, although specific nerves can produce either a yang or yin response. For example, the sympathetic branch of the autonomic nervous system is categorized as yang in function, while those of the parasympathetic branch produce yin function.

The five flavors of food and herbs belong to the general category of yin but they have both yin and yang qualities as noted in *NJSW 71* (*Great Treatise on the Six Original First Years*) (Chapter 6):

> Pungent and sweet flavors are yang because they stimulate dispersion. Sour, bitter, and salty flavors belong to yin since they produce a surging discharge. Mild or bland flavors belong to yang since they cause an oozing or leaking discharge.

Qualities associated with yin are cold, descending, material in nature (liquid or solid), storing, dark, heavy, in a lower position, causing inhibition, slow, quiescent, substantial in nature, and feminine.

Yang Function

Fire symbolizes yang due to its inherent nature of radiating heat or pouring out. The sun is considered yang because it is extremely hot and radiates (pours out) sunlight. To pour out without storing is considered a key yang property. Sunlight is considered insubstantial because it cannot be collected, saved, or carried in a container. Although not considered a material substance by the Chinese, both sunlight and fire function with yang characteristics. Functional activities of the internal organs, such as the peristaltic action of the digestive tract, are considered yang in nature.

Lightning and electrical signals are good examples of yang phenomena. Similarly, the electrochemical propagation of nerve signals is considered yang in nature. Both nerve operation and visceral function, however, depend on yin neural transmitters, hormones, and biologically active substances. With respect to the internal organs, functional activity and substance are known respectively as visceral yang and visceral yin.

Yang qualities, like the flame, are hot, bright, excited, usually rising, fast, moving, pouring out, light in both weight and color, hollow, insubstantial, upper or exterior, moving in an upward or outward direction, and masculine.

Anatomical Notation in the Yin-Yang System

The ancient Chinese were among the first to recognize the need to develop a standard nomenclature by which to describe various anatomical features, locations, and regions of the body. By adopting a common system for naming areas of the body, the early Chinese physicians were able to communicate with each other using the same terminology. This led to improved documentation and formalization of Chinese medicine, and enhanced the education process by permitting standardized training. Before adopting the yin-yang system to describe regions of the body, anatomical features, such as blood vessels, were described by the name of the region through which the vessel traveled. Some vessels originally had anatomical names such as the "ear," "tooth," or "shoulder" vessels. Eventually vessels were named by the peripheral body region (noted in yin-yang terms) that they traversed and the extremity of origin or termination. Some two thousand years later the West developed a similar approach to describing anatomical features, using either Latin or Greek words as the standard.

In comparing the two approaches, the radial artery is so named because it travels close to the radial bone of the arm in the extremity. The Chinese named this same artery the "hand taiyin vessel." Here, "hand" is the final destination of this artery, which traverses the anatomical region of the arm that is designated "taiyin" in the Chinese system. The Chinese went a step further by assigning the internally related yin or yang organ (somatovisceral relationship) known to be affected or stimulated by nodes along specific vessel pathways. The taiyin vessel was determined to be internally related to the lungs. Consequently, the full name of the radial artery in the Chinese system is the "hand anterior medial (taiyin) vessel related to the lungs."

Climatic conditions known to preferentially attack a particular region of the body, vessels traversing these regions, their related internal organs, organ pathologies, and major dysfunction of the body are all viewed in terms consistent with yin-yang notation.

Body Surface and Anatomical Position

The first step in developing standardized anatomical nomenclature was to classify the superficial regions of the body as yin or yang. As with the use of Western terms such as internal, external, posterior, and anterior, a reference is needed to clearly understand what position is being described. The standard Chinese anatomical reference position involves a living person standing erect with head and feet pointing straight ahead, and the arms hanging down the sides with the palms facing inward and toward the legs (Figure 4.2). This is the familiar "at attention" military position. This is in contrast to the Western anatomical position, which is derived from a cadaver lying on its back with the palms of the hands facing upward.

As a general classification, the entire outside or external surface of the body is considered yang, while the internal regions and the organs are considered yin. When the body surface is viewed relative to itself, the posterior regions are considered yang while the abdomen pertains to yin. The body area above the waist is classified as yang because of its upper position. The lower portion of the body is classified as yin. When discussing details of a particular extremity, the lateral aspect of the arm or leg is considered yang, while the inner aspect is yin. These relative classifications are used when referring to various parts of the body and are not necessarily the same as anatomical yin-yang nomenclature.

The Chinese already had an understanding of the vessel, muscle, and nodal routes before adopting the yin-yang anatomical notations. These pathways distribute longitudinally along the body. Consequently, the general yin-yang designators are not useful in describing the vertical pathways. Yin-yang anatomical classifications were derived by considering incident sunlight striking the body while facing east in the standard Chinese anatomical position. During the sunrise period (5:00–9:00 A.M.), the face, anterior portions of the body, and the anterior lateral aspect of the arms and legs are illuminated. This area of the body is then named the sunrise yang (*yangming*, 阳明). After the noon period (1:00–5:00 P.M.), the intensity

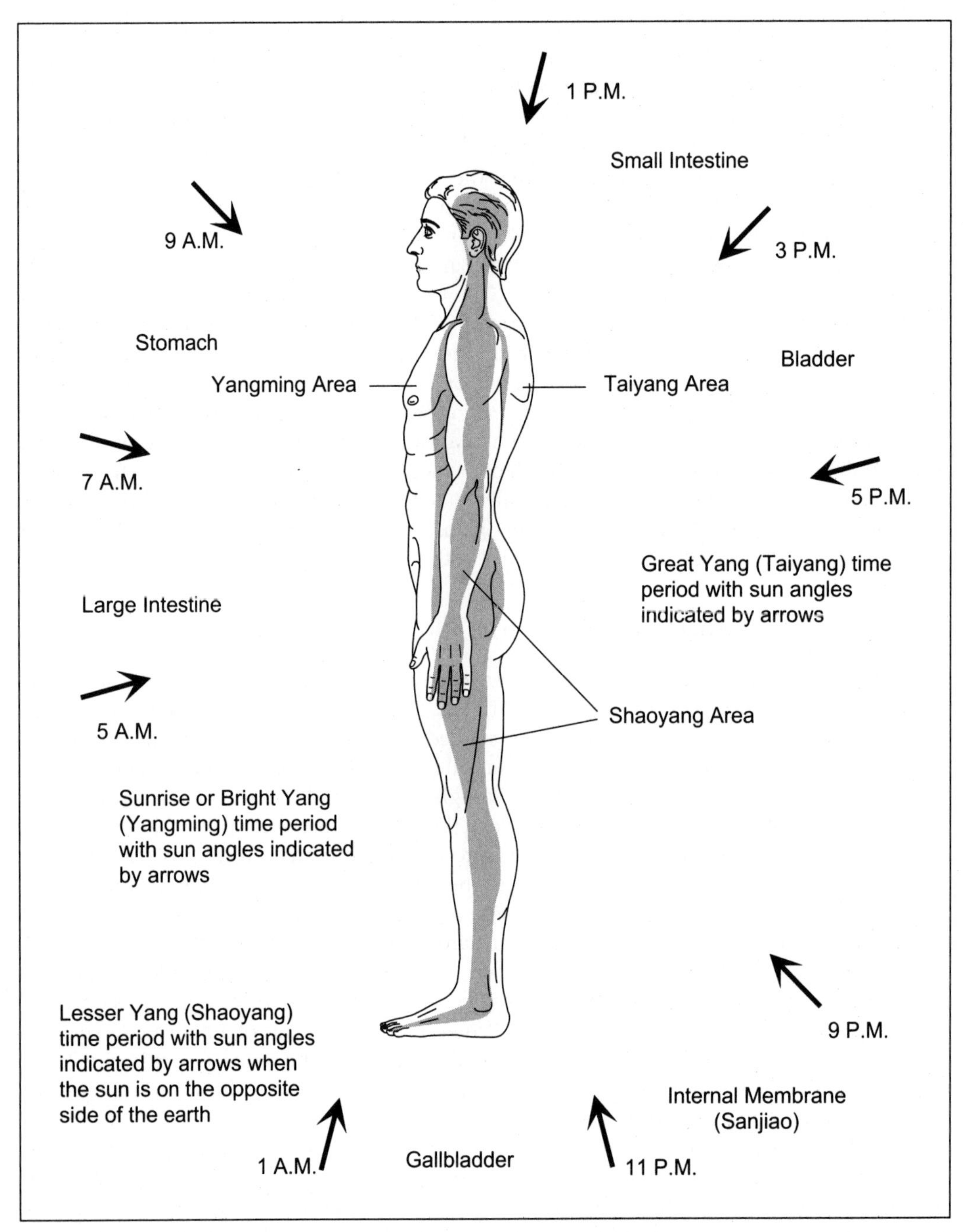

Figure 4.2 Standard Chinese anatomical orientation showing the body regions based on the yang classification system.

of the sun's rays is greatest. While still facing east, sunlight strikes the top of the head, the posterior head, neck, shoulders, and the back. The posterior lateral regions of the arms and legs are also illuminated. This time period is named great yang (taiyang), after the sun, and the name is likewise applied to these regions of the body. When the sun is shining during each of these two yang periods, little direct sunlight falls on the lateral aspect of the body. These areas, involving the side of the head and neck, and the lateral portion of the shoulders, arms, hands, legs, and feet, are called lesser yang (*shaoyang*, 少阳), referring to the stars (9:00 P.M.–1:00 A.M.). The main yin regions then lie on the inside surfaces of the arms and legs. The anterior medial aspect of the arms and legs is assigned to the great yin (taiyin), while the posterior medial aspect belongs to the lesser yin (*shaoyin*, 少阴). The medial aspect of the arms and legs is assigned to the transitional or decreasing yin (*jueyin*, 厥阴).

Six Yin-Yang Divisions

Classifying fixed longitudinal pathways along the body surface in terms of yin and yang was a major step for the ancient Chinese. Recognition of the longitudinal organization of the body, as defined by the six yin-yang regions on each side of the body, is fundamental to most physiological aspects of Chinese medicine. The upper and lower portions of the six main regions on each side of the body are further subdivided into hand and foot assignments. This results in twelve specific regions on each side of the body, each related to a particular distribution vessel and internal organ (Table 4.3). The distribution vessels, their related nodal routes (Chapter 11), and the muscle pathways (Chapter 12) are named after the yin and yang

Table 4.3 Classification of the twelve organ-related distribution vessels in matched yin-yang pairs of outflowing arteries and return veins for specific anatomical divisions of the body and extremities, along with environmental factors affecting these regions.

Anatomical Division	*Body Orientation*	*Extremity Aspect*	*Extremity*	*Vessel Type*	*Associated Internal Organ*	*Attacked By*
Taiyin	Anterior	Medial	Hand	Artery	Lungs	
Yangming		Lateral	Hand	Vein	Large Intestine	Dryness
Yangming		Lateral	Foot	Artery	Stomach	
Taiyin		Medial	Foot	Vein	Spleen	Damp
Shaoyin	Posterior	Medial	Hand	Artery	Heart	Heat
Taiyang		Lateral	Hand	Vein	Small Intestine	
Taiyang		Lateral	Foot	Artery	Bladder	Cold
Shaoyin		Medial	Foot	Vein	Kidneys	
Jueyin	Lateral	Medial	Hand	Artery	Pericardium	
Shaoyang		Lateral	Hand	Vein	Internal Membrane	Fire
Shaoyang		Lateral	Foot	Artery	Gallbladder	
Jueyin		Medial	Foot	Vein	Liver	Wind

regions through which they traverse. The net result is an anatomical notation system that is consistent with the organization and distribution of blood vessels, nerves, muscles, and their related tendons.

The six main divisions are well delineated on the arms, legs, head, neck, back, and lateral aspects of the body. How yin patterns distribute along the abdomen and chest was not made clear by the ancient doctors. Under the relative classifications, the abdomen is considered yin. However, under the orientation classification, the anterior portion of the body belongs to the sunrise yang (yangming). The yangming distribution vessels and associated nodes traverse longitudinally down the front of the body. The foot yangming (stomach) muscle distributions traverse up the abdominal regions. The six yin distribution vessels and nodal pathways (from hand and foot) terminate in the chest region. There are no yin regions on the head or face, although collateral vessels assigned to the yin distributions do reach the head. Of the yin muscle distributions, the kidney muscles lie deep in the back and do not traverse the abdomen. There are no liver-related muscles on the trunk of the body. The major spleen-related muscles on the trunk are the intercostal muscles. Only the lungs and heart have significant muscle distributions over the upper chest. It is possible that the yin divisions were considered to lie below the yang divisions on the chest and abdomen areas.

Six Atmospheric Airs

The six dominant environmental airs related to specific periods of the solar year are named after the three yin and three yang distribution regions (Table 4.3 and Chapter 6). The name of each dominant atmospheric condition is derived from the longitudinal distribution regions and associated anatomical features (vessels, nerves, and muscles) that are most likely to be attacked by these particular forces. There is a distinct advantage in relating environmental factors to specific body regions, vessels, muscles, and organs. When a person is exhibiting symptoms consistent with one of the six airs it provides important information concerning the affected vessel and organ, as well as how deeply the body is affected (Tables 6.1 and 6.2).

Yin and Yang Terms in Naming and Locating Nodes

The Chinese names for many nodal sites provide information about their anatomical location on the body. Yin and yang terms are also used in some names to indicate their location. For example, Zhiyang (DU 9) is located in the middle of the upper back. The back is classed as yang, and this node is located below the spinous process of the vertebrae at the highest region of the thoracic curve. Hence, *zhiyang* (至阳) refers to the "most (*zhi*, 至) posterior (*yang*, 阳)" location on a yang surface (the back). The lower part of the body is classed as yin, with the toes representing the terminal extremities of yin. One node located at the lateral nail margin of the small toe, Zhiyin (BL 67), is the terminal site of the bladder vessel and is the "most yin" location. The nodal sites Huiyin (RN 1), located in the perineum, and Huiyang (BL 35), located on each side of the coccyx, respectively indicate the meeting (*hui*, 会) of yin and yang.

Some nodal names give accurate descriptions of their location. Consider Yanglingquan (GB 34) and Yinlingquan (SP 9), located on each side of the leg below the knee. Here, yang refers to the lateral aspect of the leg while yin refers to the medial aspect. The word *ling* (陵), which means mound or hill, refers to the tibial tuberosity where the patellar (kneecap) ligament attaches to the tibia. The word *quan* (泉) means a spring, which is a common designator assigned to several different locations. Hence, Yanglingquan (GB 34) indicates the location of a node (called a spring) situated on the lateral aspect of the leg at the level of the tibial tuberosity. Yinlingquan (SP 9) refers to a node (also a spring) located on the medial aspect of the leg at the level of the tibial tuberosity.

Another example of using yin and yang terms to indicate specific node locations is illustrated in the region behind the knee, the popliteal fossa. One site, located in the middle of the popliteal fossa, is named Weizhong (BL 40). Here, *wei* (委) refers to the popliteal fossa, while the word *zhong* (中) means center. The name *weizhong* (委中) (center of the popliteal fossa) gives an accurate description on the node location. Other nodes are located respectively on the lateral and medial aspect of the popliteal fossa. These are named Weiyang (BL 39) and Yingu (KD 10). Weiyang (BL 39) is located at the same level as Weizhong (BL 40), but as its name implies, is located on the lateral (yang) aspect of the popliteal fossa (wei). In the case of Yingu (KD 10), which is located at the same level as Weizhong (BL 40), yin refers to the medial aspect of the popliteal fossa. The second character (*gu*, 谷) refers to a valley or gorge, and metaphorically describes the space between the tendons of the semitendinosus and semimembranosus muscles.

View of Internal Organs

All the internal regions and organs are under the general classification of yin, because everything that is hidden inside the body is considered yin with respect to the outside. However, within this yin category the organs are further differentiated into either yin or yang depending on their characteristic nature, function, or position within the body cavities.

Yin-Yang Classification of Internal Organs

The bowels, comprising the gastrointestinal and alimentary track, are hollow, have a direct communication with the outside world, and tend to pour out, and hence are yang in nature. The urinary bladder is also categorized as yang, since it too is hollow, communicates with the outside world, and pours out. The internal membrane system (sanjiao), especially the portion that encloses or surrounds the entire alimentary tract organs, is likewise considered to be a yang bowel. The gallbladder, which stores bile fluid for release when food is present in the duodenum, does not continuously pour out, and so is sometimes referred to as a special yang organ.

The heart, lungs, liver, kidneys, and spleen are solid organs, and with the exception of the lungs, have no communication with the outside world. Since these organs are internal, store for long periods, and are solid, they are classified as yin in nature. An exception is the pericardium surrounding the heart. It is not considered to be an organ, but nevertheless is classed as belonging to yin. The pericardium is internally-externally related to the internal membrane system (sanjiao).

Position Within the Body

The viscera are also classified as either yin or yang based on their anatomical location within the body. Location is considered both in terms of the relative upper and lower positions, as well as the depth within the body with respect to relative anterior and posterior position. The internal body cavities are also given specific yin and yang assignments. Other classifications relate to both the position and function of the organs. The space above the diaphragm (thoracic cavity) contains the heart, pericardium, and lungs, and is considered to be yang because of its superior position. This is also the location of the upper portion of the internal membrane system (upper *jiao*), including the pleura. The region below the diaphragm consisting of the abdominal cavity is classed as yin because of its inferior position in the body. The upper portion of this region contains the liver, spleen, kidneys, and middle jiao. Below this is the lower abdominal cavity and location of the lower jiao.

In terms of position within the thoracic cavity, the lungs are sometimes referred to as the most yang organs because they sit above and cover all the other organs as the sky covers the earth. Sometimes the lungs are referred to as the great yin within yang because of their relative location within the thoracic cavity. The heart is also classified in terms of its functional characteristics and its position in the body. Because of its critical yang function of rhythmic contractions to continuously circulate blood, the heart is classified as the great yang within yang. Here, "within yang" refers to it being located within the thoracic cavity, which is in the yang position.

With respect to the abdominal cavity, the liver is often classified as lesser yang because of its upper position tucked under the ribs and diaphragm, and its proximity to the inside abdominal surface. The kidneys are considered great yin because they lie deep within the body and against the posterior wall of the abdominal cavity. The spleen is nested between the left medial posterior area of the stomach and the internal body wall, and because it is considered to be hidden it is therefore is classified as extreme yin.

Diurnal Order

The Chinese viewed the daily variations in sunlight and darkness in several different ways (Table 4.4), one of which was to divide each day into specific yin and yang periods. Also, since seasons have yin and yang qualities, with summer being yang and winter being yin, each day is considered similar to a four-season solar year. This is noted in *NJLS 44* (*Obeying Sequence of Four Daily Seasons*). Early morning is thought to correspond with spring, noontime corresponds with summer, sunset corresponds with autumn, and midnight corresponds with winter. Just as the four seasons respectively produce birth, growth, harvest, and storage, a patient may recover or decline during each daily season. Patients typically feel better in the morning (spring), improve at noontime (summer), start to decline at sunset (autumn), and worsen at midnight (winter). Selecting the most appropriate time to provide treatment necessarily considers these characteristics for optimal clinical results.

In terms of yin and yang classifications for daily time periods, each day is divided into twelve time increments. These daily time intervals are related to the diurnal periods of the heavenly bodies. Names assigned to distribution regions of the body are also the names of celestial objects and time periods. The earth's star, the sun, is called the great yang (taiyang) and is assigned to the time period from 1:00 to 5:00 P.M., when the effect of the sun is the greatest. The lesser sun (shaoyang) refers to the background stars of the night sky, and is assigned to the period of 9:00 P.M. to 1:00 A.M. The sunrise yang (yangming) period from 5:00 to 9:00 A.M. is not related to a heavenly body, but does have a specific time period. These three yang periods set the timing of the diurnal order.

Table 4.4 Daily yin-yang time periods, and chronobiological relationship of the internal organs, heavenly bodies, daily seasons, and daily relative yin-yang conditions.

Time	*Name*	*Internal Organ*	*Heavenly Bodies*	*Six-Hour Season*	*Daily Season*	*Six-Hour Periods*	*Yin-Yang Condition*
5:00 A.M. 7:00 A.M.	*Yangming*	Large Intestine Stomach	Sunrise	Early Morning	Spring	Sunrise to Noon	Yang within Yang
9:00 A.M.	*Taiyin*	Spleen	Moon				
11:00 A.M.	*Shaoyin*	Heart	Planets	Noontime	Summer	Noon to Dusk	Yin within Yang
1:00 P.M. 3:00 P.M.	*Taiyang*	Bladder Small Intestine	Sun				
5:00 P.M.	*Shaoyin*	Kidneys	Planets	Dusk	Autumn	Dusk to Midnight	Yin within Yin
7:00 P.M.	*Jueyin*	Pericardium					
9:00 P.M. 11:00 P.M.	*Shaoyang*	Internal Membrane Gallbladder	Stars	Midnight	Winter	Midnight to Sunrise	Yang within Yin
1:00 A.M.	*Jueyin*	Liver					
3:00 A.M.	*Taiyin*	Lungs	Moon				

Unlike the sun, the moon does not radiate (radiating is a yang quality), rather it reflects sunlight and is named great yin (taiyin). The planets in a similar fashion also do not radiate like the sun or the stars, and therefore have yin qualities like the moon and the earth and are hence called lesser yin (shaoyin). The transitional yin (jueyin) does not relate to a particular heavenly body, but does have its specific time periods during the day. Daily yin periods logically bound the yang intervals. The lesser yin periods of two hours each (11:00 A.M.–1:00 P.M. and 5:00–7:00 P.M.) are appropriately placed before and after the great yang period. The transitional yin periods (7:00–9:00 P.M. and 1:00–3:00 P.M.) are logically placed before and after the lesser yang four-hour interval. Finally, the great yin periods (3:00–5:00 A.M. and 9:00–11:00 A.M.) are placed on each side of the sunrise yang four-hour interval. This overall scheme provides a logical transition of daily yin and yang periods (Table 4.4).

Associating the longitudinal yin-yang body regions with time periods of the day resulted in the development of the Chinese chronobiology theory. The daily yin and yang periods were correlated with the longitudinal regions and their related internal organs, vessels, and muscle distributions. What resulted from this correlation was the first-known effort to set forth a periodic relationship for the internal organs. The ancient Chinese endeavored to understand the key time periods during the day and the seasons that influenced certain organ functions.

Visceral Yin and Yang

Internal organs are classified as being yin or yang by their overall nature (storing, pouring out, solid, hollow), and by their function and position in the body. Each has other yin and yang properties associated with its functional activities, as well as related vital fluids and substances. Organ functional activity is referred to as visceral yang. Since the word *qi* (气) is also used to denote function, visceral yang is also known as visceral qi or *yangqi* (阳气). Visceral yin is the classification of biologically active materials and refined substances (now known to include hormones and neurotransmitters), and nutrients critical to the function of an organ. The fundamental concept is that yang function is derived from yin substance.

Consider the stomach for example. Its primary function is to break food down and pass the resulting products on to the small intestine. The normal peristaltic action (yang function) is to pass the dietary material downward. When the stomach is full the small intestine is empty. When its contents are passed on, the stomach is empty and the small intestine is full. Stomach yin consists of the vital fluids to break down food, which is now understood to involve digestive enzymes and hydrochloric acid. Other yin substances (including hormones and neurotransmitters) are critical to the function of the stomach, and either enhance or inhibit stomach yang. When there is a disturbance in stomach yang that impedes its normal function, disease results. If the stomach yang is reversed (*niqi*, 逆气), stomach acid reflux or vomiting results.

The remaining organs all have visceral yin and yang properties.

Differentiation of Visceral Symptoms

Disease manifestations are distinguished in terms of yin and yang qualities, the organs, and environmental and emotional factors. These relationships are consistent with the principles of the five phases and follow the principles of yin and yang. From *NJSW 5*, for example:

> When yin qualities predominate, yang is diseased. When yang qualities predominate, yin is diseased. Predominance of yang causes fever, and predominance of yin causes cold. Severe cold produces heat and severe heat produces cold. Cold is harmful to physical shape and heat is harmful to vital substance. Harm to vital substance causes pain, and harm to physical shape causes swelling. When wind predominates it results in symptoms characterized by movements; when heat predominates, it causes symptoms characterized by swelling; when dryness predominates it causes symptoms of dry skin and dry stools; when cold predominates it causes symptoms of edema; when dampness predominates it causes symptoms of damp diarrhea. Joy and anger are harmful to vital substance; cold and summer heat are harmful to physical shape. Frenzy is harmful to yin and wild joy is harmful to yang.

Organ Yin and Yang Mediated by the Autonomic Nervous System

The ancient Chinese only provided a rudimentary understanding of the nervous system, as previously discussed (Chapter 3). They may not have recognized that nerves mediate yin and yang characteristics of internal organ function. This mediation is now known to be provided by the autonomic nervous system (ANS) that controls the viscera and the blood vessels. The ANS is divided into the sympathetic nervous system (SNS) and the parasympathetic nervous system (PSNS), which provide the main innervation to the organs. The SNS also innervates the blood vessels. The auricle is the only place on the body where PSNS fibers—small sprigs of the vagus nerve, or tenth cranial nerve—have a superficial distribution.

The ANS contains both sensory and motor fibers. The sensory nerves are afferent fibers that provide signals to the autonomic ganglia, spinal cord, and brain on pain, pressure, temperature, and information pertinent to organ function. The autonomic motor nerves are efferent fibers that provide control signals to the vessels and organs. The processes of needling therapy depend greatly on the interaction between these nerve fibers and those that innervate the muscles and superficial regions of the body (Chapter 14).

The functions of the body that were classified by the ancient Chinese as yin or yang are consistent with presently understood PSNS and SNS activity, respectively. Most of the physiological changes due to SNS outflow are yang in nature. Changes mediated by PSNS stimulation are yin in nature (Table 4.5). Therefore the fight or flight stress response is yang, while meditation, on the other hand, is a yin response. Since the ANS dominates the function of the internal organs, visceral disorders often reflect some imbalance of this system. Many of the yin or yang qualities of disease can be understood in terms of the relative balance between the SNS and PSNS.

Dynamic Interplay between Yin and Yang

The classification of substances and phenomena in terms of yin and yang are usually fixed, and normally do not change their characteristics. Many other entities have yin and yang properties only by virtue of their relationship to each other. This interdependent association creates conditions of yin and yang. Without the earth's orbital velocity creating a centripetal force in opposition to the gravitational pull of the sun, the earth would inevitably be drawn into the sun and cease to exist. Without an up direction there can be no down. Without day there can be no night.

This interdependent relationship is a component of physiological processes. Substance is yin; function is yang. Substance is the basis of function and function itself is viewed as a reflection of substance. Function is also the motive force for utilizing substance. For example the functional activities and health of the internal organs can only be achieved if adequate nutrients are available. On the other hand, nutrients cannot be broken down and properly utilized by the body if the internal organs are not functioning properly.

There is a promoting, declining, and transforming dynamic aspect of yin and yang. Some conditions or situations can be viewed as yin or yang when compared to a dominant counterpart. Later the balance of this relationship can change when either feature is strengthened or transformed, or its counterpart declines. The yin or yang nature of a situation or condition is thus dependent on the relationship of each yin-yang component to the other at any given moment.

Interdependence and Opposition

Yin and yang are normally present in equal measures, providing a harmonious counterbalance. The earth orbiting around the sun is a good example. The sun is yang and the earth is yin. The gravitational pull between the sun and earth is yin. The centripetal force as a result of the

Table 4.5 Western physiological correlation of yin and yang responses of the five organ systems mediated by the autonomic nervous system.

Target Organs	*Yang Response*	*Yin Response*
Lungs	Bronchial and Blood Vessel Dilatation, Increased Breathing Rate	Bronchial and Blood Vessel Contraction, Decreased Breathing Rate
Thyroid Gland	Thyroxine Increased	Calcitonin Increased
Parathyroid Glands	Parathyroid Hormone Released	Parathyroid Hormone Inhibited
Skin	Localized Contraction	Relaxation
Mucus	Decreased	Increased
Sense of Smell	Impaired	Enhanced
Large Intestine	Inhibition of Secretion and Motility	Stimulation of Secretion and Motility
Spleen	Capsule Contraction	Normalization
Pancreas	Insulin and Digestive Fluid Inhibited, Glucagon Stimulated	Stimulated
Salivary Glands	Inhibited	Stimulated
Sense of Taste	Impaired	Enhanced
Thymus Gland	Inhibited	Stimulated
Stomach	Inhibition of Secretion and Motility	Stimulation of Secretion and Motility
Heart	Increased Rate, Contractility, and Pressure	Decreased Rate, Contractility, and Pressure
Pituitary Gland	Release of ACTH, TSH, and MSH	Normalization
Blood Vessels	Mostly Constricted with Some Specific Dilatation	Dilatation
Sweat Glands	Localized Secretion	Generalized Secretion
Speech	Impaired	Normalization
Small Intestine	Inhibition of Secretion and Motility	Stimulation of Secretion and Motility
Kidneys	Decreased Blood Flow	Normalization
Adrenal Glands	Epinephrine, Norepinephrine, and Corticosteriod Release	Normalization
Calcium Demand	Increased	Decreased
Hearing	Impaired	Enhanced
Testes/Ovaries	Inhibited	Stimulated
Sexual Function	Ejaculation/Orgasm	Erection/Stimulation
Urine	Increased Formation	Normalization
Bladder	Increased Capacity	Normalization
Liver	Glycogenolysis	Normalization
Pineal Gland	Increased Synthesis of Melatonin	Normalization
Adipose Tissue	Lipolysis	Normalization
Blood Fat Levels	Increased	Decreased
Eyes	Improved Far Vision	Improved Near Vision
Tears	Decreased	Increased
Gallbladder	Inhibited	Stimulated
Autonomic Outflow	Sympathetic	Parasympathetic
General Adaptive Reaction	Stress Response	Calming, Relaxation, Meditation, Taijiquan, Qigong

earth's velocity around the sun that opposes gravity is yang. These two forces are in perfect equilibrium to maintain the earth's harmonious yearly orbit around the sun.

If the earth's velocity is increased the centripetal yang force would be greater. Consequently the earth would develop an increasingly greater orbit with each velocity increase until it escaped from the sun's pull. Likewise if the earth was slowed, the gravitational yin force would dominate, eventually pulling the earth into the sun.

Transformation of Yin and Yang

The balance of yin and yang in many situations is in a continuing state of change. Because of their mutual opposition and interdependence, any change in one affects the other. If one feature is weakened or declines, the other is promoted or strengthened. This promoting, declining, or transforming of one quality over the other is one aspect of the body's internal physiological balance. Declining yin leads to the gaining or strengthening of yang. Likewise, the waning of yang leads to the gaining of yin.

A transformation in the nature of a particular illness or disease follows these same principles. Some illnesses start with a chill or cold condition: recovery often does not come about until a fever develops that eventually breaks. In other illnesses, chills and fever alternate with a cyclic dominance of one or the other. If balance is returned then recovery follows. If either yin or yang predominates, the prognosis is not favorable. A critical understanding of the health and disease process depends on a comprehension of physiological functions in terms of their yin-yang promoting, declining, and transforming relationships. This awareness provides direct information that is used in formulating a treatment approach for an identified disorder.

Under normal conditions opposite functions and processes maintain a relative internal balance in the body within certain limits. During periods of high physical activity yang predominates, while yin is dominant during sleep and relaxation. In any given situation there is an acceptable transient increase in one feature over the other, but the body's homeostatic balance is maintained. Under abnormal conditions, there is a preponderance or diminishing of yin or yang. The net effect is the manifestation of yin or yang symptoms. These are further considered in terms of excess or deficiency, and lead to at least four possible pathological situations as follows:

Preponderance of Yin
A preponderance of yin due to a deficiency of yang is a deficiency (*xu*, 虚) condition. The deficit in yang function causes yin to dominate, even though yin was not excessive, and results in typical syndromes that include deficient cold conditions, hypothyroid conditions, and depression.

Preponderance of Yang
A preponderance of yang due to a deficiency of yin substance can be classified as a heat syndrome. Since this involves a deficiency of yin as the main cause, it would also be considered a deficiency (xu) condition. Such syndromes include deficient heat conditions, urticaria, sore throat, herpes zoster, hyperthyroid syndrome, rheumatism, irritable bowel syndrome, insomnia, anxiety, and withdrawal syndrome.

Excess Yang

An excess yang condition results in anxiety and other yang syndromes. This is the most common imbalance of yin and yang observed. In a condition where excessive yang consumes yin, a heat condition is produced. Such a condition is of the excess (*shi*, 实) type, and could produce manifestations such as fever, excess heat, hyperthermia, pathogenic assault, inflammatory reaction, stress, and anxiety neurosis.

Excess Yin

Excess yin causing a decline in yang is the opposite of excess yang. Since yang is deficient it is classified as a cold condition of the excess (shi) type. Excess yin is difficult to establish, even if exposed to overabundant pathogenic cold and damp, however hypothermia is one example. What more often occurs is a suppression of yang, which then generates an imbalance causing an apparent preponderance of yin, with yin syndromes. Depression is often a major result. A possible correlation is reduced levels of norepinephrine (yang transmitter) leading to depression. Excess cortisol (a yin substance) has been implicated in depression, which may have a direct reciprocal relationship with norepinephrine. Certain medications may also contribute to conditions of excess yin. Excess yin is temporarily produced under special conditions, such as the increase of central serotonin production during the habituation or tolerance to an addictive substance. Once habituation is established, a deficiency of yin will then exist. Conditions manifesting as excess yin include excess cold, hypothermia, anti-inflammatory reactions, substance-use effect, medication-use effect, and manic depression.

5

Need for Medicine

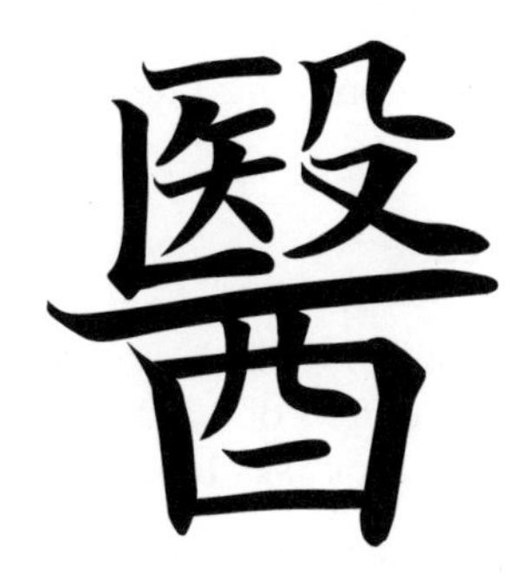

Yi: Medicine

> Therefore, the sages combined a variety of treatment approaches, each selected for its particular suitability. Consequently, in order to treat disorders prevalent to a specific geographical location and bring about a cure, the practitioner must have a feeling for the disease and knowledge of the treatment approaches, and the conditions of the patient.
>
> Qibo, *NJSW 12 (Different Methods and Appropriate Prescriptions)*

It was apparent to the ancient Chinese that the demands of living in a civilized culture adversely affected their health. When people lived in a completely natural environment, sickness was relatively uncommon. As society became more complex, the risk of disease was greater. Simple preventive health strategies no longer worked. It was then necessary to devise a practical means to treat illness. First, it was critical to understand how the body responded to adverse factors—from this information one could then identify diseases and devise treatment approaches. This effort gave rise to the development of medicine. All previous and subsequent civilized communities probably went through this process. Keeping track of basic physiological and diagnostic data, as well as treatment information, was essential. Pressures to remember this information may have been one reason that humans developed writing.

A wide range of medical approaches was developed by the early Chinese physicians; for the most part these have very ancient beginnings, dating back to before the age of writing. The emphasis was initially on the use of herbs, stone needles, and moxibustion. True needling therapy (acupuncture) came about after the introduction of metal needles. Prior to that, stone needles were employed to release a few drops of blood in what was described as draining off a solid condition. Physical medicine involving heat application, massage, manipulation, pressure, remedial exercise, and breathing exercise was also developed. Fundamental to all this was dietary therapy (Chapter 6). Different treatment schemes evolved in separate regions of Stone Age China. While similar treatment approaches were developed in other countries as well, needling therapy and moxibustion are truly unique to China. The success of Chinese medicine is evidenced by the fact that it has survived essentially unchanged for the past 2,600 years or more, and that surgery was infrequently employed prior to the introduction of Western medicine.

Disease was thought to be caused by people either not protecting themselves from environmental conditions, or living a lifestyle incompatible with normal bodily function. Initially, disease could be avoided by living in tune with nature, or through the use of meditative techniques. As life became more complex, disease was treated with cereal soups and wine. However, in later times it was noted that the strain of a more complex society resulted in lifestyles getting increasingly out of balance. Eventually intervention through herbs, diet, needling therapy, and moxibustion was considered necessary to bring about cures.

Cause and Treatment of Disease

An explanation of how changing lifestyles over the centuries directly affected health and human life span is given in the first paragraph of *NJSW 1* (*On the Simple and Unaffected Life of Ancient Times*). Here the Yellow Emperor asks his principal teacher, Qibo:

> I have heard it said that people of ancient times all lived to the extent of one hundred years of age without signs of decline in movement and motion. But people in present times all show decline in movement by the age of fifty. Is this due to influences from generation to generation, or is this due to people failing to take care of themselves?
>
> Qibo replies: People of ancient times understood the way of nature [dao], the principles of yin and yang [changes in the seasons], and appreciated the art of enumeration [using a calendar for forecasting]. They ate and drank in moderation, lived their daily lives in consistent and invariable patterns, without recklessness, and without working until fatigued. Therefore, they were able to maintain an integrated body and mind, and from beginning to end, to live out their natural life span of at least one hundred years before dying.
>
> People today are no longer like that because they consume alcohol as thick sauces, are often reckless, and have sexual intercourse while intoxicated. They exhaust their refined substances as a result of satisfying their desires, disperse their genuine vital function by overconsumption, and do not understand their limits. They take no time to manage their mental state and they devote their efforts to quick satisfaction of the heart, all of which is contrary to obtaining happiness. Consequently, they are not able to regulate their daily lives and therefore decline in health by the age of fifty.

The Yellow Emperor then inquired about how to avoid getting ill, and Qibo offered the following in *NJSW 1*:

> Sages in ancient times all taught that deficient environmental forces and stealing wind,[1] occurring now and then, should be avoided. One should remain calm and unperturbed and not be consumed by grief. One should retain genuine vital function and guard internal refined substances of vitality [including biologically active substances and hormones] to protect against disease. Hence, aspirations should be idle with few desires and the mind kept peaceful, without being alone or unfriended. Physical labor should not be undertaken to the point of becoming fatigued, and the body's functional activity therefore can remain in order. Each of these goals can be accomplished, and one can still satisfy all of one's needs.

Cure by Meditation or Prayer Alone

At one time people lived among animals and birds in complete harmony with nature. The act of contemplation could restore functional balance, and hence be used to maintain health.

This reference is provided in *NJSW 13* (*Conveying Refined Substances and Transforming Vital Function*), wherein the Yellow Emperor asks:

> I have heard that in ancient times disease could be cured by contemplation to convey refined substances and transform vital function, and meditation was all that was required. Today all diseases are treated internally by the use of toxic herbs and externally by stone needles, with the patients either becoming well or not being cured. What about that?
>
> Qibo directly replies: In the ancient past people lived a leisurely life with the birds and wild animals. They worked hard to avoid cold and their shelters were covered to avoid summer heat. Internally they had no worries or emotional attachments, nor desire to accumulate material things. Externally they had no government officials to report to for appearance sake. Theirs was a tranquil and satisfied society, so environmental pathogenic forces were not able to penetrate deeply into their bodies. Therefore toxic herbs were not needed to treat them internally, and the stone needle was not needed to treat them externally.
>
> Today the world is not like that. People suffer with worry and anxieties that affect them internally, and harsh physical labor harms them externally. In addition they fail to follow the changes in the four seasons. They live contrary to appropriate concern for environmental conditions of cold and heat. They are frequently attacked by the stealing wind and subjected to deficiency-causing pathogenic factors from morning to night. Internally these attack the five viscera, bones, and marrow, and externally they cause harm to body openings and orifices, and the muscles and skin. Consequently a minor disease becomes a serious condition, and a major disease can result in death. Hence, meditation and prayer alone cannot produce a cure.

Not Even Wine Can Cure

Later in *NJSW 13*, the topic of lifestyles deteriorating to the point where people resorted to cereal wines to treat disease is discussed. However, as civilization developed, morals started to decline and then not even wine could help. At this juncture only herbal medicine, needling therapy, and moxibustion could cure a disease. This is discussed in *NJSW 14* (*Cereal Soups and Mellow and Sweet Wine*):

> The sages of ancient times prepared mellow and sweet wine from cereal soups [but apparently didn't drink the wine], because in ancient times they only prepared rice soups for the sake of the soup, and therefore not for the purpose of serving wine. Later during the era of ancient times, the natural way and virtue [morals] declined slightly and consequently these people were frequently attacked by pathogenic environmental forces. They used mellow and sweet wine to help overcome these effects... It is necessary for people today to simultaneously be treated internally by the application of herbal medicine, and externally by needling and moxibustion to bring about a cure.

Development of Therapeutic Approaches

Medical strategies developed in ancient China formed a primary-care health system with a full range of treatment approaches. These modes of care have been used continuously from earliest times and are still employed to treat every known disease and disorder affecting humankind. Western medicine first introduced into Asia in the seventeenth century consisted of burning with hot irons and bloodletting by venesection, approaches that were not readily adopted since they offered no apparent advantage over Chinese medicine. However, as modern medical science became the dominant global influence, especially after the 1950s, conventional Western care became the treatment of choice even in China. About this time, the Chinese recognized that their time-honored medicine could complement conventional care. Since then, all hospitals provide the best of both Western and Chinese medicine, and patients are free to choose their preferred treatment approach. The emphasis is on providing patients with the most effective and safest treatment possible for his or her particular condition.

Distinctions between Chinese and conventional medicine are interesting because each places importance on different therapies. This results in part from differing views of human physiology and etiology. Chinese medicine gives great priority to environment and lifestyle considerations as causative factors in disease; conventional care, on the other hand, emphasizes either pathogenic organisms or a biomedical explanation of the problem. Both Chinese and Western medicine have developed physical therapies with much in common, and a comparison of different treatment modalities from the East and West shows a supporting overlap.

Chinese treatment strategies applied to a particular disorder are based on a diagnosis of the disorder. There are some general considerations when deciding among the various modalities. As a rule, severe and acute disorders are treated with herbs and needling. Combined use of food and herbs or a medicated diet can also be considered. In long-term chronic ailments, nutritional therapy is considered most important. All herbs have the potential for producing unexpected and unwanted side effects, and hence long-term use of any formulation is usually inappropriate. Dietary therapy, on the other hand, is safer and more forgiving, and can be maintained over longer time periods without risk of adverse reactions.

As part of its unique understanding of the causes of disease, Chinese medicine is viewed in terms of internal and external disorders. Internal problems involve the internal organs; external disorders mostly involve the musculoskeletal system. As a general rule, herbal and dietary therapy are principally used to address problems affecting the internal organs, for which needling is also applied. Conversely, needling therapy, heat application, and physical medicine are most frequently used to treat orthopedic problems, including pain, rheumatism, arthritis, muscle pathology, and joint dysfunction. In some cases, however, herbs and dietary therapy can also be considered for external disorders.

In China today, trauma victims are directed to emergency centers or hospitals where high-quality Western medical care is provided. Needling therapy can be applied early in the healing process, after appropriate emergency medical care. In cases involving surgery, needling can be used to induce analgesia or calm a patient, but is most frequently applied during the postoperative phase. In serious cases, acupuncture comes into consideration chiefly during the post-trauma recuperative and rehabilitation phase. For treatment of mild trauma and even repeated stress injuries, Chinese medicine and needling are employed as primary modalities.

Therapies and Geographical Influence

Apart from needling therapy and moxibustion, the medical strategies developed by ancient Chinese physicians are similar to many Western techniques. In most cases, however, the Chinese were the first to perfect these treatment approaches. An illustration of the diversity in treating different conditions with a wide range of modalities is provided in *NJSW 5 (Great Treatise on the Proper Representation of Yin and Yang)*, as follows:

> When the patient's body is in poor condition, his or her vitality can be improved with warm herbs. If the patient has a deficiency of refined substances, this can be strengthened by using the five flavors [herbal and dietary therapy]... When pathogenic winds attack the patient, hot baths are used to cause perspiration. When disease involves the superficial skin, the method of inducing perspiration [heat packs] is applied. If the attack results in the patient being high spirited and violent, massage therapy is used to contain the condition. If it results in a solid [excess] condition, it should be dispersed and drained off [by drawing off a few drops of blood].

Historically it is thought that various treatment modalities had their origins in different geographical locations in China. Approaches were related to prevailing climates and perhaps customs of the different regions. This meant that different methods were employed to treat similar conditions with excellent effect. Reference to the geographical development of various treatment modalities is noted in *NJSW 12 (Different Methods and Appropriate Prescriptions)*. Herbal medicine developed in western China, the stone needle in eastern China, metal needles in southern China, moxibustion in northern China, and physical medicine in central China.

Medical Departments

During various ruling periods of Chinese history, therapeutic categories and medical specialties were classified into anything from four to thirteen separate divisions or medical departments, starting with the Zhou dynasty (1128–221 BCE), which was the first to organize clinical medicine into various specialties or departments. The Tang dynasty (618–907) had four medical departments, consisting of medicine (herbal and dietary), needling therapy and moxibustion, massage and manipulation, and charms and incantations.[2] During the Song dynasty (960–1279) there were nine medical departments: internal medicine; pediatrics; ulcers, abscesses and fractures; ophthalmology; obstetrics and wind diseases (including stroke); diseases of the mouth, teeth, and throat; needling and moxibustion; war wounds; and written incantations. The Yuan dynasty (1271–1368) had thirteen departments, consisting of internal medicine; miscellaneous diseases; wind disease; pediatrics; obstetrics; ophthalmology; diseases of the mouth and teeth; nose and throat diseases; orthopedics and bone setting; needling and moxibustion; supplications; and incantations. The Ming dynasty (1368–1644) also had thirteen departments, comprising internal medicine; pediatrics, gynecology; carbuncle and ulcers; needling and moxibustion; ophthalmology; mouth and teeth diseases; nose and throat diseases; febrile diseases; orthopedics and bone setting; war wounds; manipulation and massage; and supplication. Finally, the Qing dynasty (1644–1911) had nine medical departments: internal medicine; febrile diseases; gynecology; pediatrics; ulcers and abscess; ophthalmology; diseases of the mouth, teeth, and throat; needling and moxibustion; and orthopedics and bone setting.

Medicines for Internal and External Use

Herbal remedies, ordinary food, and medicated food used to address certain symptoms are included in the category of medicines. Herbs and food are used as internal medicines, while some herbs are also applied to the superficial regions of the body. Therapeutic use of herbs and food is fundamental to the practice of Chinese medicine. It is thought that herbs and food, notably of a of particular flavor, nourish specific viscera during fetal development, while the various flavors are an important consideration in treating or preventing certain conditions (Chapter 6). The selection of herbs and food is also based on their nature, which is classified as being hot, cold, warm, cool, or neutral—this property does not refer to the temperature of the herb or food, rather to the effect it has when consumed. Specifically, the main pharmacological properties of herbs are based on their nature, while the desired physiological effect is based on their inherent flavor.

The characteristic of the herb or food is usually selected in opposition to the nature of the disease being treated; specific diseases may manifest as being either hot or cold, or deficient or excess in nature. Herbal remedies or therapeutic food that is cold in nature is considered in cases of a hot disease that is severe. Cool herbal remedies or food is considered in cases of a hot disease that is mild. Hot herbal remedies or food is considered in cases of a cold disease that is severe, whereas warm herbal remedies or food is considered in cases of a cold disease that is mild. The properties of herbs and food are also selected with respect to the prevailing climatic conditions. Certain cold foods are avoided during cold seasons; certain hot foods are avoided during hot seasons. Also, the actual temperature of an herbal decoction to be consumed is considered with respect to the nature of the disease.

Herbal Remedies

Herbal remedies developed along with dietary strategies. Consuming or applying medicinal substances, such as plants, roots, tubers, stalks, flowers, and leaves, is an integral part of Chinese medicine. Of the several thousand different plant materials available, only about six or seven hundred are commonly used as herbal medicines, along with several mineral and animal products (Cai: 1983; Bensky and Gamble: 1986; Qu, Zhang and Xie: 1990; Zhang et. al. (eds.): 1990a; Geng et. al.: 1991a; Xu et. al. (eds.): 1994a; Ling: 1995; Fan: 1996). Herbal remedies can consist of a single ingredient, although most formulas contain several herbs. Formulas are derived from the main therapeutic effect of the key herb. Other herbs are added to harmonize the ingredients, enhance the effect of the remedy, or improve its palatability. Typical formulas may contain four to eight different herbs. Normally, a particular remedy is boiled down with a certain amount of water to produce a decoction. The solid remains are removed and the concentrated remaining liquid is taken orally.

Although herbal medicines were also used in the West, most of these gave way to chemical medicines in the nineteenth century, which now constitute the field of Western pharmacology. Many drugs are still derived from herbs or have an herbal beginning. The efficacy of long-used herbal formulas has been demonstrated over the years, but few have been thoroughly investigated on a scientific basis. While it is clear that some disease conditions call for a powerful pharmaceutical drug as the treatment of choice, there are numerous other conditions where a milder approach, as might be provided by herbal remedies, is more appropriate. The application of medical substances, herbal products, and pharmaceuticals can be used in a complementary fashion.

Most herbal remedies are intended for oral consumption, although some are also used externally as a liniment, poultice, plaster, creme, paste, ointment, powder, or suppository (Bensky and Barolet: 1990; Li et. al.: 1990; Geng et. al.: 1991b; Xu et. al. (eds.): 1994b). In addition, remedies are available in ready-to-use herbal products, frequently referred to as patent medicines (Fratkin: 2001; Zhu: 1989; Zhang et. al. (eds.): 1990b; Xu et. al. (eds.): 1994e). Ready-to-use products are available as pills, powders, extracts, pellets, soluble granules, tablets, capsules, tinctures, dilutions, syrups, and oral liquids.

Dietary Therapy

Proper diet is essential to fetal and childhood development, as well as to sustain human life and prevent disease. Chinese dietetics involves a highly sophisticated system, where the consumption of food, classed by flavor, exerts an interrelated dynamic influence on the organs and tissues of the body (Chapter 6). Proper food intake is based on a well-balanced daily diet, avoiding the overconsumption or underconsumption of any particular flavor. Overconsumption eventually leads to predictable diseases. Foods with other flavors can often be used to counteract the effects of overconsumption of a particular flavor. In addition to herbs, flavors of foods are used in the treatment of primary visceral symptoms or in promoting certain visceral tendencies. Flavors are also used during different seasons to treat either excess or deficiency conditions.

Medicated Diet

Herbs can be added to various food products to create a medicated diet. Medicated diets are used to treat both acute and chronic disorders (Cai: 1988; Zhang et. al.: 1990). Both the foods and the introduced herbs are selected for their inherent flavors and basic properties, as well as for their known therapeutic effects. The most common vehicle for introducing herbs into the diet is a rice gruel or porridge, known as *xifan* (稀饭). This is preferably made from non-glutinous white rice because it is easily digested. Rice gruel is thought to protect the function of both the spleen and stomach. A gruel can also be made with wheat, millet, or maize, but these are considered inferior to rice.

Many additional food products are used to introduce herbs for the treatment of acute and chronic disorders. The particular food is selected for its ability to work with the herbal component to bring about the best therapeutic result. Different forms of medicated diet or the materials used in their production are categorized as follows: gruel or porridge; thick soups; drinks; medicated tea; specially cooked dishes; medicated wine and liquor; decoctions; juices; honey paste; honey extract; preserved fruits and vegetables, and candy; and miscellaneous items.

Needling Therapy (Acupuncture)

Needling therapy, perhaps the most distinctive treatment method in Chinese medicine, involves inserting very fine needles into specific locations of the body. The Western term "acupuncture" is called "needling therapy" by the Chinese, while the tools for its practice are referred to as *zhenjiu* (针灸), which is the word for needle (*zhen*, 针), together with the word for moxibustion (*jiu*, 灸) (Ma, J.: 1983). These two modalities frequently go together, although some practitioners exclusively use moxibustion, and others use only needling therapy.

Use of Stone and Metal Needles

Initially, fine arrow points and stone slivers called *bian* (砭) were employed for pricking the body, usually to draw a few drops of blood. These stone needles were also used for reducing abscesses and carbuncles. Ancient stone points have been found in archaeological sites in China; some made from flint, others from quartz and other materials. Needling therapy, involving the insertion of fine needles, was not possible until the metal needle was developed around 800 BCE. These were made of various metals, including gold and silver. Nine specific types of needle were employed, each with a different application. Some were blade-like instruments for reducing abscesses and perhaps for performing minor surgery, while others consisted of probes to massage the areas between the skeletal muscles.

Application of Needling

Needle stimulation is applied to critical junctures or nodes to regulate vital substances and functional activities of the body. In addition to being needled, nodes (acupoints) can be massaged, scraped, pressed, cupped, heated by moxibustion, heated by other means, or pricked to release a few drops of blood. Nodes can be palpated diagnostically for sensitivity, numbness, or minute temperature differences, and to assess effectiveness of treatment. Needle stimulation adds nothing to the body—its effect comes from its ability to bring about functional balance and to restore blood flow.

Insertion of needles into the superficial body requires knowledge both of the location of nodes and the underlying anatomical structures (Foreign Languages Press: 1975, 1980; Cheng: 1987). Each node has a nominal insertion depth that is adjusted for the size, shape, and condition of the patient. Needles are typically inserted perpendicularly to the skin, but some nodal locations require insertion to be at a specific angle. This is necessary because of local anatomical restrictions. Although node locations are found in association with nerves and blood vessels, under no circumstances are needles to be inserted into these structures. Likewise, needles are never inserted into the internal organs because of potential fatal consequences, as noted in *NJSW 64* (*On Needling with Respect or Contrary to the Four Seasons*):

> Regarding inserting needles into the five viscera: insertion into the heart causes death in one day, with the main symptomatic change of belching; insertion into the liver causes death in five days, with the main symptomatic change of talking; insertion into the lungs causes death in three days, with the main symptomatic change of coughing; insertion into the kidneys causes in death in six days, with the main symptomatic change of sneezing and yawning; and insertion into the spleen causes death in ten days, with the main symptomatic change of swallowing or gulping. Needle insertion into the human body that injures the five viscera produces symptomatic change and certainly results in death. The affected organ is determined by noting the symptomatic change in order to identify when death will result.

Modern Needles

Most of the nine types of ancient needle were used to prick, massage, bleed, or stimulate the superficial body, without being retained in the tissues, perhaps as was originally done with the bian stones. The only exception to this is the fine or filiform needle, which could be inserted and retained because it was considered small enough to cause little or no damage. This particular needle design is still in use almost unchanged since ancient times. Bloodletting associated with Chinese medicine usually involves expressing just a few drops of blood from a specific node using a three-cornered needle. The Chinese were shocked by the venesection and extensive bleeding practiced by Western medicine when it was first introduced to China. Their concern was quite valid since Western-style bloodletting of the time was sometimes fatal.

The most significant change related to needles came in the 1980s, and concerned quality control, sterilization techniques, and quality of materials. Needles most commonly consist of a thin metal shaft, extremely thin in diameter, usually from 0.5 to 2 inches in length (1 to 5 centimeters). They are almost always made of stainless steel, typically with a wire-wrapped handle, although since the 1980s some have plastic handles. The handle allows the practitioner to better manipulate the needle and prevents the needle from migrating into the body. One incident in France in the early 1800s, involving the use of a sewing needle for acupuncture, resulted in the needle migrating into the body cavity—the patient died two days later. Buttons were then attached to the needles to prevent recurrence of the problem.

With the increased concern for safety since the 1980s most practitioners, at least in the United States, use presterilized, disposable needles, available with needle guide tubes. Needling therapy, for certain conditions, still involves releasing a few drops of blood by pricking with a special three-cornered needle. This needle is also basically the same as its ancient counterpart.

Another type of needling device consists of a hammer-like instrument with a group of small needle points in the head used to stimulate the superficial skin without insertion. A very light tapping stimulates specific locations, and is frequently used to treat children and sometimes older or extremely sensitive patients. These are called seven-star or nine-star needles, depending on the number of needle points contained in the head, or plum blossom needles, after the pattern of the needle points in the head.

Percutaneous and Transcutaneous Electrical Stimulation

Critical nodes can also be stimulated by means of an electrical connection to inserted needles (percutaneous application), or to conductive pads placed on the skin (transcutaneous application). The use of electrical stimulators attached to inserted needles is commonly called electroacupuncture. This procedure is often used where profound analgesia is desired, such as in surgical analgesia. It is also employed in treating nerve dysfunction, paralysis, and substance-abuse withdrawal. Even though electroacupuncture seems to be quite modern, it has the longest history of any electrical therapy. Use of electricity to treat pain was reported in the West as early as the first century, when electric torpedo fish were used to treat gout (Stillings: 1975).

After the discovery of electricity in the late 1700s, machines of various types were developed. These involved devices using direct and alternating current, as well as those that employed galvanic and static electricity, and capacity storage techniques. Renewed interest in acupuncture in France during the early 1800s coincided with the period of research and exploration of electrical phenomena. Sarlandiere le Chevalier (1825) of France and da Camino (1834, 1837) of Italy were the first to apply percutaneous electrical nerve stimulation (PENS). By 1900 electrotherapy fell into disuse (Stillings: 1975), but was revived in the 1970s when it was discovered that electroacupuncture (PENS) was being used in lieu of anesthesia for surgery in China.

One consequence of the early use of electrostimulation was the observation that many nodal sites and other areas elicited a muscle contraction. This phenomenon peaked the interest of researchers to study and locate all the "points of election," as they were called. This led Von Ziemssen (1829–1902) and Erbs (1840–1921) to study these sites on terminally ill patients, who were dissected immediately after their deaths to observe the anatomical basis of the reactive locations. Von Ziemssen made the first Western correlation of where the motor nerve connects to the muscle (neuromuscular attachments). Unfortunately the relationship between motor point discovery and Chinese needling therapy was soon forgotten.

Heating Therapy

The heating therapy of ancient times, apart from moxibustion, has changed with the advent of newer equipment, assuring better temperature control and patient safety. Moxibustion is a specialized technique that is used to heat specific nodes or locations, or limited areas on the body. When it was necessary to heat larger areas, the ancient Chinese physicians used heat packs, or in some cases, required the patient to be seated over or near hot coals to allow radiant heat to penetrate the body. The modern equivalent to heat therapy involves the use of heat packs, infrared lamps, and ultrasound application. These devices are in common use in acupuncture clinics in present-day China, Japan, Europe, and to some extent in the United States.

Moxibustion and Warm Needle Therapy

Moxibustion is a heating therapy that involves igniting certain combustible plant fibers to heat specific areas or nodal sites, which then promotes warming in a localized area. Moxibustion can also be used to apply heat to slightly larger areas by moving a heated moxa stick, held safely above the skin, back and forth across the affected regions of the body. It is employed to treat the effects of cold attacking or invading the body, or to strengthen the body's immune or defensive system. Moxa fibers can be rolled into sticks or used as loose material to form balls ignited on needles or cones burned on the skin. Little has changed in the application of moxibustion (Zmiewski and Feit: 1989).

The word moxa derives from a Dutch transliteration of the Japanese words *mo gusa*, which means to burn a herb. The Chinese for this practice is jiu, which means the same thing, while the Chinese name for the herb used in moxibustion is *ai* (艾), consisting of the hairy fibers on the underside of *Artemisia vulgaris*, or common mugwort leaves. Many Westerners are familiar with this material as the tinder used to ignite fireworks.

Warm needle therapy refers either to heating needles after insertion using moxa ignited on the needle handle, or to preheating needles prior to insertion. This latter technique was often applied in treating rheumatism. Moxibustion and warm needle therapy are thought to have originated in northern China, perhaps by Stone Age people sitting in damp caves or campsites, fighting off winter chills.

Heat Packs

The use of heat packs has continued from ancient times to the present. Heat packs are applied in the treatment of many musculoskeletal problems, as well as a variety of other conditions. This is especially true where cold conditions are involved, or where there is impairment in the flow of blood, nutrients, and vital air. Detailed instructions on fabricating herbal heat packs for use in treating rheumatism due to cold are provided in *NJLS 6 (Longevity, Premature Death, Firmness, and Softness)*:

> Before using them in treatment, warm the heat packs over mulberry charcoal. Place the packs on the area of cold rheumatism that was needled until the heat penetrates into the affected area.

Herbal material included in the packs enhances warming by promoting superficial vasodilatation. One novel use of heat packs, used after needling treatment to resolve abscesses due to intestinal parasites, is noted in *NJLS 68 (Above the Diaphragm)*:

> After needling, one must apply herbal heat packs to warm the interior. Daily heating of the interior regions is applied to dissipate pathogenic factors and break up the large abscesses.

Modern heat packs have mostly replaced the old-style herbal packs. New technology and equipment permits uniform temperature control to assure more effective application and patient safety. Cold packs are also available, and are often used alternately with heat packs. However, the ancient Chinese did not use cold packs, and always warned of the risk of chilling any part of the body.

Radiant Heat

Radiant heat therapy in ancient times involved seating the patient near or over hot mulberry-wood coals. The *NJLS 13 (Muscle Distributions)* provides an example where radiant heat, ointment, or liniment and massage are used to treat facial paralysis (Chapter 12). The radiant heat application of ancient times was inconvenient for the patient, and neither the therapeutic results nor the patient's safety could be easily assured. Since the 1970s and 1980s, modern heat lamps are safely and efficiently used to provide radiant heat therapy equivalent to traditional methods. The use of these devices provides greater uniformity of heat distribution and temperature control than was possible with the ancient approach.

Ultrasound

The application of this technique also provides a modern means of heat application that safely duplicates traditional heating methods. It induces heat locally by mechanical vibration of the tissue and combines heat and deep massage. Ultrasound has been used in conjunction with acupuncture for more than twenty years (Oyle: 1974; Khoe: 1975, 1977). In cases where it is important to achieve a deeper heat penetration, ultrasound may be a more efficient and safer method than other heat sources.

Physical Medicine

Sophisticated physical modalities were developed by the ancient Chinese that can be generally grouped into three categories: pressure, massage, and manipulation. Physical medicine also includes exercise and breathing techniques, as well as cupping and scraping therapy (*guasha*, 刮痧). Slightly different techniques are used for adults than are applied to children. Many of these traditional approaches are similar to, but not necessarily the same as, Western physical therapy and osteopathic and chiropractic procedures. Physical modalities involve hands-on manipulation of various regions of the patient's body, which can be directed to specific nodal sites or to the head, neck, trunk, and extremities. Both orthotics and restraints were used by the early Chinese, who also performed bone setting.

Over the years, numerous physical techniques have been recorded in the Chinese texts. Very gentle specialized manipulations are used to treat problems in children under the age of twelve. For adults there are about twenty different methods that can be categorized under the general headings of pressure, massage, and manipulation (Wang, Fan, and Guan: 1990).

Physical modalities, including exercise, breathing exercise, massage, and manipulation are thought to have developed in central China. Remedial exercise routines became highly developed, and are mentioned in *NJSW 12*, as well as in other sections of the *Neijing*, including *NJSW 24* (*Blood, Vital Air, and Physical-Mental Conditions*), *NJLS 42* (*Transmission of Disease*), and *NJLS 73* (*Official Abilities*). Reference to different types of therapeutic bathing is also found in ancient texts such as the *Neijing*, including *NJSW 5* and *NJSW 19* (*Inscriptions on the Jade Astronomical Instrument and True Visceral Function*).

Physical medicine strategies are employed to treat disorders, for physical rehabilitation, and for health preservation. Many of these techniques are employed to treat musculoskeletal problems, including the aftermath of stroke. Massage and manipulation are still commonly used in China as an adjunct to treating paralysis and motor impairment. Many excellent and detailed books on Chinese physical medicine have been written from ancient times to the present.

Pressure Techniques

Pressure is often applied to specific nodal sites in the affected region of the body, or to sensitive areas that are either distal or proximal to the problem. Pressure methods are often referred to as acupressure, or shiatsu, from the Japanese (Cerney: 1974; Schultz: 1976). The magnitude and duration of applied pressure varies depending on the desired reaction. In some situations, where a sensitive site has developed in a muscle that affects that muscle and others in its longitudinal pathway, sufficient pressure is applied to cause an ischemic reaction, ameliorating the condition (Baldry: 1989). Pressure techniques, directed to particular muscles or muscle distributions, are applied to treat pain and dysfunction and to restore blood flow. Pressure methods treat serious musculoskeletal problems in both children and adults (Wang: 1991). Pressure techniques consist of: pushing; pressing; ischemic pressure; finger pressure; and finger-striking methods (Wang, Fan and Guan: 1990).

Massage

Massage is a general term for the manipulation of the muscles and tissues in a kneading motion (Wang, Fan, and Guan: 1990). Since rubbing the skin is involved, oils or other lubricants are often employed to prevent irritation. In some situations special oils are used to stimulate the skin; some massage techniques involve the use of hot water. There are massage methods that employ only the practitioner's hands, while some involve application of the fists, knuckles, arms, and elbows, providing deeper stimulation. One popular form uses a pinching and pulling technique, called *tuina* (推拿) (Xu et. al. (eds.): 1994c). Massage therapy is employed to treat pain and a wide range of musculoskeletal problems, as well as to regulate tissues,[3] relax muscles, restore blood and vital nutrient flow, and remove blockages in the superficial vessels. Common massage techniques consist of: rolling; kneading; rubbing; scrubbing; pushing; grasping; flat-pushing; patting; tapping; and vibrating (Wang, Fan and Guan: 1990).

Manipulation

Therapies classed as manipulation have a long history throughout China, and include a variety of techniques applied to the joints of the body, including spinal adjustments (Xu et. al. (eds.): 1992; Li and Zhong: 1998). Manipulation therapy includes specialized and general massage to specific areas or to the entire body, and controlled or practitioner-guided movement of the extremities, head, neck, and spine. Ancient techniques involved a gentle stepping therapy, where pressure is applied with the foot to adjust the upper and lower back in treating back pain. As described in *NJSW 12*, manipulation therapy is thought to have developed in central China. Other references to manipulation therapy are contained in *NJSW 4* (*On the Virtuous Word of the Golden Cupboard*), *NJSW 14*, *NJSW 19*, and *NJLS 42*. Many books have been written on this topic over the centuries.

The purpose of manipulation is to remove obstructions in the superficial vessels, improve circulation of blood and vital nutrients, regulate tissues, and relax muscles. Manipulation is also used to lubricate the joints, reduce swelling, alleviate pain, restore normal joint function (including range of motion), treat soft tissue injuries, correct dislocated joints, enlarge joint spaces, relieve nerve compression, and reduce adhesions. There are many specialized manipulation methods that focus on a specific effect or are directed to particular joints. Common techniques generally include: rolling-kneading; holding-twisting; shaking; wiping; rotating; pulling; and traction–counter-traction manipulations (Wang, Fan and Guan: 1990).

The degree of understanding of physical modalities by the ancient Chinese was extensive, including knowledge of contraindications, as noted by the following reference from *NJSW 4*:

> When the environmental forces of winter [cold] attack they cause disorders to the four limbs… In winter, this attack most likely results in rheumatism and cold limbs. Therefore, in winter, massage and manipulation therapy is not appropriate.

Early Chinese doctors were careful not to apply pressure or manipulation therapy in cases of internal heat conditions or infections. One example is provided in *NJSW 40* (*Abdominal Diseases*):

> This disease is called the bent beam disease… Pus and blood accumulate in the abdomen and wrap around the outside of the intestines and stomach. This condition should not be treated. If treated by pressing manipulation, death can result.

Manipulation therapy was applied by Chinese doctors to treat a wide range of problems, much as that employed by Western physical therapy specialists. They also used it to treat conditions that are not generally thought to respond to physical manipulation in the West. One novel example of shaking manipulation used to treat edema is noted in *NJSW 14*:

> The practitioner should profoundly shake the patient's four limbs and then cover and warm the patient. Reverse needling is applied to the swollen area to restore the normal

> physical shape [reduce swelling]. The patient's pores are then opened by inducing perspiration [by use of heat packs].

Cupping

This therapeutic technique involves using a vacuum in a suction cup placed on various parts of the body; the ancient Chinese originally used hollow animal horns. By briefly heating the air in an inverted cup, a vacuum is produced when the air cools after the cup is quickly applied to the skin. The resultant low pressure under the cup causes a localized expansion of tissue, which produces a profound vasodilatation reaction. Thus, cupping is used to increase blood flow to painful constricted areas, resupplying vital nutrients and vital air. Sometime later, cups of various sizes and shapes were fashioned from bamboo, while some were made of glass or ceramic. Cups are now available that can be mechanically evacuated using a small pump.

Cupping has been part of both the Chinese and Western therapeutic arsenal. Cups of all sizes are employed to treat a wide range of disorders. Small cups may be applied to the face to treat facial paralysis, whereas larger cups placed in the lumbar region are used to treat lumbago. Cupping is frequently applied over nodal sites, but can be used in non-nodal regions as well. Cups can also be applied over inserted needles, but in some cases this can result in blood oozing into the cup space—in all such cases, the proper handling and disposal of blood products is essential.

Scraping Therapy

Scraping therapy, known as guasha, is a technique involving scraping skin covered with oil with a smooth-sided object. The side of a typical Chinese porcelain spoon or other small, smooth object is used. The oil can contain herbs that, along with the scraping action, enhance superficial vasodilatation. This technique is used to remove stagnation and improve circulation in the superficial region; it produces a reddening of the skin that may last from several hours to a full day.

Exercise Therapy

The Chinese developed a wide range of exercises, some of which involve guided stretching of tendons and muscles, such as *daoyin* (导引) and others involving slow-motion martial arts movements as in *taijiquan* (太极拳). Many exercises are taught to patients to address specific muscle or articulation joint problems. Sometimes the therapy is directed to strengthen particular muscle groups, or those associated with a particular joint or muscle distribution. Exercises are included as part of the therapeutic approach in treating many musculoskeletal problems during rehabilitation. Some exercises are directed to general problems, such as tight tendons or general weakness.

Breathing Exercise

Breathing exercises are called *qigong* (气功), where *qi* (气) is air or vital air/breath and *gong* (功) means exercise. This practice originally derived from Daoist breathing exercises, and from the ancient practice of guided stretching (daoyin). Since the proper circulation of blood and vital nutrients, including vital air, is indispensable in Chinese medicine, it is understandable that breathing exercises would be included as a therapeutic method. Qigong is noted in many ancient sources as being a fundamental part of health preservation strategies, including *NJSW 1*, where the Yellow Emperor says:

> I have heard it said that in ancient times there were genuine people who could give guidance and understanding concerning the interaction of the sky and earth, and they could grasp the principles of yin and yang. Also, they did breathing exercise to take in the critical essence of air on their own, guarding their vitality [spirit]. They kept their muscles and flesh so strong that it was like all their muscles were one. Consequently, their longevity could wear out heaven and earth, because of their seemingly endless lives, since they followed the way [dao] of nature.

Qigong therapy involves instructing patients in breathing exercises appropriate to their condition (China Sports Magazine: 1985; Zhang and Sun: 1988; Bi et. al.: 1990; Xu et. al. (eds.): 1994d). There are various levels of breathing exercise; some of the simplest techniques require learning to breathe properly with the diaphragm, others are used to promote overall health and well-being. Some approaches are much more complex, involving movement and the directing of vital air to specific parts of the body, or addressing specific problems and diseases.

Baths and Water Therapy

Therapeutic bathing is still practiced in China, but the techniques are not generally taught in Chinese medicine or acupuncture schools in the United States or Europe. Modern therapeutic bathing equipment is presently available in most Western hospitals and physical therapy clinics, but this therapy is not normally used in modern acupuncture clinics—techniques are usually limited to instructing the patient on how to use therapeutic bathing at home.

Orthotics and Restraints

In treating musculoskeletal problems, simple splints and restraints are sometimes necessary to temporarily immobilize a joint and allow the healing process to proceed. Some of these orthotic approaches involve temporary soft casts made of herbal material, which further promotes healing. Today, modern devices are also employed with the emphasis on short-term use.

Bone Setting

Manipulation to correct a dislocated joint, or bone setting in the case of a fracture, is still a standard element of Chinese medicine in various parts of Asia (Xu et. al. (eds.): 1992). Bone setting was one of the major departments of standard medical practice in China. While these skills are still taught in some schools in Asia, they are not typically included in Western training programs in Chinese medicine (Zhang: 1996). The widespread availability of modern emergency clinics and hospitals in most countries easily accommodates these types of emergency problems.

Prevention and Rehabilitation

Prevention and rehabilitation is a crucial area of Chinese medicine—throughout Chinese history, these have been common themes (Sun et. al.: 1990). It is far more effective to prevent a disorder than treat the expression of disease. The basic ideas of health preservation include living a calmer life, reducing stress, avoiding excess physical activity, paying attention to diet, considering the condition of one's residence, and avoiding extremes of climatic conditions.

Prevention, health preservation, and rehabilitation all rely on the application of dietary strategies, medicated diets, remedial exercises, breathing exercises, relaxation techniques, and protecting oneself from harmful environmental exposure. In the case of rehabilitation, it is also necessary to consider the therapeutic use of herbs, needling, moxibustion, heat therapy, hot baths, cupping, pressure, massage, and manipulation appropriate to the condition of the patient.

In addition, the practitioner has the major task of attending to the patient's lifestyle and providing guidance where necessary. This aspect of the practitioner–patient relationship may involve examining the main sources of stress and disharmony in a person's life. The primary requirement, however, is that the practitioners themselves conduct their lives by the same principles—otherwise the individual has no credibility and will find it difficult to be a good practitioner.

6

Interaction of Sky and Earth

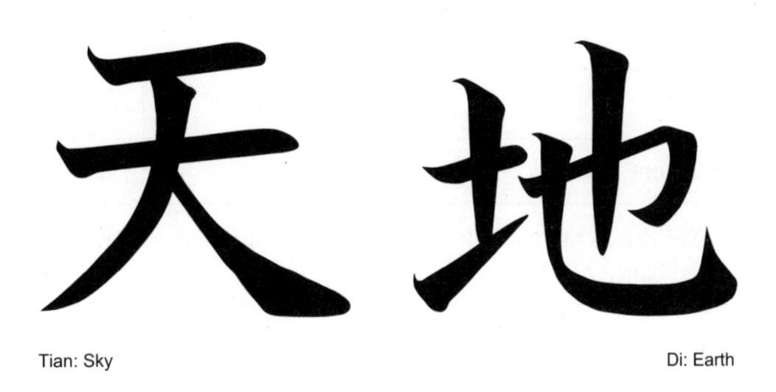

Tian: Sky | Di: Earth

> The mutual interaction between physical shape [earth] and environmental conditions [sky-airs] allows transformation, which gives birth to everything. So the sky and earth are the top and bottom of everything, left and right are the streets of yin and yang. Water and fire are the symbols of yin and yang. Metal and wood are the endings and beginnings of growth.
>
> Gui Yuqu, *NJSW 66 (Primary Periods of the Sky)*

Every primitive culture observed the change in the annual seasons. They also observed the cycles of the moon, planets, and stars. These celestial motions were correlated with the weather, growing seasons, and animal migrations. Moving from a hunter-gatherer culture to an agrarian society required a keen ability to predict climatic patterns and growing seasons. Most early people, including Chinese cultures, developed elaborate and sophisticated systems for recording celestial events and forecasting climatic conditions. In 2254 BCE, according to legend, Emperor Yao ordered that the timing of the four solar seasons be determined so farmers might know when to plant their crops. Solstices (extreme limits of the sun angle) and equinoxes (equal day and night periods) were then identified.

Solar seasons were noted to have an influence on atmospheric changes, which resulted in certain weather conditions prevailing during six specific annual periods. These environmental forces were simply called the six airs or sky-airs. The interaction of these airs with the physical earth, as influenced by the sun, produces five distinct climatic seasons or annual growing phases. These are the five earth phases. Since airs are transitory, move around, and constantly change, they are thought of as guests. The earth, on the other hand, is stable, relatively immobile, and changes slowly, and thus is considered host to the sky-airs.

The geophysical model defined by four solar periods, six environmental forces (sky-airs), and five climatic or growing phases (earth phases) was considered fundamental to everything on earth. It provided the Chinese with a means of predicting climatic conditions to assure success in growing food to sustain the people. In addition, most phenomena, notably attributes and relationships, were viewed in terms of five-phase concordances, including flavors, emotions, vitalities (spirits), anatomical features, internal organs, and physiological relationships. Environmental conditions (Tables 6.1 and 6.2), overconsumption of certain flavors (Table 6.5), and emotions (Table 7.1) were identified as potential disease-causing factors.

Table 6.1 Patterns of transformation for the three yin atmospheric airs (from *NJSW 71*: *Great Treatise on the Six Original First Years*).

Atmospheric Airs	Jueyin	Shaoyin	Taiyin
Primary Attribute	Wind	Heat (Monarch Fire)	Damp
Seasons	Harmony and Peace	Warm	Dusty and Damp
Atmospheric Forces	Gives rise to birth and disturbance of wind	Gives rise to flourishing and visible shape	Gives rise to transformation, clouds, and rain
Transforming Duty	Birth	Flourishing	Moistening
Disease Manifestations	Internal acuteness	Carbuncle, skin rash, and hot sensations in body	Indigestion, sputum, and blockage
	Pain in ribs on both sides	Shock, dislike of cold, shivering, and talking in dreams	Accumulations and fullness
	Muscle weakness and twitching	Sadness, nosebleed, and dirty blood	Fullness in middle region, cholera, vomiting, and diarrhea
	Pain in ribs and vomiting	Talking and laughing	Heaviness of body and swelling of the skin

Table 6.2 Patterns of transformation for the three yang atmospheric airs (from *NJSW 71*: *Great Treatise on the Six Original First Years*).

Atmospheric Airs	Shaoyang	Yangming	Taiyang
Primary Attribute	Fire (Minister Fire)	Dry	Cold
Seasons	Flaming Summer Heat	Cool and Quick	Cold and Foggy
Atmospheric Forces	Gives rise to growth and beautiful freshness	Gives rise to constriction, and fog and dew	Gives rise to storage and tight closure
Transforming Duty	Dense plants	Firmness	Storage
Disease Manifestations	Sneezing, vomiting, itching, and carbuncle	Skin edema	Lumbago
	Jumpiness associated with shock, dizziness, and acute disorder	Nasal discharge, and disease occurring along the hip, thigh, knee, calf, tibia, and foot	Immobility of joints, difficulty in flexing and extending
	Sore throat, ringing in ears, vomiting	Dry and withered skin	Perspiration at night in chest, throat, neck, and armpit, and convulsions
	Acute diarrhea, shaking and tics, and sudden death	Nasal discharge and sneezing	Cool diarrhea, suppression of urination, and constipation

Dynamic Forces of Evolution

The concept of environmental transformation due to the interaction of sky and earth indicates that the Zhou people had a profound appreciation for the forces of nature, and reflects the importance of the idea of spirit. The Zhou believed the sky represented the true spiritual reality; to them the mutual interaction of sky forces with that of the earth was responsible for the creation, evolution, and even destruction of all things. In the sky, spirit was believed to consist of atmospheric forces that gave rise to the five phases. On earth, spirit is physical shape. This is noted in *NJSW 66* (*Primary Periods of the Sky*), where Gui Yuqu, an advisor of the Yellow Emperor, says:

> The circulation of the five phases and yin and yang are the way [dao] of the sky and earth. They are fundamental to everything; they are the father and mother [parents] of evolution, the basic beginnings of birth and destruction, and are the official home of the spirits... The utility of change or evolution is the subtle and profound nature of the sky. In man, it is the way that gives birth to wisdom, and it is the subtle and profound that gives birth to the spirit.
>
> The spirit in the sky becomes the wind and on earth it is wood. In the sky it [spirit] becomes heat and on earth it becomes fire. In the sky it becomes dampness and on earth it is soil. In the sky it becomes dryness and on earth it is metal. In the sky it is coldness and on earth it is water. Therefore, in the sky the spirit is atmospheric forces but on earth it is physical shape.
>
> The mutual interaction between physical shape and environmental conditions allows transformation, which gives birth to everything.

Six Sky-Airs

The life-supporting and protecting atmosphere is viewed in terms of six environmental forces of wind, heat, damp, fire, dryness, and cold that follow a specific order of circulation (Figure 6.1). There is little question that life on earth is totally dependent on power radiated from the sun, and the resulting climatic conditions are due to interaction with the atmosphere. No animal or plant life existed on the earth landmasses until organisms within the oceans metabolically produced and released enough gases into the atmosphere to form the protective ozone barrier to ultraviolet light. The earth is thought to be supported by the atmosphere, and the six airs have specific roles as noted by Qibo in *NJSW 67* (*Motion of the Five Phases*):

> The atmosphere [*daqi*, 大气, big air] holds up the earth. Atmospheric forces of dryness can dry up all things and heat can cause everything to be steamed. Wind can move all things [blow things around] and dampness can moisten everything. Climatic cold can harden all things and fire can warm everything... These forces work upon the earth so that birth and transformation are possible in the universe.

The Chinese word *tianqi* (天气) consists of two characters, *tian* (天, sky) and *qi* (气, vital air), and literally means sky-air. This term is still used to mean weather or atmospheric conditions. Airs are named after the anatomical locations of the body as designated by yin and yang nomenclature (Chapter 3). Considered in terms of six environmental forces, the sky-airs influence each other during their own periods of dominance, and each opposite factor can reinforce the ruling air. When wind occupies the dominant position (Figure 6.1) during its annual period (Figure 6.3) it can be reinforced by fire; when heat occupies the dominant position it can be reinforced by dryness; the period for damp can be reinforced by cold, and so on.

Atmospheric conditions are considered the most important external dynamic in health and disease. In addition, changes in the annual seasons, including the adjustment in daylight availability and variations in daily (diurnal) time periods, significantly influence behavior, health, and physiological function of the internal organs. When excessive, or when the influence of the airs penetrates the body (Figure 13.2), environmental forces become primary external factors in disease. Key transforming duties and disease manifestations of the six airs—from *NJSW 71* (*Great Treatise on the Six Original First Years*)—are summarized in Tables 6.1 and 6.2. Disease conditions that mimic the environmental factor are thought to be related to that factor, or at least are named after that factor. As an example, wind causes things to be blown around, sometimes in an erratic fashion. Thus, conditions involving muscle spasm, contractions, twitching, and even paralysis are termed internal wind conditions.

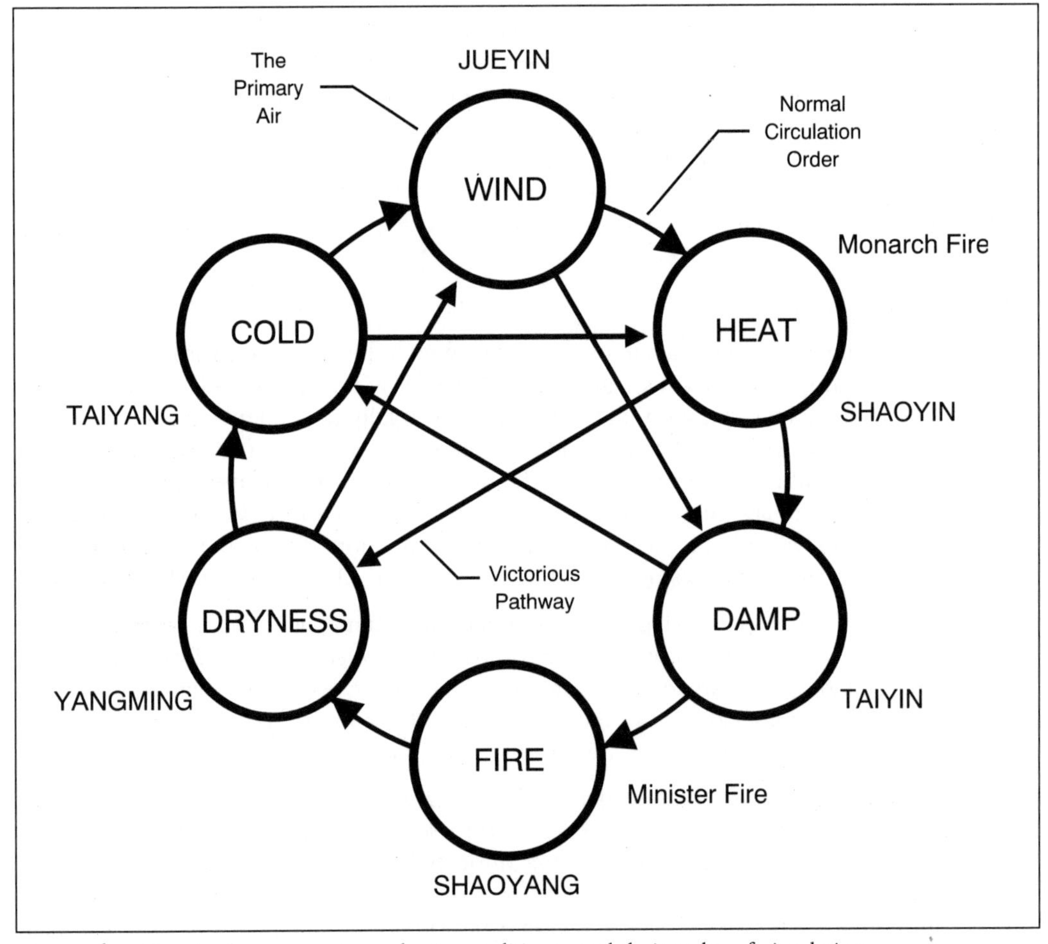

Figure 6.1 The six sky-airs or atmospheric conditions, and their order of circulation.

Five Phases of the Earth

Climatic seasons represented by wood, fire, soil, metal, and water are called phases because each represents a different period of the development and growth of plants. Expected annual changes are viewed in terms of cycles of budding, growing, transforming, harvesting, and storing crops (Figure 6.2). When viewed in this light, the function of the earth phases can be correlated with expected variations throughout the year. Spring, for example, represents the birth (*sheng*, 生) or creation phase, as evidenced by the budding of plants and sprouting of seeds. This is followed by the significant growth (*zhang*, 长) phase of plants during the summer climatic season. Plants then go through a transformation (*hua*, 化) during the long summer phase from the growing to the mature stage. This period is characterized by plants obtaining their full growth and grain reaching its fully developed state. During the autumn phase, green plants such as rice and wheat change to their straw-colored state, and it is the time of harvesting and gathering (*shou*, 收). Finally, the winter phase is the storage (*zang*, 藏) period for the collected grain.

The first earth phase of each year begins in spring and is related to plants and grasses. The Chinese character for this first earth phase generally refers to wood, so this phase is now known as the wood phase. The remaining four phases follow in a set sequence through the rest of the year.

Because of its familiarity with the Greek idea that the universe is composed of the basic elements of earth, fire, water, and air, the West has erroneously compared the five earth

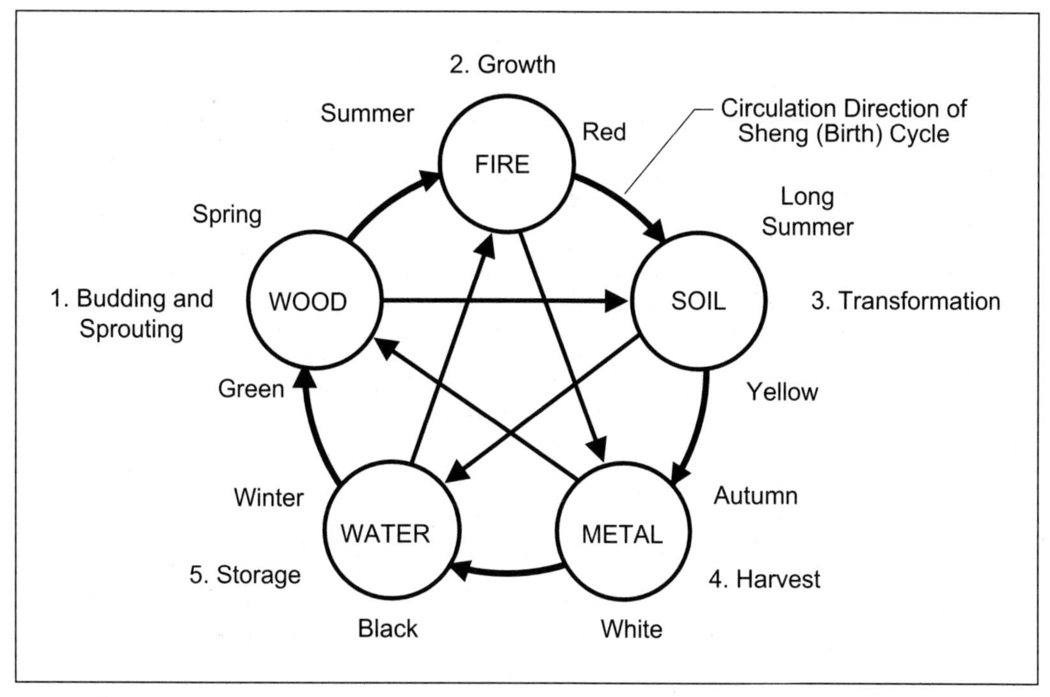

Figure 6.2 Order of circulation of the five earth phases, starting with wood in spring and rotating clockwise.

phases to the concept of elements. The Chinese character for phase is *xing* (行), which denotes movement, such as walking, marching, or circulating, and therefore indicates an active process. Translating xing as element gives the erroneous impression that phases have a static rather than dynamic nature. From their basic understanding of annual climatic cycles, the ancient Chinese carefully worked out a practical theory to view a constantly changing physical world, referred to as the theory of the five phases or *wuxing* (五行). This model provides a logical approach to accessing the complex relationships between environmental transformations and their potential impact on health and disease.

Timing of the Seasons

Early Egyptian, Indian, and Chinese cultures all appreciated the fact that plants require good soil and water for growth. These civilizations understood that reliable crop yield depended on predicting year-to-year and seasonal weather conditions. Of these three cultures, the Chinese developed the most detailed geophysical model for determining dominant future environmental conditions, involving the dynamic relationship between the four solar periods, six sky-airs, and five earth phases. Both the solar periods and earth phases are associated with specific viscera, while the six sky-airs represent environmental conditions (Figure 6.3). Each day, month, and year is assigned a specific earth phase and sky-air. Repeating patterns of five earth phases and six sky-airs results in sixty-day, sixty-month, and sixty-year cycles. The

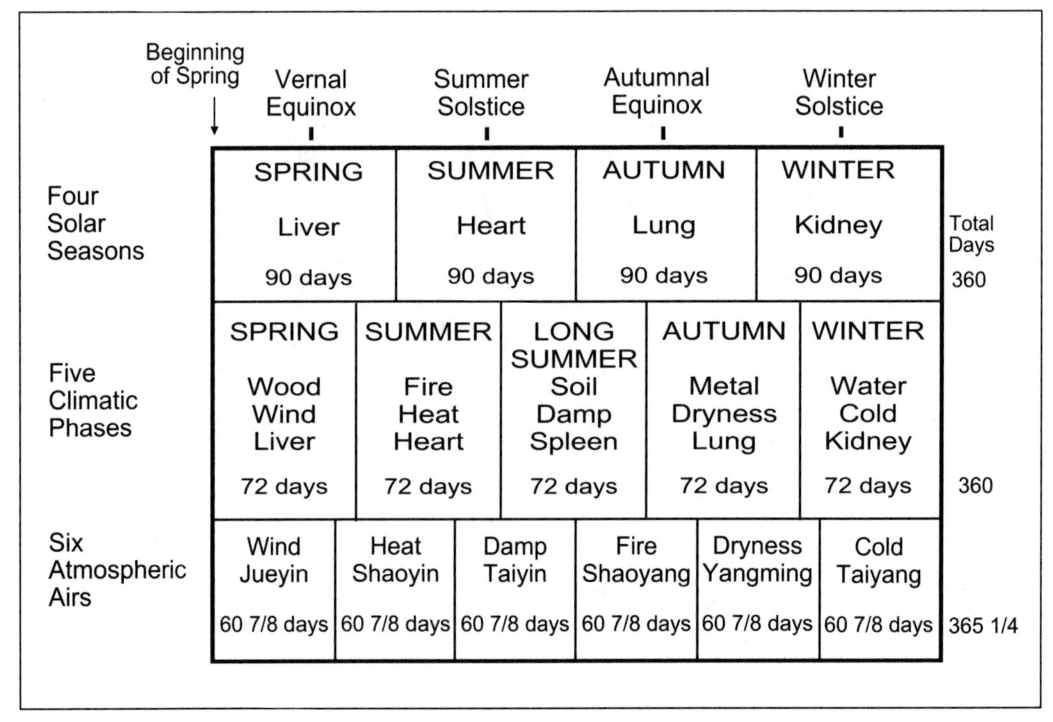

Figure 6.3 Relationship between the four Chinese seasons, five earth phases, and six atmospheric airs, with the solstices and equinoxes and the beginning of Chinese spring.

sixty-year cycle is an almanac that predicts the dominant weather condition for each year and forms the basis of the Chinese calendar. Climatic changes during each year are viewed in terms of basic five-day periods. Three such five-day periods are considered one seasonal juncture or solar term, resulting in twenty-four unique climatic periods each year. Calculations of expected seasonal patterns are reassessed at the beginning of each year, sky-air period, and seasonal juncture for earliness or lateness, and for severity or deficiency. From this, the timing of certain events can be predicted, including planting, growing, and harvesting times, as well as any possible impact on health.

The ability to calculate periods or times of seasonal influence was mandatory for the ancient practitioners. This is noted by Qibo in *NJSW 69* (*Great Treatise on the Meetings and Changes in the Sky-Airs*):

> The *Upper Classic* (*Shangjing*) notes that a person with knowledge of the way [dao] should know about the theory of astronomy in relation to the sky [upper region], the theory of geography in relation to the earth [lower region], and the affairs of people in relation to life on earth [middle region] in order that one may live a long life.
>
> Study of the affairs of people concerns the transformation and changes brought on by the atmospheric conditions. Therefore excess is the result of atmospheric airs arriving ahead of their assigned sky period and deficiency is the result of them arriving after their scheduled time.

The appreciation of relatively small (five-day) environmental periods constituting the fundamental sequence of climatic phases is considered important when assessing the possible impact of local and general weather on health. This is illustrated in *NJSW 9* (*The Six Junctures and Manifestations of the Viscera*):

> The order of the five phases continues like a ring without end. The sequence of basic climatic periods [five-days] follows a rotating pattern by the same rules. Therefore it is said if one does not understand the yearly variations in the seasons, and the flourishing or decline of the climatic conditions, as well as the deficiency and excess brought on by their arrivals, one cannot be considered a skilled practitioner.

Astronomical sightings are used to accurately gauge the beginning of months, annual cycles, sky-air and earth phase periods, and the solar periods. The Chinese zodiac contains twenty-eight constellations, with seven in each of the four quadrants of the celestial sphere. Ten specific star sightings are used to determine the beginning and end of the five phases—these positions are referred to as the "ten sky stems." Twelve star sightings, designated the "earthly branches," are used to determine the twelve months of the year. Each basically corresponds to one of the lunar months. A day is similarly divided into twelve equal periods, also designated by the earthly branches. A period of two earthly branches makes sixty days and approximately corresponds to a sky-air interval, which contains sixty and seven-eights of a day. The sum of the six sky-air periods give a relatively precise measurement of the year at 365.25 days. The Chinese year starts with the first new moon of the lunar month at or near the beginning of their spring. This nominally occurs during the early part of February in the Western calendar. The two solstices and two equinoxes fall in the middle of the Chinese solar seasons, while in the West they are taken as the beginning of the four solar seasons (Figure 6.3).

Interaction of Earth Phases

Most aspects of existence—including the viscera, related tissue, vitality (spirit), nature, virtue, utility, color, flavor, senses, and emotions—are viewed in terms of the five-phase concordances and interactions. Each of the five phases relate to each other through three specific modes: the promoting (creation or *sheng*, 生), subduing (victory or *sheng*, 胜, or controlling or *ke*, 克), and counteracting (insulting or *wu*, 侮) functions (Figure 6.4). The promoting mode is also referred to as the birth cycle, since each phase is viewed as having been created by its preceding phase through what is called the mother-son relationship. Certain communication (*shu*, 输) nodes or acupoints are assigned to specific earth phases, and the use of these sites influences vessels and related organs in accordance with the five-phase dynamic relationships.

Ideas relating physiology to the interaction of atmospheric airs and earth phases are discussed in *NJSW 67*, where the Yellow Emperor asks:

> How do cold, heat, dryness, dampness, wind, and fire combine in the human body, and how do they give birth and transformation to everything?

The answer to this question involves a detailed discussion about how each direction (in China) creates its own dominant atmospheric factor, which in turn creates a related earth phase, flavor, viscus, body tissue, and next-phase organ. As an example, the direction of the

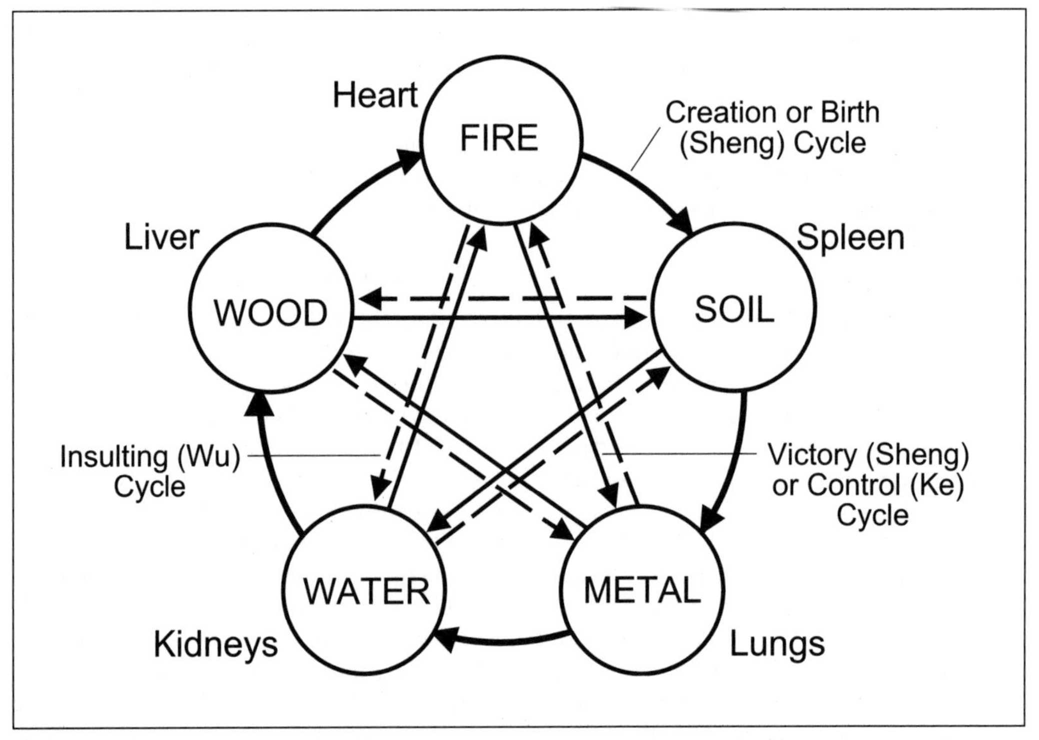

Figure 6.4 Dynamic relationships between the five phases, as represented by the birth (creation or *sheng*), subduing (victory or *sheng*, or controlling or *ke*), and counteracting (insulting or *wu*) cycles or modes.

east creates wind, which in turn creates wood, wood then creates the sour flavor (herbs and food of a sour flavor), which in turn creates the liver, which creates muscles, and muscles then create the heart. Creation cycle concordances are summarized in Table 6.3, along with the nature of each phase and other general characteristics.

Dynamic Interplay between Earth Phases

Earth phases have a fixed cyclic relationship, thought of as rotating to the right in a clockwise fashion. This sequence is the primary order, and constitutes the promoting or birth (sheng) cycle. Earth phases also interrelate through a victorious or controlling (sheng/ke) and insulting or counteracting (wu) mode (Figure 6.4). These three interacting modes are used to explain the five-phase active relationships involving most geophysical, physiological, and emotional phenomena. This dynamic system represents a continually changing process that follows certain predictable and interdependent rules.

Birth Cycle

The promoting or creation cycle is also called the mother-son sequence, since one phase is thought of as the mother of the following phase in the sequence. Wood, which is considered the son of water, is in turn the mother of fire, and conversely fire is the son of wood. Taking wood as the first phase, it can be burned to create fire. Fire then creates soil, perhaps as fire created earth with the formation of the solar system. Fire continues to create soil just as volcanoes spew up molten earth, rocks, and even mountains from their fiery interiors. Fire also creates soil from the ashes of things burned. Fire is the mother of soil, and soil is the son of fire. Soil gives rise to metal, because the earth yields metal ores. Soil is the mother of metal, and metal is the son of soil. Metal then gives rise to water, because ditches and wells are dug with metal implements. Metal is the mother of water. Finally, water, son of metal, gives the necessary moisture for plant growth, and therefore gives rise to wood. Thus, water is the mother of wood, completing one repetition of the birth (sheng) cycle.

Table 6.3 Creation cycle concordances and the nature of the five earth phases (from *NJSW 67: Motion of the Five Phases*)

Phase	*Wood*	*Fire*	*Soil*	*Metal*	*Water*
Direction	East	South	Center	West	North
Climatic Air	Wind	Heat	Damp	Dryness	Cold
Flavor	Sour	Bitter	Sweet	Pungent	Salty
Viscera	Liver	Heart	Spleen	Lungs	Kidneys
Bowel	Gallbladder	Small Intestine	Stomach	Large Intestine	Bladder
Related Tissue	Muscles	Blood	Flesh	Skin and Hair	Bones and Marrow
Nature	Warmness	Heating	Peacefulness	Coolness	Shivering
Utility	Movement	Fierceness	Transformation	Solidness	Cracking
Function	Dispersing	Brightness	Tranquilizing	Strength	Clean
Color	Green	Red	Yellow	White	Black
Will	Anger	Joy	Pensiveness	Worry	Fear

Victory or Control Mode
Each of the five phases can influence or restrain each other in a victorious manner. This is illustrated in Figure 6.4 by solid straight lines connecting each phase to form a five-pointed star. Because the character for victorious is also sheng, although written differently than the sheng character for birth and spoken in a different tone, in the West this mode is usually referred to as the ke (control) cycle.

Influence is exerted by one phase over another; fire for example is victorious over metal, in that most metals cannot be forged or molded without being heated by fire. Metal, in turn, is victorious over wood, because metal axes, saws, and tools cut and carve wood. Wood is victorious over soil, in that plants, bushes, and trees help stabilize earth, especially on hillsides and mountains. Soil, in turn, is victorious over water by providing ditches and earthen embankments to direct streams, rivers, and irrigation water. Finally, water is victorious over fire by being able to extinguish flames.

Insulting Mode
Phases can also exert a counteracting influence on each other. Usually this mode comes into play when there is an excess or deficiency in one phase. If one phase becomes excessive it can exert control over its normally subdued phase through the victorious pathway. Being in excess, the phase can also insult (wu) the phase that it is normally controlled by. This insulting or counteracting mode functions in an opposite direction to the victorious mode. Figure 6.4 notes this relationship with dashed straight lines in the reverse direction to the victory or control cycle. When an earth phase, such as soil, is in deficiency, it is at risk of provoking an insulting or counteracting response from the water phase it normally controls, and also of bringing on a victorious response from the wood phase that it is normally controlled by.

Relationship to Disease

Environmental conditions and transformations have an obvious affect on human physiology. However, *NJLS 66* (*Origins of All Disease*) points out that pathogenic climatic forces do not cause disease unless the person is already in some weakened condition. It is noted that not all people get sick after a single exposure to an intense weather situation, such as a gale or rainstorm. When weather conditions are severe or long term, or if the timing of the sky-airs and earth phases is early or late, excess or deficient conditions will exist, thus impacting human health.

Disharmony in Sequence
Major problems resulting from the five climatic seasons occur when they are out of sequence, or are either overly abundant or lacking. This is also noted in *NJSW 67*:

> The five climatic conditions change one to another in sequence. When they do not conform to their sequence, pathogenic conditions result. When their sequence is proper, healthy balance can result… When atmospheric conditions maintain their mutual relationships, disease is insignificant. If they are not in proper sequence or relationship, disease is severe.
>
> When the climatic condition of a particular phase is in excess it regulates or restrains the phase that it normally subdues. It also insults the phase by which it is normally subdued. When climatic conditions of a specific phase are deficient, the phase that normally

> subdues the deficient phase can attack it. The phase normally subdued by the deficient phase can take advantage of the situation and insult the deficient phase. If attack by the subduing phase is moderate, the insult by the subdued phase is moderate. The insulting phase attacks in the opposite direction, which makes it weak and subject to pathogenic assault. The insulting phase is friendless and has a dread of being at the receiving end of a pathogenic assault.

Further information on the consequences of environmental factors affecting the viscera and causing disease is provided in *NJSW 9*:

> When a climatic season arrives early, this is called excessive. Normally, a slight or meager excess will not cause a victorious [subduing] situation. Nevertheless, an ascending excess [an increasing condition] results in a victorious situation. This is known as an atmospheric excess. A seasonal condition occurring out of its own proper time period results in unhealthy environmental influences, causing internal disorders. The resulting condition cannot be contained [cured], even by a skilled practitioner. When a seasonal condition does not arrive on time, it is called deficient. Ordinarily this causes subduing and disorder among the phases, resulting in suffering and disease. If there is no subduing or victory over a phase, the attack is moderate. This is known as atmospheric urgency.

Timing of Excess and Deficiency

Atmospheric airs frequently arrive later or earlier than their nominal schedule. Early arrival causes excess, late arrival causes deficiency. A variation as great as 30 percent from the norm is not considered harmful; however, a variation of 50 percent or greater is considered pathogenic. The earth phases can be either flourishing or in decline compared with the expected, as discussed in *NJSW 66*, where Gui Yuqu notes:

> To say physical shape may be flourishing or in decline means that the order or reign of each phase may be in great excess or deficiency. At the beginning there may be a surplus, and although it is presently an excess it is followed by a deficiency. Later the deficiency is replaced by an excess. When the cycle of these patterns [excess and deficiency] is understood, environmental conditions can be predicted for a specific period. When they correspond to the sky, it is said they are in harmony with the sky. When they support the harvest, the harvest is said to be just or is said to be straight with the earth. When all three are in harmony, peace and order will prevail.

The importance of harmony or balance is perhaps the fundamental premise of Chinese medicine. The first of the three factors that must be in harmony is that the atmospheric conditions of the sky are consistent with the expected seasonal conditions. Second, the conditions on earth (available food, lifestyles, and so on) are consistent with the prevailing five phases. Finally, dominant conditions are consistent with or fit the physical shape on earth.

Diagnostic Value of Concordances

Pathological conditions can reflect characteristics and symptoms associated with specific earth phases. These are useful in diagnostic evaluation and may indicate a possible disorder in the related vessel or organ. When specific atmospheric factors penetrate the body and become pathogenic winds, they attack particular areas, causing related symptoms. Furthermore, the transmission of environmental factors to the interior of the body is influenced by the internal organ–related superficial distribution vessels (Figure 13.2). This is noted in *NJSW 4* (*On the Virtuous Word of the Golden Cupboard*), as noted by Qibo:

> When the eight winds become vicious [pathogenic], they are considered winds of the distribution vessels, and move on to strike the five viscera. Then pathogenic climatic conditions cause disease.

Products of the Soil

The original impetus for understanding sky and earth interactions was to predict weather conditions to support success in agriculture and to gauge the best time to collect herbs. Flavors of herbs and food were eventually categorized into five groups, with each being assigned a specific earth phase. These flavors are sour, bitter, sweet, pungent, and salty, corresponding to wood, fire, soil, metal, and water, respectively. Classifying herbs and food according to flavor or fundamental taste is based on the idea that the viscera are predominantly nourished by one of the five basic flavors. It is thought that specific flavors give rise to or create their related viscera. Presumably this occurs as the fetus develops in the womb, being nourished by various flavors consumed by the mother. In addition to carbohydrates, fats, proteins, vitamins, and minerals, plants contain thousands of secondary compounds that influence their taste, physiological action, and pharmacological properties. These compounds, which could be the basis in Western physiological terms for the Chinese belief in the importance of flavor, are classed under the general categories of glycosides, complex polysaccharides, alkaloids, peptides, phenylpropanoids, terpenoids, steroids, and others (Figure 6.5). High-food-value plants may have fewer of these secondary constituents, while medicinal herbs may contain more. Chinese herbal and dietary concepts represent a detailed system to enhance health and treat disease. Only a summary of the basic theories is provided in this and the final section of this chapter.

Perhaps the most significant aspect of the sky and earth interactions involves human bioenergetics (Figure 6.5). Plants absorb water (H_2O) through their roots and carbon dioxide (CO_2) from the atmosphere. Sun-powered plant photosynthesis converts H_2O and CO_2 to sugars (carbohydrates), with the release of oxygen (O_2) into the atmosphere. Carbohydrates are consumed by humans and delivered to the mitochondria in the body cells as glucose, where, along with oxygen breathed in from the atmosphere, adenosine diphosphate (ADP) is converted to adenosine triphosphate (ATP), releasing CO_2 and water in the process. ATP is then used in the body cells to fuel all energetic processes, while CO_2 is exhaled into the atmosphere. Plants then convert atmospheric carbon dioxide and water through photosynthesis to produce nutrients and secondary compounds, and to release oxygen into the atmosphere. Humans must continuously breath in the oxygen contained in the atmosphere to support metabolism and sustain life.

Considering herbs and food in terms of flavor is a convenient method of classification, providing of course that the basic dietary approach supplies all essential needs. Although the early Chinese, along with other primitive cultures, had no detailed knowledge of food composition, they nevertheless understood that food satisfied different nutritional needs. A review of the ancient Chinese diet shows that it provided an excellent balance of critical nutrients—most important of which was an optimum availability of essential amino acids, especially tryptophan. Chinese food groupings provide a high level of this essential amino

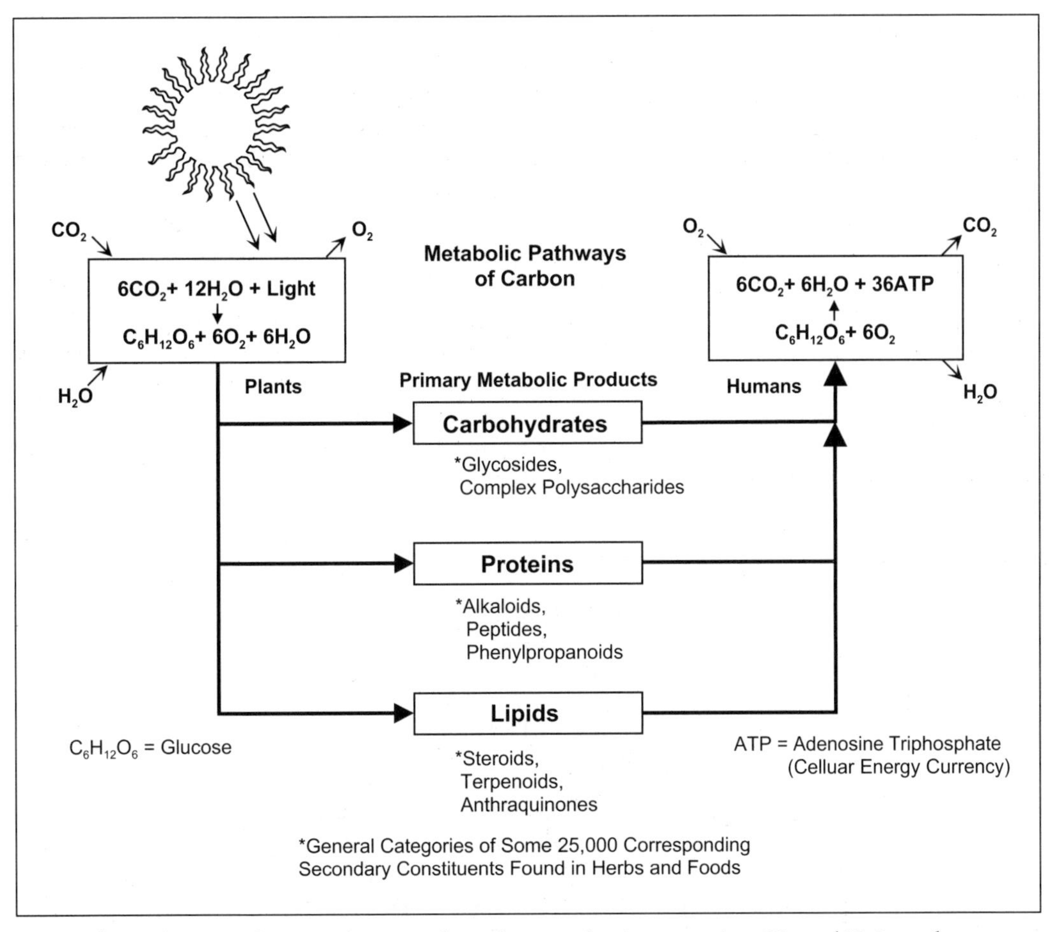

Figure 6.5 Schematic diagram showing plant photosynthesis converting CO_2 and H_2O to glucose (stored as carbohydrate) with the release of oxygen, used as the primary bioenergetic source for humans, along with the primary and secondary constituents of herbs and food.

acid, as well as dietary bulk, vitamin A, and calcium. A low caloric intake of fat and the avoidance of excessive total calories is also recommended.

The Five Flavors

As the stomach is the first bowel to receive ingested food, and the spleen controls the pancreas and deep lymphatics, these two organs are considered essential in controlling digestion and assimilation of flavors, as noted in *NJSW 8* (*Canon of Precious Secrets*):

> The spleen and stomach are the officials in charge of food storage, from which the five flavors are derived.

It is thought that each of the flavors has an affinity or relationship to a particular internal organ. The viscera in turn are responsible for certain physiological functions and processes.

Flavors are also believed to exercise an influence over visceral roles. Food and herbs in each flavor group preferentially distribute their special nutrients to the tissues dominated by the viscus that corresponds to the flavor. This preferential distribution is thought of as a traveling route, where sour flavors distribute to tendons and muscles, bitter flavors to blood, sweet flavors to flesh, pungent flavors to vital air, and salty flavors to bones (Figure 6.6), as noted in *NJSW 23* (*Comprehensive Treatise on the Five Atmospheric Influences*).

Some of these relationships make logical sense in present times, such as glucose (sweet) supplied to the muscles having an impact on flesh. Also, the fact that pungent flavors affect breathing is easily demonstrated by eating a raw onion, or taking a warm-pungent herb like *Ephedra* (*mahuang*, 麻黃). The relationship between salty flavors and the kidneys is due to their role in sodium, potassium, and fluid balance—the Chinese were the first to note the relationship between hypertension and salty flavors. The kidneys also have a role in maintaining calcium levels, which correlates with their relationship to bones. The impact of sour flavors on tendons and muscles results from the liver's control over the spleen and pancreas through the victorious cycle. The influence of bitter flavors on blood has long been appreciated,

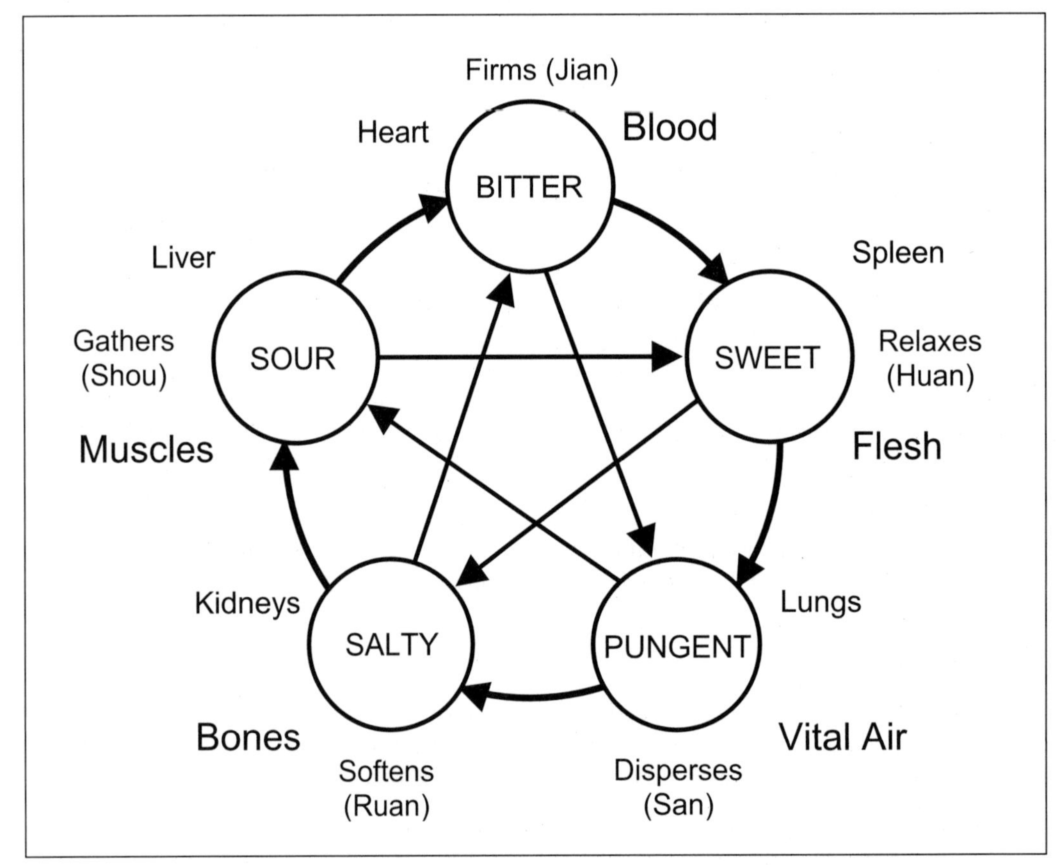

Figure 6.6 Relationship between the five flavors of herbs and food, indicating the preferential traveling routes to particular body tissues or vital air (in the case of pungent), and their therapeutic properties.

evidenced by the use of bitter melon in winter to purify and clean the blood, and the fact that many herbs used to invigorate blood and improve circulation (such as *Salvia root* or *danshen*, 丹参) are bitter or pungent-bitter.

Because the five flavors interrelate in the same pattern as do the earth phases, it is expected that the normal consumption of a particular flavor nourishes its corresponding viscus and tissue. However, overconsumption of a flavor can be harmful to its related phase, as well as to the phase it normally controls. Conversely, a significant deficiency of a particular flavor can result in an impairment of the corresponding viscus and tissue, and provoke an insult (wu cycle) from the phase it controls. These ideas comprise one of the basic principles of Chinese herbal and dietary therapy. Particular flavors are recognized as having specific therapeutic potential.

The Five Moderations

Although flavors have special relationships with specific viscera, under particular pathological conditions the flavor must be avoided. Restrictions on eating and drinking certain flavors that directly affect their related viscera is noted in *NJLS 78* (*The Nine Needles*):

> Regarding the five moderations: sour flavors are not to be consumed in diseases of the tendons and muscles; pungent flavors are not to be consumed in diseases involving vital breath; salty flavors are not to be consumed in diseases of the bones; bitter flavors are not to be consumed in diseases affecting the blood; and sweet flavors are not to be consumed in diseases of the flesh. Even if there is a strong desire to eat these flavors, consuming them to excess is avoided by applying self-restraint. These are called the five moderations.

Life Nourished by the Flavors

Although the basic flavors are limited to five categories, it was acknowledged that these are combined in food and herbs to produce an endless combination of tastes, as noted in *NJSW 9*:

> Herbaceous plants give rise to five colors, but these five colors undergo changes and it is not possible to see all of their variations. Herbaceous plants give rise to five flavors. The five flavors have many delicious combinations and so it is not possible to experience [taste] them all. Individuals develop specific strong preferences in tastes [literally, become addicted to particular tastes] and these are not all the same [for all people]. However, each flavor, to some extent, has its specific transmission to a particular viscus.
>
> The five flavors enter [the body] through the mouth and are stored in the intestines [small and large] and stomach. The five flavors, to some extent, distribute to specific viscera to nourish the functional activity of the five viscera. When functional activity is harmonious and saliva and body fluids are mutually supportive, this gives rise to life and animation.

Food in Ancient Times

A wide variety of food existed in ancient times, although only a limited list is provided in the *Neijing* for the five flavor categories (Table 6.4), perhaps selected for their therapeutic properties.

Some food, such as fish and milk, is mentioned in ancient texts but the flavor categories are not discussed. Thus, confusion exists today about which food belongs to each flavor category. Further, it is not always clear what food is represented by some of the old written characters. For example, the Chinese character used for rice in some sections of the *Neijing* refers to a growing field of rice, and not necessarily to a grain available for consumption.

Another complication is that many varieties of food have been introduced into China since ancient times, including much from the Americas, such as corn, beans, peanuts, potatoes, and tomatoes, all of which were unknown to the ancient Chinese. Other foods were introduced from Persia and India.

Perhaps the most important aspect of the Chinese diet involves the basic food categories contained within each flavor group—each group lists five selections, including grain, solid fruit and vegetables, green leafy vegetables, ordinary fruit, and meat, of which only a limited amount was consumed (Table 6.4). Food within a particular flavor group represents a balance of items to be consumed on a daily basis.

The most important quality of each flavor is its influence on the functional activity of its own related viscera (Table 6.4). Flavors have specific physiological effects as well as influencing the phases. Thus, the application of each flavor has to be carefully evaluated. Although there are five flavors, each associated with a particular earth phase, a mild or bland flavor, sometimes associated with the soil phase, can also be assigned to foods and herbs. A bland flavor is also mentioned with respect to yin and yang qualities. Reference is occasionally made to six flavors, such as noted in *NJSW 71*:

> Pungent and sweet flavors stimulate dispersion and belong to the yang classification. Sour and bitter flavors produce a surging discharge and belong to yin. Salty flavors

Table 6.4 Flavors of the five phases and viscera with related foods, including vegetable greens, solid fruit and vegetables, grain, fruit, and meat, along with the physiological action promoted by each flavor of food and herbs.

Phase	*Wood*	*Fire*	*Soil*	*Metal*	*Water*
Viscera	Liver	Heart	Spleen	Lungs	Kidneys
Flavor	Sour	Bitter	Sweet	Pungent	Salty
1. Green Leafy Vegetables	Leeks, Chives	Shallots	High Mallow Greens	Onions, Scallions	Leafy Greens
2. Solid Fruit and Vegetables	With Pit	Fibrous, Pithy	Fleshy, Pulpy	Hard Surface, Shelled	Soft, Moist
3. Grain	Lentils, Sesame	Wheat, Barley	Non-glutinous Rice	Yellow Millet	Soya Beans, Peas
4. Fruit	Plums	Apricots, Almonds	Dates	Peaches	Chestnuts
5. Meat	Dog	Mutton	Beef	Chicken	Pork
Physiological Action Promoted	Gathers (*Shou*)	Firms (*Jian*)	Relaxes (*Huan*)	Disperses (*San*)	Softens (*Ruan*)

produce a surging discharge and belong to yin. Mild or bland flavors cause an oozing or leaking discharge and belong to yang. The six flavors result in either constricting or dispersing, either slowing or quickening, either drying or lubricating, and either softening or firming. These are the benefits to induce changes in order to regulate vital substances and function, and to bring about balance.

Vital Air and Flavors

The role of vital air in the metabolism of food-derived nutrients is discussed in some detail in *NJSW 5* (*Great Treatise on the Proper Representation of Yin and Yang*):

> Water [a material substance] represents yin qualities, while fire [nonmaterial] represents yang qualities. Therefore, yang is the category or classification of vital air [gases], and yin is the quality of flavor [food and drink]. Flavors give rise to the physical body [food nourishes growth] and the physical body gives rise to vital air [since the body is required to breathe air from the atmosphere]. Vital air in turn comes together with refined substances [oxygen is required to convert absorbed refined foods to usable energy] and refined substances are the result of digestion. Thus, refined substances feed on vital air and the physical body feeds on the flavors. Digestion creates the refined substances and vital air gives life to the physical body.

Flavors in Health and Disease

The five flavors of food and herbs are consumed to ensure a balanced diet, to maintain health, and to treat illness, consistent with the prevailing seasons and other variables. Flavors have particular benefits, produce certain physiological responses, and enhance visceral tendencies. These features are viewed in terms of the five earth phase modes (promoting, subduing, or counteracting). Either overconsumption or underconsumption of a particular flavor causes problems for its related earth phase, which also affects the other phases. Certain flavors can be consumed to correct a problem of dietary deficiency, or counteract the problems induced by overconsumption. Specific flavors are also used to enhance visceral tendencies, treat visceral disorders, or address conditions of excess and deficiency. These are the principal pharmacological properties associated with herbs and food. Herbal and dietary therapy also involves selecting flavors that benefit the ruling sky-air and earth phase. In addition, flavors are applied during different seasons to address chronic disorders. Good dietary and herbal practices are essential to assure a long and healthy life.

Pathology due to Overconsumption

People tend to prefer certain foods and herbs, which can lead to overconsumption of specific flavors. Overconsumption impairs the functional activity of the related organ corresponding to the flavor in disharmony, and damages the dominant tissues (Table 6.5). It also affects the organ belonging to the phase that it normally controls. These are the theoretical rules involved in pathogenesis due to flavors. Examples exist in the West of disease due to overconsumption that are consistent with those described by the ancient Chinese. Foods of certain flavors can also be underconsumed, thereby failing to nourish the dominant tissue corresponding to a

Table 6.5 Harm to the body due to excess consumption of specific flavors from food and herbs, along with conditions in which flavor is avoided or used to overcome excess.

	Sour	*Bitter*	*Sweet*	*Pungent*	*Salty*
1. Condition in which flavor is avoided	Disease of muscles and tendons	Blood disease	Diseases of flesh	Disorders of vital breath	Disease of bones
2. Harm by excess consumption on functional activity	Accumulation of liver fluids, and exhaustion of spleen functional activity	Failure of spleen to moisten, impairing stomach function, causing it to thicken	Shortness of breath, heart fullness with dark complexion, and imbalance of kidney functional activity	Injures muscles and tendons causing flaccidity, and depletion of endocrine gland vital substance	Bone-related fatigue and shortening of the muscles, restraining of heart function
3. Effect of excess consumption	Thickening of flesh and protrusion of lips	Withering of skin and body hair falls out	Pain in bones and falling out of hair on head	Cramps in tendons and muscles, and withering of fingernails and toenails	Stiffening of blood vessels (hypertension) and change in their color
4. Flavor used to counteract excess consumption	Pungent, except when liver disease is present	Salty, except when heart disease is present	Sour, except when spleen disease is present	Bitter, except when lung disease is present	Sweet, except when kidney disease is present

particular viscus. A deficiency in a particular flavor provokes an insult from the phase it normally controls. Caution is applied not to overconsume food or alcohol, as noted in *NJSW 3* (*On Communication with Life-Giving Atmosphere*):

> As a result of overeating, the muscles can become flabby and there can be bloody stools due to hemorrhoids. As a result of drinking excessive alcohol there can be an upsurge of functional activity.

The Chinese observed that a diet excessive in calories and fatty foods was unhealthy. Rich fatty food was recognized in ancient times to be a major factor in heart and vascular disease. One detailed account of an apparent stroke is provided in *NJSW 28* (*Comments on Hollowness and Solidness*):

> Normally the controlling factors related to the affliction of falling down prostrate, like being beaten, with hemiplegia, syncope with flaccid paralysis and cold limbs, along with chest fullness and an upsurge of vital air, occurs in very fat [obese] rich people. This disease is due to overeating rich and fatty foods.

Harm to Functional Activity
The mechanism of injury due to an excess of certain flavors is via the direct impact on the refined substances (*jing*, 精), which then impact the organ's functional activity (Table 6.5, Row 2). This is noted by Qibo in *NJSW 3*, along with advice on eating a balanced diet:

> The production of yin substances [*ying*, 营, and *wei*, 卫] have their origins in the five flavors, as does the yin material of the five senses [biologically active substances]. But this yin material can also be damaged by the five flavors.
>
> Therefore, a careful and harmonious selection of food of the five flavors results in straight bones, soft and pliant muscles, the free flow of vital substances and blood, and fine textured skin. Similarly, the bones will normally be vibrant due to refined substances [jing derived from food]. If one carefully abides by the prescribed laws of nature [dao], it can be one's destiny to live a long life.

Harm by Victorious Flavors
Overconsumption of a flavor adversely impacts the body via the victorious cycle (Table 6.5, Row 3). Resulting physical manifestations are consistent with a phase being impaired by attack from a normally controlling phase. These manifestations provide diagnostic clues to determining which flavor is impacting health and causing disease. Details of the effect of overconsumption are provided in *NJSW 10* (*Development of the Five Viscera*):

> This is the way the five flavors cause harm to the body: the heart craves bitter flavors; the lungs crave pungent flavors; the liver craves sour flavors; the spleen craves sweet flavors; and the kidneys crave salty flavors. This is the correspondence between the flavors and the viscera and their harmonious relationship with each other.

Counteracting Flavors
The effect of overconsumption of a particular flavor can be countered therapeutically to some extent by eating the flavor of its controlling earth phase (Table 6.5, Row 4). However, caution must be applied when using flavors of the victorious cycle to counteract an imbalance due to overconsumption. The principal concern is not to control a phase that is already in a state of disease. This is noted in *NJLS 56* (*The Five Flavors*):

> Concerning the five restraints: pungent flavors are prohibited in liver disease; salty flavors are prohibited in heart disease; sour flavors are prohibited in spleen disease; sweet flavors are prohibited in kidney disease; and bitter flavors are prohibited in lung disease.

Herbal and Dietary Therapies

In terms of therapeutic application, herbs and food are selected for their ability to counteract overconsumption or to influence specific organs, and may include the effect of a particular flavor on the functional activity or tissue dominated by the corresponding viscus. The use of flavors for specific visceral problems can be viewed in terms of the treatment of acute symptoms or the need to stimulate the fundamental tendency of the organ. The acute presentation of organ symptoms gives an indication of the flavor that can be employed most beneficially to treat the particular problem (Table 6.6A). Clinical situations also occur where it is necessary to stimulate the basic tendency or disposition of an affected organ, such as using a pungent flavor to enhance liver dispersion. In these cases, the appropriate flavor known to provoke the desired response is selected (Table 6.6B). Flavors are used for their therapeutic ability to drain off (*xie*, 泻) a solid or excess condition, or mend (*bu*, 补) a hollow or deficiency disorder (Table 6.6C). Colors are associated with each of the viscera and can manifest on the skin, face, or eyes in certain clinical conditions. These are observed with respect to diagnostic interpretation. A dominant coloration may indicate the possible therapeutic application of the particular flavor associated with each specific organ (*NJLS 56*).

Most ailments, including heart and vascular diseases, can be treated using herbal and dietary strategies, as described throughout the *Neijing*. The degree of knowledge of the early physicians is illustrated by many examples, including the following reference to heart pain due to lack of vital air (myocardial ischemia) in *NJSW 21* (*Distribution Vessel Pulse Differentiation*):

> Heart pain due to deficiency should be treated with proper diet and herbs.

Table 6.6 Therapeutic application of flavors from food and herbs to treat visceral symptoms and tendencies, and to address solid (excess) and hollow (deficiency) conditions, from *NJSW 22* (*On Visceral Function and Seasonal Rules*).

	Liver	*Heart*	*Spleen*	*Lungs*	*Kidneys*
A. Visceral Symptoms					
Primary Acute Symptom	Irritability	Weakness	Dampness	Congestion	Dryness
Suitable Flavor for Treatment	Sweet	Sour	Bitter,[1] also Salty	Bitter	Pungent
Principal Therapeutic Action	Relaxes (*Huan*) Liver irritability	Gathers (*Shou*) Heart weakness	Dry (*Zao*) Spleen dampness	Vents (*Xie*)[2] Lung congestion	Moistens (*Run*) Kidney dryness
B. Visceral Tendencies					
Tendency	Dispersion	Weakness	Relaxation	Constriction	Firmness
Enhancing Flavors	Pungent	Salty	Sweet	Sour	Bitter
Therapeutic Action of Flavor	Disperses (*San*)	Softens (*Ruan*)	Relaxes (*Huan*)	Gathers (*Shou*)	Firms (*Jian*)
C. Excess and Deficiency					
Flavors to Mend (*Bu*) or Reinforce	Pungent	Salty	Sweet	Sour	Bitter
Flavors to Drain Off (*Xie*) or Reduce	Sour	Sweet	Bitter	Pungent	Salty

1. Bitter has the effect of impairing the function of the spleen to moisten, and hence is considered primary in drying spleen dampness; however, *NJSW 22* further notes that salty is also suitable for drying spleen dampness.
2. This character *xie* (泄) means to vent, and is different from the character *xie* (泻) meaning to drain off or reduce.

Dietary therapy is a basic modality of Chinese medicine, and emphasis is placed on the prudent use of food, as well as herbs, to prevent the development of disease. However, if a disease condition requires the intervention of dietary strategies, the therapy is only continued until recovery, as noted in *NJSW 70* (*Great Treatise on the Normal Affairs of Five Phases*):

> When grains, meat, fruits, and vegetables are used to treat a disease, their application should be discontinued as soon as the disease is cured, otherwise excessive application can cause harm to homeostatic balance or antipathogenic factors.

Therapeutic Benefit of Flavors

The therapeutic impact of specific flavors of herbs and food is derived from the special physiological role of each. The food groups—grains, fruit, meat, and vegetables—have the roles of maintaining, assisting, benefiting, or filling, respectively. Details are provided in *NJSW 22* (*On Visceral Function and Seasonal Rules*):

> Pungent flavors disperse [*san*, 散], sour flavors gather [*shou*, 收], sweet flavors relax [*huan*, 缓], bitter flavors firm [*jian*, 坚], and salty flavors soften [*ruan*, 软]. Whereas herbal medicines can be used to attack pathogenic conditions directly, the five grains [cereals] can be used to maintain the body. The five fruits assist the body, the five domestic meats can benefit the body, and the five vegetable greens can fill the body.
>
> Vital air and the flavors combine in order to serve and reinforce [mend] refined substances [absorbed refined nutrients], which in turn benefits functional activity. These five flavors include pungent, sour, sweet, bitter, and salty. Each has its particular benefit, either to disperse [san] or gather [shou], either to relax [huan] or tighten [*ji*, 急], either to firm [jian] or soften [ruan]. Each should be applied in accordance with the four seasons and the five viscera. Also, they should be applied in accordance with particular diseases associated with the five flavors, consuming those herbs and food suitable for that purpose.

Counteracting Overconsumption

Excessive consumption of certain flavors leads to problems that are often of a chronic nature (Table 6.5), usually developing over a long period of time. Treatment involves using flavors from herbs and food to counteract the previous use of offending flavors, by eating flavors related to the phase that subdues the original flavor (Table 6.5, Row 4). For example, excess consumption of sour flavors, which affects the liver (wood), can be counteracted by consuming pungent (metal) flavors, because pungent (metal) subdues sour (wood) through the victorious mode. Care is taken not to overconsume the victorious flavor, since this causes additional imbalance. Using a flavor of the victorious phase to control overindulgence is not applied if the affected viscus is suffering from an acute disorder (Table 6.5, Row 1).

Treating Prime Acute Symptoms

Specific flavors can be employed to treat symptoms of the five viscera. For example, irritability is a fundamental acute symptom related to the liver, which can be relaxed by the use of sweet flavors (Table 6.6A). Employing flavors for prime acute symptoms does not follow the victorious or insulting cycles. Here they are employed based on the physiological property of the flavor. Use of flavors to address primary symptoms is discussed in *NJSW 22*:

> When a patient suffers with liver-caused irritability it should be quickly treated by consuming sweet flavors to relax [huan] the condition... When a patient is suffering heart weakness, it should be quickly treated by consuming sour flavors in order to strengthen or to gather [shou] the condition... When a patient suffers with spleen dampness it should be treated by quickly consuming bitter flavors to dry [*zao*, 燥] the condition... When a patient is suffering with an upsurge of breath [congested chest] it should be quickly treated by consuming bitter flavors to vent [*xie*, 泄] the condition... When a patient is suffering with kidney dryness, it should be quickly treated by consuming pungent flavors to moisten [*run*, 润] the condition, to open the pores, to stimulate the flow of body fluids and promote the circulation of vital substances.

Treating Visceral Tendencies

Each of the five viscera has a fundamental tendency that is unique, and the five flavors have similar specific physiological tendencies. Flavors can be employed to enhance visceral tendencies. The liver, for example, has a function to disperse nutrients that are absorbed from the gut, so its specific tendency is to disperse. Pungent herbs and food have the property of dispersing, and hence are employed to aid the liver in its dispersing function (Table 6.6B). The lungs are responsible for breathing and tend to constrict. Sour flavors tend to gather and are used to address deficient conditions where the lungs need to be constricted.

Many diseases affecting the heart cause the heart to be weak. Thus, the tendency of the heart function is toward developing weakness. Salty-flavored herbs and food tend to soften, so in the case of conditions that result in firming the heart, salty flavors can be applied to soften the heart condition. Salty flavors refer to the basic taste of the food or herb, and should not be confused with salt itself—the use of salt to flavor dishes is thought to have an influence on increasing blood pressure. The Chinese assigned the tendency of firmness to the kidneys. Bitter flavors tend to firm, and so in conditions where the kidneys need to be firmed bitter flavors are employed.

Flavors for Excess and Deficiency

Flavors that are employed clinically to enhance visceral tendencies also reinforce or mend a deficiency. In the case of a deficiency resulting in impaired liver dispersion, pungent flavors are appropriate to reinforce or mend the liver condition. When the lungs have a deficiency of failing to constrict, sour flavors are used to reinforce or mend the situation. Kidney softness is addressed by using bitter flavors to produce firmness, and hence reinforce or mend the deficient condition. Salty flavors mend a weak heart deficiency, and sweet flavors are used to address spleen deficiencies. For excess conditions that need to be drained off, sour is used for liver, sweet is applied for heart, bitter is used for spleen, pungent for lungs, and salty for kidneys (Table 6.6C).

7

Spirit, Vitality, and Emotions

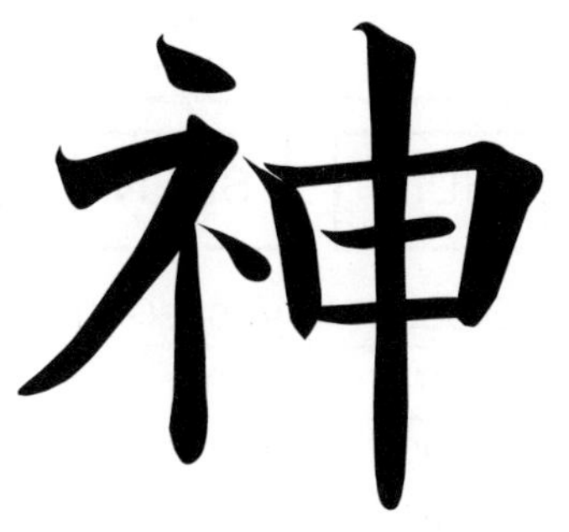

Shen: Spirit

> It is said that which causes life to come about is called refined substances [mother's ovum and father's sperm]; that which is produced due to the mutual struggle [conception] between these two refined substances is called spirit.
>
> Qibo, *NJLS 8 (Origin of the Spirit)*

Ancient people recognized that humans and other animal species have a special quality that distinguishes them from the inanimate world. This property, vital force, vitality, or animation was called "spirit," or at least a word that is translated as such. When applied to human beings, the Western interpretation is frequently associated with an immortal soul. The Chinese idea of spirit, however, equates mostly accurately with "vitality." The early Chinese—and later the Greeks—endeavored to explain all physiological processes, and associated the idea of spirit with animation, natural abilities, mental faculties, personality, determination, temperament, mood, and emotions. These early physicians keenly understood that the spirit, mind, and body are fully integrated and do not exist as separate entities in a living being. There is an emotional component to all physical stimuli, just as there is a physical response to psychological stimuli. Everyone is endowed with these normal interactions for the purposes of defensive responses, survival, procreating, and sustaining life.

After the initial spark of life is provided at conception, the spirit is mediated by physical means. This mediation involves substances circulating in the blood supply that are derived from the intake of food, water, and air. These refined substances of vitality (essence of the spirit)—equivalent to what in the West are termed biologically active materials—could include hormones, neurotransmitters, and other substances. In the Chinese schema, these substances are associated with each of the five visceral systems and are important to the organs' functional role in the body. This idea represents the first attempt to describe something akin to the endocrine system function, although individual glands were not described. Each of the organ vitalities (spirits) is accorded a predominant emotional component, and is also associated with sensory and nerve function. All this results in a complex organization of spirit that is unique to Chinese medicine (Figure 7.1). Of the organ vitalities, drive (*zhi*, 志) and intent (*yi*, 意) are considered the most important in defining an individual's physical and emotional status.

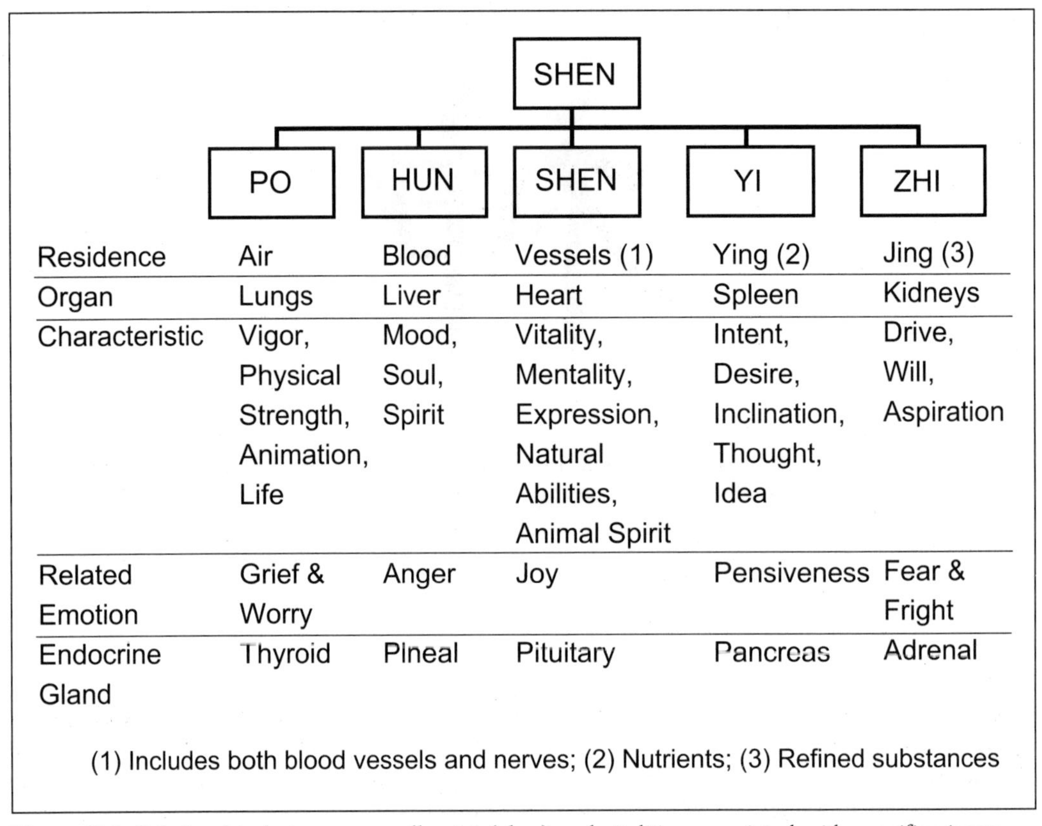

	PO	HUN	SHEN	YI	ZHI
Residence	Air	Blood	Vessels (1)	Ying (2)	Jing (3)
Organ	Lungs	Liver	Heart	Spleen	Kidneys
Characteristic	Vigor, Physical Strength, Animation, Life	Mood, Soul, Spirit	Vitality, Mentality, Expression, Natural Abilities, Animal Spirit	Intent, Desire, Inclination, Thought, Idea	Drive, Will, Aspiration
Related Emotion	Grief & Worry	Anger	Joy	Pensiveness	Fear & Fright
Endocrine Gland	Thyroid	Pineal	Pituitary	Pancreas	Adrenal

(1) Includes both blood vessels and nerves; (2) Nutrients; (3) Refined substances

Figure 7.1 Relationship between overall spirit (*shen*) and vitalities associated with specific viscera, indicating principal residence, traditional characteristics, related emotions, and possible linked endocrine gland.

Role and Meaning of Spirit

Refined substances of vitality are associated with the five viscera and their related characteristics, namely drive, intent, vigor, mood, and overall vitality. These components interrelate through the five earth phases. Thus, vitalities and emotions can relate with each other through the five-phase creation, victorious, and insulting modes. In addition, both vitalities and emotions can be affected by environmental factors, seasonal influences, and diet. Emotions themselves are thought to be the primary internal factors in disease. Consideration of an individual's spirit or vitality is crucial in the diagnosis and treatment of disease (Chapter 13).

Each of the internal organs has a specific functional role, while spirit or vitality is in charge of the dynamic function and homeostatic control processes in the body, thus permitting the body to respond and adapt to both external and internal stimuli alike. The Chinese noted that the bowels contain food to be digested, and that the viscera contain the refined substances that mediate vitality or spirit. This is presented in *NJSW 9* (*The Six Junctures and Manifestations of the Viscera*) as follows:

> The number nine corresponds to the nine districts of China, the nine districts correspond to the nine organs of the body. Therefore, four of these [stomach, small intestine, large intestine, and gallbladder] store physical substances, and five [liver, heart, spleen, lungs, and kidneys] store refined substances of the spirit.

This indicates that the material that mediates vitality is a physical substance. Further reference in *NJSW 9* explains that vitality or spirit and body fluids are important to the functional activity of the organs as follows:

> The five flavors to some extent distribute to specific viscera to nourish the functional activity of the five viscera. When functional activity is harmonious and the body fluids are mutually supportive, this will give rise to life and vitality [spirit].

Spirit and Refined Substances

On a physiological basis, the Chinese idea of spirit or vitality is mediated by the two great control mechanisms of the body, the endocrine glands and the nervous system, which includes the motor, autonomic, and sensory neural systems. Endocrine glands release substances into the bloodstream to influence visceral activity and emotional response. The heart dominates the vessels of the body, associated nerves, and the brain. Since refined substances of the spirit circulate in the bloodstream, the vessels are considered the residence of overall vitality.

Given that vital essences of the spirit (*shenjing*, 神精) are defined as refined physical substances critical to the functional activity of each organ, an obvious parallel can be drawn with the Western conception of biologically active substances, including hormones—which clearly fall within the general Chinese category of refined substances (*jing*, 精) that mediate vitality or spirit. Most bodily functions require an interaction with hormones or other biologically active vital refined substances. In the Chinese physiological organization, specific endocrine functions are related to particular organs, although as previously mentioned, the actual glands were never discussed. Vitality substances have a direct effect on emotions and mental activity, which in turn have an effect on these critical substances as well.

Source of the Seven Emotions

The ancient Chinese recognized seven basic emotions, each of which is associated with a specific earth phase, organ, and corresponding visceral vitality (Figure 7.2). Each emotion represents the specific will of each of the sky-airs. Seasonal and environmental forces that affect their related viscera are considered the underlying factor in stimulating emotions. There is little question that warm, balmy temperatures produce relaxation and a pleasurable feeling (joy). This is especially true if someone has just traveled from a cold, harsh climate, which produces shivering and fear. The correlation between sky-airs or environmental forces and the generation of emotions is not always obvious. Part of the process involves an analysis of correspondences; fear, for example, can produce a shivering-like shaking, similar to the shivering produced by cold. Exposure to cold also provokes the stress reaction mediated by the adrenal glands, and can result in feelings of fear and fright.

Emotions are affected both by specific organ vitalities (spirits) and by mental activity, providing a close relationship between the viscera, their individual vitalities or spirits, and emotions. Emotions are also influenced by seasonal conditions, with prevalent emotions in

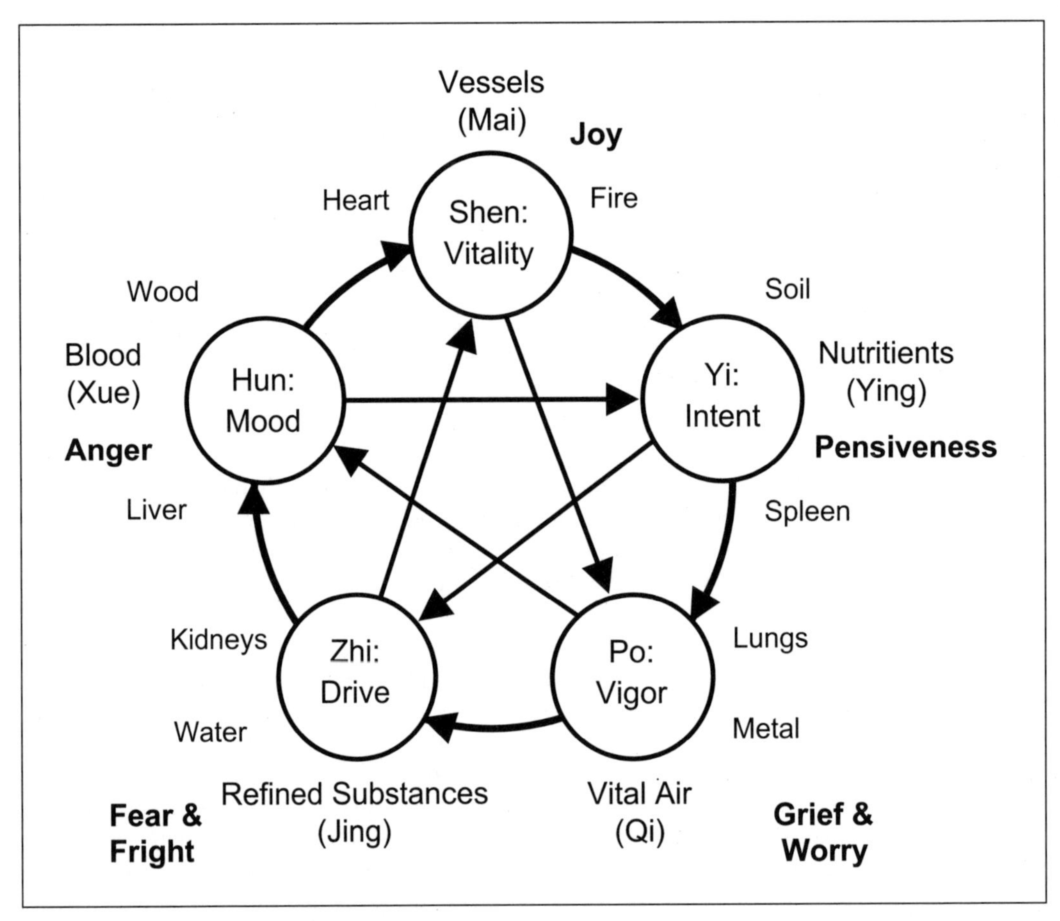

Figure 7.2 Relationship of the five-phase organ vitalities (*shen*, *yi*, *po*, *zhi*, and *hun*) indicating principal material residence, and related emotion.

each of the climatic seasons, and by flavors. Organ vitalities directly influence emotions; when excessive, emotions cause harm to vitalities, which then impairs the functional activity of the organs, which results in disease.

Five-Phase Relationships of Vitalities and Emotions

Since organ vitalities or spirits are associated with particular visceras, they can be viewed in relationship to the five phases (Figure 7.2). The vitality of mood is considered the mother of overall vitality (*shen*, 神) while at the same time exerting a controlling influence on intent (yi), since the wood phase controls soil. An individual's mood gives rise to overall vitality through the mother-son relationship. One's vitality, outward expression, and mental function is greatly influenced or nurtured by a healthy mood. A bad mood can easily repress desires and intentions.

Overall vitality (shen) belongs to the fire phase and is the mother of intent. A healthy heart and vessels result in excellent vitality, which is necessary for intent through the mother-son association. Fire controls metal, vitality (shen) controls vigor. The heart controls the vessels, including the nerves to the bronchial tubes and blood vessels associated with the lungs, and thus influences the amount of air that can be breathed into the lungs. Therefore vitality has a direct influence on vigor. This relationship seems obvious, since individuals are more physically alive when their vitality and spirits are high, and they dislike or avoid physical activity when their vitality is low.

Intent is the mother of vigor. On a physical basis the fundamental energetic processes of the body involve the absorbed nutrients controlled by the spleen. Thus, a healthy intent or desire has a direct affect on an individual's vigor and physical strength through the mother-son association, because there can be no vigor or physical strength without these nutrients. Soil controls water. Intent exerts a potentially controlling influence on drive. An individual's intentions, inclinations, or goals have a direct impact on their will or drive.

Vigor is responsible for the utilization of vital air and has an obvious effect on the use of refined substances (jing). Vigor is the mother of drive and refined substances, themselves the residence of drive. Hence, vigor has a direct affect on drive via the mother-son relationship. In addition, vigor controls mood, since metal controls wood. An individual's vigor has a definite controlling effect on their mood.

Drive, along with intent, has a role in managing the refined substances of vitality (biologically active substances, including hormones). When these spirit substances are focused, mood and vigor are not dispersed. A person's drive gives rise to mood consistent with the five-phase relationships. Water controls fire, which indicates that drive controls overall vitality. Drive has an influence on vitality, mental activity, outward expression, and natural abilities.

The *NJSW 67* (*Motion of the Five Phases*) discusses the five-phase emotional relationships. One emotion can potentially counteract the effect of another emotion through the victorious mode (see straight arrows in Figure 7.2). Anger (liver) overcomes pensiveness[1] (spleen). Fear and fright (kidneys) subdues joy (heart). Joy of the heart subdues worry and grief (lungs), which in turn overcomes anger (liver). Pensiveness (spleen) subdues fear and fright (kidneys). The creation cycle associations of emotions may not correlate well in all cases (see circular pathway in Figure 7.2). It is perhaps understandable that joy, for example, might give rise to pensiveness, and pensiveness itself can certainly lead to worry. Grief and worry can clearly lead to fear and fright, and the latter two emotions can obviously give rise to anger. However, it is not clear how anger gives rise to joy, unless there is joy in reducing anger, or joy in expressing anger openly and calmly.

Origin of the Spirit

Vitality or spirit is provided to the embryo at conception. As the viscera start to form, each makes a physiological contribution to the overall spirit, mediated by refined substances. It is thought that the mother and father contribute unique genetic features to the vitality of the offspring. Vitality is a normal human attribute; each living person is endowed with spirit regardless of their situation or status in life. Because spirit or vitality involves physical substances, it must be sustained by nutrients and normal bodily function. Whenever nutrients are depleted, such as by starvation, or visceral function is significantly impaired or exhausted, vitality cannot be sustained and life comes to an end.

Spirit Created at Conception

The virtue of the sky is the driving force of the atmospheric airs that interact with the earth to give life to everything, including plants, animals, and people. The human spirit produced at conception results from the contribution of reproductive vital essences from both parents. This is noted in *NJLS 8* (*Origin of the Spirit*), where the Yellow Emperor asks Qibo:

> The principles of needling are primarily based upon the source or origin of spirit or vitality. Blood [*xue*, 血], vessels [*mai*, 脉], nutrients [*ying*, 营], vital air [*qi*, 气], refined substances [jing], and vitality [shen] are stored in the five viscera. When they are excessive or overflowing, and leave their storage, it causes a loss of refined substances, a dispersion of mood [*hun*, 魂] and vigor [*po*, 魄], a sudden disorder or confusion of drive [zhi] and intent [yi], and a departure of wisdom [*zhi*, 致] and thought [*lu*, 虑]; how can this be correct? Are these faults offered by the sky, or are they inherent in people? What is meant by virtue, vital air, birth, refined substances, vitality, mood, vigor, mind, intent, drive, pensiveness, wisdom, and thought? Please may I hear your response?
>
> Qibo replies: The sky is the source of our virtue [*de*, 德] and the earth is the source of our vital air. Virtue flows to combine with vital air to create life. It is said that which causes life to come about is called refined substances [mother's ovum and father's sperm]; that which is produced due to the mutual struggle [conception] between these two refined substances is called spirit or vitality; that which comes and goes together with vitality is called mood; that which combines with refined substances, moving in and out [breathing], is called vigor; and that which appoints activities is called the mind. The ability of the mind for recalling and recollecting is called intent.
>
> Intent [yi] exists because of the presence of drive [zhi]. Because drive undergoes changes, this is called thinking or deliberating. Because thought can promote yearning, this is called planning, pondering, or worry. Because planning, pondering, or worry are involved in all things, this is called wisdom.
>
> Therefore, wisdom can support living, especially if one obeys the changes in the four seasons, properly adjusts for cold and hot weather, and lives with a harmonious balance between joy and anger to maintain a peaceful and cooperative home life, separating yin and yang in order to regulate strength and softness.
>
> If one lives in this manner, attacks of pathogenic forces will normally be rare and not reach extremes, and the person can look forward to a long life.

Contribution From Parents

The ancient Chinese description of an individual's life beginning at conception was quite advanced for its time and is consistent with most Western thinking. These theories may not be unique to the Chinese, but they certainly had considerable understanding about this topic. This is further illustrated in *NJLS 54* (*Natural Life Span*), where the Yellow Emperor asks Qibo:

> I desire to hear about the beginning of life for a person, and what vital principle is responsible for building the foundations of life? What establishes and supports people's external defenses? What is lost which then causes death? What is needed to support life?

> Qibo replies: That which is contributed by the mother supports the foundation of life, and that which is contributed by the father supports external defenses. Loss of vitality [spirit] will result in death, and the spirit is what life depends on.
>
> The Yellow Emperor asks: What supports the spirit?
>
> Qibo replies: When blood and vital air [qi] are already circulating harmoniously, and nutrients [ying] and defensive substances [*wei*, 卫] are already in communication, and after the five viscera have already formed, vitality [shen] resides in the heart, and mood [hun] and vigor [po] are fully present, this then becomes the human being.

The idea that the mother and the father each provide a unique genetic property was very advanced; this belief included the insight that the mother's genetic contribution supports the foundation of life. This correlates well with Western understanding in the 1990s that it is the mother who is solely responsible for contributing mitochondrial DNA, although both parents contribute to the cellular DNA of their offspring. The reference to the father contributing to external defenses could conceivably be to do with immune system function—although nothing is known presently in the West about whether either parent contributes anything genetically unique to the immune cells or immune system function. Suggesting that the father contributes to defense may also be a reference to the father's role in protecting the family.

Spirit as a Natural Human Attribute

Every living human being without prejudice or bias is endowed with spirit. This vitality is necessary to support birth, growth, and development, and is intimately involved in the normal function of the body. The complex association of spirit and normal physiological function is discussed in *NJLS 47* (*Root of the Viscera*), where the Yellow Emperor notes:

> A person's blood, vital air [qi], refined substances [ying and wei], and refined substances of vitality [shenjing] are necessary to respectfully support birth and growth, and circulate throughout the body to sustain life. The distribution vessels are required to circulate blood and vital air [qi], nourish body function [yin and yang], moisten the muscles and bones, and facilitate articulation of the joints. Defensive substances [wei] are necessary to warm the striated muscles, serve the skin—including the fat between the skin and flesh [adipose tissue], and manage the closing and opening of the pores. Drive [zhi] and intent [yi] are necessary to manage refined substances of vitality [biologically active materials, including hormones], and gather mood [hun] and vigor [po] to adjust cold and warm, and harmonize joy and anger.
>
> Therefore, when blood is in harmony it flows through the distribution vessels. Body function [yin and yang] is nourished. The muscles and bones are strong and powerful, and the joint articulations are completely functional. When defensive substances are harmonious, the striated muscles are smooth and functional, the skin is regulated and soft, and the pores are fine and dense. When drive and intent are harmonious, the refined substances of vitality are focused, mood and vigor are not dispersed, regret and anger do not arise, and the five viscera are immune to attacks of pathogenic forces. When cold and warm are harmonious, the six bowels can digest food, wind rheumatism does not occur, the distribution vessels communicate, and the joints of the extremities are free of problems. These are natural human attributes.

> With respect to the five viscera, they store refined substances [jing], vitality [shen], blood [xue], vital air [qi], mood [hun], and vigor [po]. With respect to the six bowels, they digest water and food, and cause circulation of body fluids. Each person without bias receives these natural attributes from the sky, no matter whether a person is foolish or wise, or virtuous or not.

Sustaining the Spirit

Since the organ vitalities or spirits have a major physiological basis, they need to be sustained with nutrients. An adequate dietary intake is therefore necessary to support the body and maintain proper function of the internal organs in order to process the nutrients. The importance of maintaining vitality through adequate food intake is illustrated by the effects of long-term fasting. Unlike the so-called developed countries, where being overweight is common, the Chinese carry little stored fat. Consequently the effects of fasting for several days on a naturally thin person are more dramatic. Therefore, fasting is considered potentially dangerous because it depletes the essential material that sustains the spirit (Chapter 3).

Maintaining vitality is more difficult as one ages and the functional activity of the internal organs declines. During the final stages of life the internal organs weaken to the point of being unable to sustain the spirit with refined substances. This is noted by Qibo in *NJLS 54* after discussing the developmental and aging process through each decade of a normal life span:

> By the age of one hundred years, the five viscera are all hollow [deficient], the vital function of the spirits are all gone, only the physical body and bones remain, and life comes to an end.

Organ Vitalities and Emotions

Individual organ spirits have a major task in mediating or assisting in the primary functional activity of specific viscera. While all the organ vitalities affect the entire body, vitalities or spirits associated with the spleen, lungs, and kidneys have a primarily physiological role, while those related to the heart and liver have a significant influence on behavior and emotions. The impact of the heart and liver systems on emotional health is partly related to their effect on the flow of blood to the brain. Here, the internal carotid artery is assigned to the heart distribution vessel, while the internal jugular vein belongs to the liver distribution vessel (Chapter 11). Although the heart is responsible for overall vitality, drive and intent play the most crucial role because they manage the refined substances of vitality (shenjing). Drive and intent are further responsible for gathering mood and vigor, adjusting body temperature, and balancing joy and anger in order to provide immunity to attack by environmental factors. These roles can mostly easily be understood with reference to the function of the adrenal glands associated with the kidneys and the pancreas related to the spleen. There is a special relationship between intent and drive, just as there is one between mood and vigor. A dispersion of intent and drive results in mental confusion, while a dispersion of mood and vigor results in regret and anger. Organ vitalities can also be deficient or in excess, reflecting certain disturbances in functional activity (Table 7.1).

Table 7.1 Effects on the organ vitalities of either hollowness (deficiency) or solidness (excess) in functional activity, and corresponding emotions.

Organ Vitality	*Hollowness*	*Solidness*	*Emotion*
Liver Mood (*Hun*)	Reduced blood storage suppresses mood, causing fear.	Increased blood storage agitates mood, causing anger.	Anger
Heart Vitality (*Shen*)	Depresses vitality, leading to sadness.	Overstimulates vitality, leading to incessant laughter.	Joy
Spleen Intent (*Yi*)	Impairment in four limbs and imbalance in five viscera.	Abdominal distension and diminished urine flow.	Pensiveness
Lung Vigor (*Po*)	Decreased lung capacity, causing a deficiency of vigor leading to unproductive nasal blockage, breathing difficulties, and shortage of vital air (*qi*).	Increased vigor, causing short and harsh breathing (asthma), congested chest, and panting with face held upward.	Worry and Grief
Kidney Drive (*Zhi*)	Deficiency of refined substances (*jing*), causing coldness in limbs, fainting, loss of consciousness, or coma.	Abdominal distension and disharmony in the viscera.	Fear and Fright

Each of the five organ vitalities directly dominates a specific emotion. Hence, organ dysfunction directly affects its own vitality and corresponding emotional behavior. The effect can also be a reflection of environmental or seasonal conditions, dietary influences, or emotional and physical stress. Excessive emotions impair bodily function, which can then cause disease through the primary mechanism of disruption of metabolic and functional processes of the body. Furthermore, the outward manifestation of any of the seven emotions, especially if they are expressed either to an excessive degree or as a dominant characteristic, indicates possible pathology. Because flavors relate to the earth phases, these can also be involved in emotional behavior. Further, an emotion that is not appropriate to any given situation can provide a clue to a possible visceral dysfunction.

Pathological conditions that can result when emotions impact organ vitalities are noted in *NJLS 8*. The following is a summary of the overall influence of emotions on each viscera and refined substance (Table 7.2):

> Thus, fear, cautiousness, deliberating, anxiety, and pondering injure vitality [spirit]. When vitality is harmed it can cause an excess outflow of fear and dread. Grief and sorrow affect the internal circulation [internal organs], cutting off and exhausting vitality, leading to loss of life. Joy and happiness cause the spirit to have a fear of dispersing and not storing. Worry and anxiety can block vital air so it cannot circulate. Flourishing anger [rage and frenzy] leads to confusion and loss of self-control. Fear can cause the spirit to have an agitated dread about not gathering [fear of dispersing].

Table 7.2 Pathological manifestations as a result of emotions causing injury to organ vitalities (from *NJLS 8: Origin of the Spirit*).

Organ	*Emotions*	*Injures*	*Manifestations*	*Season*[2]
Heart	Fear, cautiousness, thinking, pondering, and planning	Vitality	Dreadful fear of losing one's self, damage to prominent muscles, wasting of flesh, thin pallid hair, and looking close to an early death.[1]	Winter
Spleen	Inseparable worry and anxiety	Intent	Deception and confusion, unable to raise limbs, thin pallid hair, and looking close to an early death.	Spring
Liver	Grief and sorrow impairs internal circulation	Mood	Mania with depletion of refined substances (*jing*), causing person to feel that things are not as they should be, atrophy of sexual organs, muscle contractions, inability to raise ribs on either side, thin pallid hair, and looking close to an early death.	Autumn
Lungs	Joy and happiness, even though not extreme	Vigor	Madness, which affects consciousness and threatens person's survival, with skin like shriveled leather, thin pallid hair, and looking close to an early death.	Summer
Kidneys	Incessant frenzy or rage (flourishing anger)	Drive	Person happily forgets spoken remarks, unable to bend, flex, or stretch lumbar spine, thin pallid hair, and looking close to an early death.	Last Month of Summer
All five organs	Unresolved fear and dread	Refined substances	Aching bones, flaccid paralysis with cold limbs, seminal emissions, loss of natural defenses, deficiency of organ yin, impaired functional activity. Loss of organ functional activity results in death.	

1. Refers to a morbid condition that puts the person at risk of dying early, usually before the age of 30.
2. Indicates likely time during the year that the individual will die.

In addition to their impact on organ vitalities, emotions can disrupt the functional activity of the body, which then results in injury to the body itself. Emotions are the primary internal pathological factors involved in disease and dysfunction: their mechanism of action is to disrupt the flow of nutrients and vital breath, and to impair the functional activities of the body. Emotions can also disrupt the normal balance of yin and yang attributes in the body. Any of these changes can then result in physiological damage or injury to the body. A detailed account of the effect of emotions on vital air, nutrients, defensive substances, and functional activity being a primary cause of disease is presented in *NJSW 39* (*On Various Types of Pain*), and is summarized in Table 7.3. An additional reference to some of these relationships is noted in *NJSW 5* (*Great Treatise on the Proper Representation of Yin and Yang*):

Table 7.3 Pathological conditions resulting from the effects of emotions on functional activity and vital substances (from *NJSW 39*: *On Various Types of Pain*).

Emotion	*Impact*	*Manifestations*
Anger	Functional activity moves upward	In severe cases this causes vomiting blood, along with watery diarrhea containing undigested food.
Joy	Relaxes functional activity	Results in harmonious vital substance that benefits circulation of blood and defensive substances.
Pensiveness	Congeals vital substances	Results in mind having a place to remain, vitality a place to converge, and antipathogenic forces are in reserve, but not circulating.
Grief	Depletes vital substance	Tightens heart connections (nerves and blood vessels), and lobes of lung expand and touch, restricting pleural cavity, with blood and defensive substances not dispersing, producing heat in the thorax.
Fear	Vital substances move downward	Decrease in refined substances, causing blockage in pleural cavity, with vital substances moving down, resulting in lower abdominal distension with vital substances not able to circulate.
Cold	Constricts vital substances	Causes pores to close, vital substances cannot circulate in superficial regions.
Heat	Outflow of vital substances	Opens pores, allowing blood and defensive substances to circulate, resulting in profuse sweating.
Shock	Disorders functional activity	Results in mind having nothing to rely on, vitality no place to converge, and thoughts no place to focus.
Physical Labor	Consumes vital substances	Causes panting and perspiration, exceeding limits of the musculoskeletal system and internal organs.

> Therefore, joy and anger damage functional activity, and cold and heat injure the physical body. Wild anger [rage and frenzy] damages yin and wild joy harms yang... When joy and anger are not restrained, and cold and heat are excessive, the stability of life is impaired.

Also, irregular or chaotic periods of joy and anger cause injury to the internal organs, as noted in *NJLS 66* (*Origins of All Disease*):

> Irregular joy and anger are harmful to the internal organs.

Acute worry also has the result of contracting the diaphragm, which can impair the circulation of vital air, nutrients, and defensive substances, as noted in *NJSW 28* (*Comments on Hollowness and Solidness*):

> Squeezing the diaphragm and cutting off the communication of vital substances and function between the upper and lower body is a disease caused by acute worry.

Mood, Wind, and Anger

Mood (hun) is the spirit or vitality of the liver. The liver has a major role in the storage of blood, and blood itself is the residence of mood. Hence, conditions of the liver have a direct influence on a person's mood. There is a correlation between mood and the emotion of anger. A bad mood can predispose an individual to being easily irritated, causing anger. Hence anger, which includes rage and fury, associated with the liver is consistent with the influence of mood. Anger does not directly give rise to joy through the mother-son relationship, however a good mood does.

Intense environmental conditions involving wind are often referred to as "angry" or "evil" winds, and are most often associated with destructive or angry situations. Anger is related to the liver, and is derived from windy environmental conditions affecting the liver. Wind has a direct physical influence on the body, producing symptoms of motion or moving around. In a similar manner, anger is characterized by movements, motions, twitching, and shouting, such as may be typical of a fit of anger.

Vitality, Heat, and Joy

Overall vitality (shen), residing in the vessels, is dominated by the heart and is reflected in outward expression. A bright, cheerful, and joyful expression is normal for a healthy individual. Joy is the emotion related to the heart, and is derived from the environmental condition of heat. Heat has a direct influence on the physical body, causing relaxation and comfort, and producing joy. The heart controls all other organ vitalities. Overall vitality is also closely related to the functioning of the mind. The Chinese theory holds that the heart has a close relationship with the mind. The word for the heart (*xin*, 心) is also used to indicate the mind.

The heart is of greatest importance to vitality because it dominates the vessels, including blood vessels and nerves, the most crucial being those that directly supply the brain and the heart itself. Interruption of blood supply to the brain can result in paralysis, loss of speech, impaired mental function, and even death. Impaired blood flow to the heart can result in physical and emotional problems, and in instant death in severe cases.

Intent, Dampness, and Pensiveness

The spirit or vitality of the spleen is intent (yi), and can include desire, wishing, inclination, thought, idea, expectation, and sentiment. The spleen is the storage area for nutrients (ying), which are in turn the residence of intent. The spleen is also the residence of wisdom, resourcefulness, and wit. Intent has a direct influence on the pensiveness associated with the spleen, which involves excessive thinking or contemplation. Since intent resides in nutrients, disorders in spleen function have an effect on their availability and hence an impact on intent. Pathology associated with spleen dysfunction is primarily related to effects on nutrients themselves.

Pensiveness, associated with dampness and the spleen, involves thinking or thinking to excess, and is different from worry. Pensiveness correlates directly with the spleen vitality or spirit of intent, and is derived from the environmental condition of dampness. The spleen is responsible for maintaining water balance and controlling edema. The accumulation of body fluids is considered to be influenced by dampness.

Vigor, Dryness, Grief, and Worry

The spirit or vitality of the lungs refers to vigor (po), and can include reference to physical strength, life, form, shape, body, or animation. The lungs are the storage place for vital air (qi), which is itself the residence of vigor. The overall vigor of an individual includes the life-sustaining principle associated with the utilization of vital air. The lungs are related to the skin and therefore perspiration is sometimes referred to as "po sweat," since the pores are considered the gate (*men*, 门) of vigor. However, the anus is also called *po men* (魄门) or the gate of vigor, because flatulence is the release of gas that is believed to be related to inhaled air.

Grief and worry related to the lungs are derived from the environmental condition of dryness. It is not clear how dryness induces grief or worry—the mechanism could involve hyperventilation, which can bring on extreme worry or panic. The process involves the effect of dryness on the lung organ vitality of vigor and the utilization of vital air. Physical labor induces a similar effect to grief and worry by consuming vital air and nutrients. Worry and grief, on the other hand, have a direct affect on the lungs: being extremely nervous or worried, or the experience of sorrow and grief with sobbing or crying, impacts breathing. The two emotions of worry and grief, which also includes sorrow, anxiety, and concern, directly impact the organ vitality of vigor via the lungs.

Drive, Cold, Fear, and Fright

The kidney spirit or vitality is drive (zhi), will, or aspiration. The kidneys store refined substances (jing), which in turn are the residence of drive. Fear is related to the kidneys and is derived from the environmental condition of cold, producing chills and shivering. The kidneys are also associated with the emotion of fright (*jing*, 惊), which includes shock, surprise, and alarm.

There is an excellent correlation between the kidney organ vitality of drive, emotions of fear and fright, and the environmental factor of cold. Exposure to cold stimulates the adrenal glands, which are anatomically and physiologically related to the kidneys. This produces a stress reaction that results in the expression of fear, fright, shock, and alarm. This reaction is mediated by the refined substances of vitality of the kidneys, involving catecholamines and other hormones associated with the adrenal glands and with the kidneys themselves. Fear and fright also includes dread, terror, and intimidation.

Organ Vitalities and Endocrine Glands

The refined substances of vitality or spirit of each organ are released into the blood circulation to mediate a wide range of organ and bodily functions. This concept correlates with the Western understanding of endocrine glands. This is particularly true for the adrenal glands, pancreas, and thyroid glands, which relate to the kidneys, spleen, and lungs, respectively. The ovaries and testes were specifically described as being associated with the kidneys. The two endocrine glands that fit the heart and liver attributes are the pituitary and pineal glands, respectively. Assigning endocrine attributes to specific organ systems is unique to the Chinese.

Endocrine glands are essential for development, sexual maturation, and sexual function. Their primary role is the control of body metabolism under a wide range of external and internal stimuli. Carbohydrate metabolism is controlled by insulin, glucagon, and somatostatin from the pancreas (spleen), epinephrine and glucocorticoids from the adrenals (kidneys), thyroid hormones from the thyroid gland (lungs), and growth hormone from the pituitary (heart). These hormones and what they produce or modify have the net effect of stimulating processes in the liver, which in both Chinese and Western science are recognized to disperse metabolic products to the body cells. The pineal gland, associated with the liver, has a major influence on diurnal activities and behaviors associated with carbohydrate intake and processing, as well as sexual activity. The endocrine glands are associated with the characteristics mediated by the vitalities (organ spirits) related to each organ.

Overall Vitality and the Pituitary Gland

The heart dominates the vessels, blood circulation, nerves, brain, and overall vitality. For these reasons the heart is considered master of all organs. The pituitary gland, which is directly controlled by the hypothalamus of the brain, is the only endocrine gland that has an equivalent function to the heart in mediating or controlling overall vitality. Just as the heart controls the other viscera, the pituitary is the master endocrine gland, which controls the organs by secreting hormones and hormone releasing factors that affect all other endocrine glands. The pituitary has an influence on the release of refined substances of vitality from the organs.

There are a number of hormones released by the anterior pituitary: thyroid stimulating hormone (TSH) causes the thyroid gland to release thyroxine; adrenocorticotropic hormone (ACTH) causes the adrenal cortex to release cortisol; follicle stimulating hormone (FSH) and luteinizing hormone (LH) influence the testes to release testosterone and the ovaries to secrete estrogen, progesterone, and prolactin, which stimulates milk production (lactation). Growth hormone, which influences body, skeletal, and internal organ growth and metabolism, and melanocyte stimulating hormone (MSH) are also released from the anterior lobe. The posterior lobe, controlled via neural input from the hypothalamus, releases oxytocin, which causes uterine contraction and milk release. The posterior pituitary is the source of arginine vasopressin (AVP), which influences the kidneys to reabsorb and retain water.

Vigor and the Thyroid Gland

Thyroid gland hormones have a relationship to vigor since they stimulate oxygen consumption in most cells in the body. They also help regulate fat and carbohydrate metabolism, and are essential for normal growth and development. When in low supply, as in hypothyroid conditions, the individual is physically and mentally lethargic. When in oversupply, as in hyperthyroidism, the individual is hyperactive and sometimes agitated. Other important thyroid hormones involve calcium utilization, which affects vigor and the bones. The relationship of the lungs to bones is by means of the birth cycle, where the lungs are considered mother of the kidneys, which in turn are responsible for bones.

The principal refined substances released into circulation associated with the lungs are thyroid hormones. Anatomically the thyroid gland is closely positioned on each side of the trachea, the air tube that connects and belongs to the lungs. Thyroxine (T4) and triiodothyronine (T3) are the main hormones of the thyroid gland; their principal role involves the utilization of oxygen. Without thyroid hormones, the air breathed into the lungs and absorbed into the blood cannot be utilized by the cells of the body.[2] The relationship of thyroid hormones to vigor is through their influence as general regulators of body metabolism, which can increase oxygen consumption, body temperature, pulse rate, systolic blood pressure, and lipolysis,[3] and can decrease serum cholesterol levels. Thyroid hormones control physical vigor and mental alertness, which are major features of the lung visceral vitality (po).

Four small parathyroid glands are contained within the thyroid gland. These principally release parathyroid hormone, which liberates calcium stored in the bones and is essential for life. This hormone also reduces calcium loss from the body through the urine by stimulating the kidneys to reabsorb calcium back into circulation. Calcium is needed for muscle function and proper response to environmental and emotional stress, as mediated by the kidneys and adrenals. When plasma calcium levels decrease there is an increase in the amount of parathyroid hormone released. Similarly, an increase in calcium levels results in a decreased output of this hormone. When serum levels of parathyroid hormone fall there is a corresponding decrease in plasma calcium. The thyroid gland also produces the hormone calcitonin (thyrocalcitonin), which has the opposite effect to the parathyroid hormone and which promotes calcium storage. The parathyroid hormone and calcitonin, along with the kidneys and the active form of vitamin D, help maintain plasma calcium levels within a normal range, even under severe conditions such as stress.

Mood and the Pineal Gland

The fact that the liver has a related endocrine gland is not necessarily apparent. Gallbladder (matched *fu*, 腑 organ of the liver) contractions can be initiated by the hormone cholecystokinin released from tissue in the duodenum when dietary fat is detected. Stomach peristalsis is also inhibited at the same time by this hormone. Bile from the gallbladder helps break fat down into finer particles. Cholecystokinin seems to have little if any effect on the liver.

Ultimately the liver is essential for metabolism because of its role in converting, processing, and breaking down nutrient-based materials and biologically active products used by the body. Perhaps the highly energetic nature of the liver in breaking down carbohydrates, fats, and proteins resulted in the observation of a relationship between liver function and mood. Functional activities of the liver are influenced by diurnal cycles where liver metabolic processes are inhibited at night and reactivated the next morning by daylight. These events are now known to be mediated by melatonin, which is produced by the pineal gland's conversion of central serotonin. Central serotonin levels have a direct influence on mood. Overproduction of melatonin or diets low in tryptophan (from which serotonin is produced) depresses central serotonin levels, leading to many problems, including mood disturbance, depression, seasonally adjusted depression, inability to concentrate, mental fatigue, premenstrual syndrome (PMS), carbohydrate craving, obesity, reduced libido, and chronic pain. Many of these disorders are aggravated during the winter, especially in the higher northern and southern latitudes where incident sunlight is much lower. The pineal gland establishes the body's internal clock based on incident light. The liver dominates the eyes and is also the abode of mood through its association with the pineal gland.

Melatonin rhythm has a diurnal clock and annual calendar function (Reiter: 1993; Laakso et. al.: 1994). Melatonin also has a lunar or monthly cycle that possibly triggers the luteinizing hormone releasing hormone (LHRH) pulse generator that resides in the arcuate nucleus (ARC) of the hypothalamus. In a sense, the pineal functions in the endocrine system in a way that matches the Chinese idea of the liver functioning as a commander-in-chief responsible for planning and strategies (*NJSW 8*). Here, the pineal can be regarded as a regulator of the other regulators (endocrine glands and organ vitalities). This is especially true in optimizing reproduction and metabolic processes with respect to daily, monthly, and annual environmental influences, involving the production and secretion of LH and other adenohypophyseal hormones such as prolactin, growth hormone, FSH, TSH, and ACTH.

Intent and the Pancreas

The pancreas has both exocrine and endocrine functions. Exocrine activity involves releasing substances directly into the gastrointestinal tract to aid digestive processes. The endocrine function involves the release of hormones, including insulin, into the circulating blood supply. These hormones are the refined substances of vitality associated with the Chinese function of the spleen, which are associated with nutrients (ying). The spleen organ system vitality is intent. This is affiliated with the mental and physical activity of moving the body, especially the four limbs. Lack of desire or inability to articulate the body indicates an impairment of intent. Impairment in articulating the limbs is associated with poor utilization of nutrients by the muscles. This is the result of a problem in supplying the refined substances of intent, which in this case is insulin. This condition is distinct from the situation found in flaccid paralysis.

Insulin plays a major role in the uptake of glucose by the body cells. Without adequate insulin there is an impairment in nutrients available to the cells for energy metabolism. Insulin also plays a major role in the storage of glucose, fatty acids, and amino acids in the form of fat. Almost all cells have insulin receptors, their number and affinity for insulin are affected by the insulin itself, other hormones, food intake, exercise, and other factors. As blood insulin levels increase, receptor concentrations decrease, and conversely lower insulin levels increase the affinity of receptors.

Intent involves a major mental component and is also under the influence of insulin, but not necessarily for the purpose of utilizing glucose. Most cells require insulin in order to use glucose; this is not the case with brain cells—large amounts of glucose are taken up by the brain, where it is the ultimate source of energy under normal conditions. There may be some utilization of amino acids from blood circulation, but their transport into the brain is minute. One of these amino acids is tryptophan, which is converted to serotonin (5-hydroxytryptamine or 5HT). Brain uptake of this amino acid is enhanced by the presence of insulin. Impairment in the process of supplying serotonin to the central nervous system (CNS), either by diets chronically deficient in tryptophan or overactivity of the pineal gland, results in loss of intent, depression, and carbohydrate craving.

The pancreas also produces three other hormones, including glucagon, somatostatin, and pancreatic polypeptide. Glucagon and insulin are the most important regulators of intermediate metabolism of carbohydrates, proteins, and fat. These two hormones have opposite effects and under most circumstances are secreted from different islet cells of the pancreas. Glucagon and somatostatin are instrumental in islet cell secretion regulation; however the role of pancreatic polypeptide is not yet understood.

Drive and the Adrenals Glands

The principal refined substances of vitality released into the bloodstream that mediate the vitality of drive are the catecholamines of the adrenal medulla. These hormones correlate with kidney yang. They consist mainly of epinephrine and norepinephrine, along with a small amount of dopamine and endogenous opiate peptides. These hormones emanate from the medullary tissue in response to splanchnic nerve stimulation. Medullary output can be stimulated by a number of emotional and physical stimuli, including emergency and survival responses, stress, cold, surgical trauma, febrile infections, and competitive drive. Epinephrine increases metabolism, heart rate, blood pressure, blood flow to the legs, lung function, and metabolic functions of the liver. Epinephrine also inhibits many digestive functions during a stress or competitive response, shifting the task of nutrient supply to liver-dominated processes.

The output from the adrenal cortex consists mainly of corticosteroids that influence mineral and glucose metabolism, and correlate with kidney yin. Androgynous sex hormones are also released, and are secreted from the cortex under the influence of ACTH released by the pituitary gland. The principal mineralocorticoid is aldosterone, which has a major role in sodium, potassium, and fluid balance. Cortisol is the main glucocorticoid hormone secreted and has an anti-inflammatory function. Impaired output of cortisol produces a clinical manifestation of "false heat," or an inappropriate inflammatory condition that the Chinese characterized as kidney yin deficiency. Cortisol plays an important role in mediating the anti-inflammatory effects produced by needling therapy.

8

Basic Substances and Metabolism

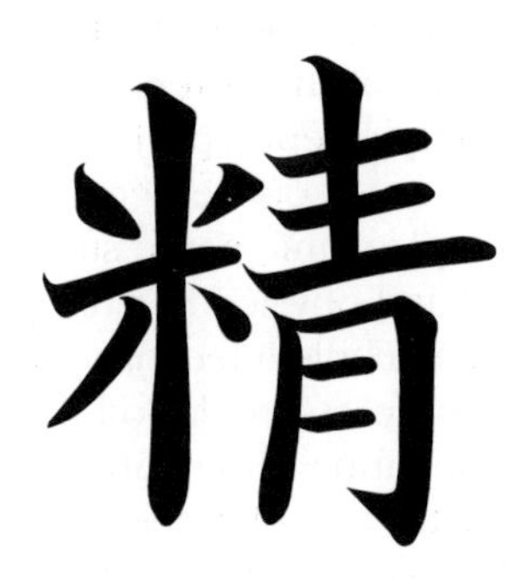

Jing: Refined Substances

> The abdominal peritoneum [middle jiao] converges at the stomach, and issues forth after the thoracic membranes [upper jiao] from where the stomach receives food [via the esophagus]. From here [stomach] waste material gushes forth, from which the body fluids are evaporated, and from which digestion yields the minute refined substances [jing].
>
> Qibo, *NJLS 18 (The Meeting and Interaction of Nutrients and Defensive Substances)*

Nutrients (*ying*, 营), defensive substances (*wei*, 卫), and organ vitality substances (*shenjing*, 神精) are together classed as refined substances or essence (*jing*, 精), and are carried in the bloodstream (*xue*, 血). These are the basic materials that support and maintain life, and along with body fluids (*jinye*, 津液), and vital air (*qi*, 气) containing oxygen, they supply the metabolic or energetic source for bodily function and maintenance for all tissues, internal organs, vessels, brain, and nerves. These critical materials are derived from ingested food and water, and the inhalation of air from the atmosphere. The internal organs (*zangfu*, 脏腑) are responsible for processing and distributing these materials, and the organs also require nutrients and vital air in order to function. Hence, an interdependence always exists between essential substances and organ functional activity. The ancient Chinese theories on these topics are close to Western concepts, even including the idea that certain metabolic processes are under the influence of genetically controlled determinants. Many of these functions are also greatly influenced or controlled by specific endocrine glands and their related organs, as discussed in Chapter 7.

Collectively, nutrients (ying), defensive substances (wei), and vital air (qi) are sometimes referred to as "vital substance qi," which can create confusion. Even the Yellow Emperor asked for clarification of the meaning of qi, as noted in *NJLS 30* (*Deciding on Vital Substances*), where he says:

> I have heard that the human body has refined substances [jing], vital substances [qi], clear and thin fluids [*jin*, 津], unclear fluids [*ye*, 液], blood [xue], and vessels [*mai*, 脉]. I thought there was only one vital substance [qi], and now we must differentiate between six specific names. I do not know which is correct.

Qibo replies: When the two vitalities [mother's ovum and father's sperm] mutually struggle, they combine and take shape to create the fetus. These two vitalities are called refined substances [jing].

The thoracic cavity [lungs and heart] opens up to direct flavors of the five grains to warm the skin, supply the body, and moisten the hair, like irrigating by fog and dew. These materials are called vital substances [qi, used collectively to represent ying, nutrients; wei, defensive substances; and qi, vital air].

When the tissue between the skin and flesh [pores] vents out, it produces abundant perspiration. This is called clear and thin fluid [jin].

Ingested grains fill the stomach with vital food, from which muddy fluids pour into the bones, so the bones can flex and extend. The flowing fluids beneficially strengthen the brain and spinal cord, and moisten the skin. These muddy fluids are called thick or unclear fluids [ye].

The abdominal cavity receives the vital food from which the juices are taken and transformed into red fluid. This red fluid is called blood [xue].

Structures that constrain flowing nutrients [ying] so as not to escape are called vessels [mai].

The Yellow Emperor then asks: The six vital substances may be in a state of surplus or deficiency, there may be plenty or less, the brain and spinal cord may have hollow or solid conditions, the blood vessels may be clear or turbid, how do we know about this?

Qibo replies: When refined substances [jing] are dissipated, it results in deafness. When vital substances [qi] are dissipated, vision will be blurred. When clear and thin fluids [jin] are dissipated, pores will be open causing profuse perspiration. When unclear fluids are dissipated, bones will not be able to flex and extend, there is withered complexion, decreased brain function, aching pain along the tibia, and frequent ringing in the ear. When blood [xue] is dissipated, there is a pale complexion that is withered and dull, and the blood vessels are empty. These are the indications when vital substances are dissipated.

Each of the six vital substances has a specific body region it is in charge of. Its high or low value, its satisfactory or unsatisfactory condition, can be understood by the region it is in charge of. However, the stomach is the great sea of the five grains.

Vital Substances

Nutrients (ying), defensive substances (wei), organ vitality substances (shenjing), and vital air (qi) that provide the essential metabolic basis for bodily maintenance and function correspond to Western ideas with few exceptions. These substances are distributed via the blood, and only the defensive substances can leave the blood circulation to mount a protective reaction (Chapter 10). Defensive substances are then returned to the venous circulation by means of the lymphatic vessels. Impaired supply of vital substances causes deficiencies, leading to disease and dysfunction (Table 8.1), while proper supply results in good health. The main role of vital substances is often categorized by the Chinese with respect to general physiological functions and includes: promoting, related to growth and development of the human body from the embryonic stages to early adulthood; warming, which under normal conditions

Table 8.1 Abnormal conditions of vital substance qi (nutrients, defensive substances, refined substances of vitality, vital air, and function) and related syndromes.

Syndrome	*Etiology*	*Manifestations*
Qi deficiency	Hypofunction of the internal organs due to protracted illness, overstrain, or improper diet, leading to deficiencies in vital substances, and vital air in the case of lung hypofunction.	Dizziness, blurring of vision, shortness of breath, dislike of speaking, lassitude, spontaneous sweating, all of which are aggravated by exertion.
Sinking or collapse of qi	Continued worsening of functional deficiency, or overstrain leading to further impairment in visceral function and autonomic tone.	Dizziness, blurring of vision, lassitude, a bearing-down distending sensation in the abdominal region, prolapse of anus or uterus, gastroptosis, and renal ptosis.
Qi stagnation	Obstruction or impaired flow and dispersing of vital substances by functional disturbances of the internal organs by emotional upset, improper diet, and by invasion of pathogenic factors.	Distention and pain in the particular regions of specific internal organs.
Perversion of qi (Inverse or abnormal function)	Inverse function of internal organs mainly involving the lungs, stomach, and liver, as a result of external pathogenic factors, or to stagnation of phlegm.	Upward disturbance of lung function manifests as cough, dyspnea, and asthmatic breathing. Upward disturbance in the stomach function causes belching, hiccups, nausea, acid reflux, and vomiting. Excessive ascending in liver dispersion causes headache, dizziness and vertigo, coma, hemoptysis, and hematemesis.

maintains the body at a constant temperature; defensive function, to fight off invading pathogenic organisms, usually by mounting an inflammatory reaction, and also to protect the body surface against excessive environmental forces; nourishing, to keep the body supplied to support overall bodily activities; transforming, related to digestion and conversion of materials to produce biologically active substances; and regulating, involving most critical processes, tissues, and organs in the body to maintain overall physiological balance (*zheng*, 正) or homeostasis over a wide range of external factors and internal conditions.

Vital Air

Of the metabolic components, vital air (qi) may be the most critical because survival without it is extremely brief. The ancient Chinese never apparently knew that the indispensable element in air was oxygen. However, they did comprehend that vital air absorbed into the blood supply via the lungs was necessary to activate nutrients (ying) and defensive substances (wei). A person can be deprived of food for a number of days and water for perhaps a few days and still survive. Deprivation of air for just a minute is usually life threatening. Almost all metabolic processes in the human body use oxygen as the primary reactive agent. Only a few anaerobic energetic mechanisms of short duration operate in the absence of oxygen. The principal role of oxygen is now known to take place in the mitochondria in conjunction with nutrient-derived glucose to activate the high-energy compound adenosine triphosphate (ATP), which serves as the energy currency of the body (Chapters 1 and 6).

Nutrients

Basic nutrients (ying) absorbed from digested food are considered by the Chinese to be the most precious of substances that are circulated in the body, and are crucial to sustaining life. Presently, these nutrients are classed in terms of carbohydrates, proteins, vitamins, and minerals. Nutrients are absorbed into the venous blood supply from the small intestine. This process is discussed in *NJSW 43 (Rheumatism)*:

> Nutrients [ying] are the vital essences of water and grains, harmoniously regulated by the five viscera. Nutrients are broken down into fine particles in the bowels and then absorbed into the blood vessels [mesenteric veins]. Thus, nutrients flow up and down [circulate] within the vessels, passing through the five viscera, and in the vessels that form collaterals with the six bowels.

Evidence that the early Chinese had a clear understanding of the absorption of nutrients from the gut into the blood vessels is further illustrated in *NJLS 71 (Invasion of Pathogenic Forces)*:

> With respect to nutrients [ying], they are secreted in the body fluids to pour into the blood vessels. Here nutrients are transformed in order to benefit blood and nourish the four extremities, and internally concentrate in the five viscera and the six bowels. All of this takes place in accordance with fixed time periods.

Because nutrients, which are absorbed into the venous supply and distributed to the arteries, are not entirely used up as they are circulated to the body tissues, the venous supply has about 70 percent as much circulating nutrients as does the arterial blood supply. The role of nutrients is to nourish and maintain the body, and promote the functional activity of various tissues and organs. Nutrients also maintain the complex blood coagulation system that keeps the blood circulating in the vessels.

Defensive Substances

Defensive substances (wei) are also derived from food and water. While nutrients are absorbed into the veins of the gut, defensive substances are not. Defensive substances flow from the gut into the deep lymphatic vessels, which also carry absorbed dietary fat and lymph fluid. The deep lymphatics are drained into the venous blood supply at the subclavian vein. A description of this is noted in *NJSW 43*:

> Defensive substances [wei] are the fierce or brave vital substances of water and grains. Defensive substances are high spirited, travel quickly, are smooth or sliding in nature, and are not directly absorbed into the blood vessels. Thus, defensive substances flow between the skin and striated muscles [superficial lymphatics], vaporize in the membranes, and spread or disperse in the chest and abdomen [deep lymphatics].

The identification of defensive substances and their role by the ancient Chinese provided the first description of the body's immune system. They understood subtle details, such as the fact that defensive substances leave the arterial circulation to mount a protective reaction and then drain back into the venous supply from the lymphatic vessels. The defensive function (*weiqi*, 卫气) has both a yin and a yang characteristic, with inflammatory reactions classed as yang and anti-inflammatory functions as yin.

In addition to normal immune functions, defensive substances also have a role in warming the superficial body and in controlling the pores and sweating. Defensive functions include control over superficial vasodilatation and the immune complement system.

Relationship between Nutrients and Defensive Substances

Many functions in the body depend on the interplay between nutritive and defensive reactions. Perhaps most important is the interaction between the blood coagulation and immune complement systems. This is a fundamental process that responds to even the smallest of assaults on the body, including the insertion of acupuncture needles (Chapter 14). The early Chinese had a clear concept of this since they accurately described diverse phenomena such as swelling, formation of pus, and tissue reactions to needling. Even the specific vessels involved in these responses and the mechanism by which pathogenic factors penetrate into the body were correctly noted. They also recognized that reactions that cause heat, such as an inflammation or infection, usually result in the formation of pus. Attack by cold pathogenic forces results in rheumatism. One important discussion of these details is noted in *NJSW 58* (*Vital Nodes*):

> It is by means of these vessels [arterioles, capillaries, venules] that pathogenic forces can overflow into the body, and also by which nutrients and defensive substances are distributed.
>
> When nutrients and defensive substances are delayed or obstructed [by pathogenic forces], defensive substances are dispersed and nutrients overflow. This results in the exhaustion of vital substances and accumulation of blood, causing external fever and internal impairment of vital substances [or functional activity].
>
> When pathogenic forces overflow [into the muscles], vital substances are obstructed, resulting in heat in the blood vessels and withering of the muscles. Nutrients and defensive substances are then unable to circulate, resulting in the formation of pus. Internally there is depletion of the bones and marrow and externally there is damage to the knee joints. When pathogenic factors accumulate in the joints, it results in withering of the muscles.
>
> Accumulation and retention of cold results in restricting the availability of nutrients and defensive substances. This causes a curling of the flesh, and contraction of muscles and tendons. The ribs and elbows cannot be extended. Internally there is bone rheumatism, externally there is loss of sensation [numbness]. This is a deficiency due to retention of great cold in the streams and valleys [small and large muscles].

The Chinese also explained some characteristics of swelling resulting from the interaction of nutrients (ying) and defensive substances (wei). This was an attempt to differentiate swelling due to possible assault or injury, and swelling due to localized edema. This is explained in *NJLS 35* (*Swelling*), cited in Chapter 10.

Organ Vitality Substances

The five viscera contain refined substances that mediate organ vitality or spirit (shenjing), as presented in *NJSW 9* (*The Six Junctures and Manifestations of the Viscera*), and cited in Chapter 7. Refined substances of vitality (shenjing) are refined physical substances critical to the functional activity of each organ, a concept which seems to correlate with the Western understanding of biologically active substances, including hormones. Most bodily functions require an interaction with hormones or other biologically active refined substances. Although the heart is responsible for overall vitality, in the Chinese view, drive (related to the kidneys) and intent (related to the spleen) have the most crucial role because they manage the refined substances of vitality. Specific physiological activities associated with each viscus can only be fully understood in relation to a particular endocrine gland (Chapter 7).

Substance and Function

Since the vital air (qi) that contains oxygen is essential for activating energetic processes it is thought to provide vital function. Also, vital air can mean providing vitality to something. The Chinese word qi can denote both material substance and/or function, which are closely related and cannot be entirely separated, and it can also mean vitality. It is often difficult to determine from written Chinese when the term qi is used to mean substances, including vital air, and when the concept of function or vitality is intended.

After nutrients and defensive substances are circulated through the lungs, they are then accompanied by oxygen in the arterial blood supply. The character qi is then often added along with the characters ying and wei. So *yingqi* (营气) becomes vital nutrients or nutrient function, and *weiqi* (卫气) becomes vital defensive substance or defensive function. In some situations, particularly involving the internal organs, qi is used to denote functional activity. Organ activity is also referred to as organ qi.

The character qi is used in conjunction with other terms to indicate vital air, vitality, or function. When qi is used in conjunction with ancestral or primordial (*zong*, 宗), true or genuine (*zhen*, 真), and righteous or straight (*zheng*, 正), these words then take on a more functional connotation. *Zongqi* (宗气) becomes the primordial function that provides the contractile nature of the heart and its relationship to breathing, *zhenqi* (真气) becomes the true or perfect function at the lowest tissue levels, and *zhengqi* (正气) becomes righteous function or physiological balance.

When used in conjunction with the word qi, terms such as spirit (shen) and distribution vessel (*jing*, 经) take on a new significance. The term *shenqi* (神气) becomes spirit function or vitality, and *jingqi* (经气) becomes vessel function or vitality. Both of these words are used to indicate nonmaterial transmission of function, which is equivalent to a nerve response. The word jingqi (vessel function) can also be used to denote the motive force of the heart in circulating blood. When qi is combined with the word jing, meaning refined substances (different from the character for distribution vessel), it forms the word *jingqi* (精气), meaning vital substances.

Body Fluids

Body fluids are one of the most basic constituents of humans and animals, since our cells are surrounded by an internal sea of extracellular fluid (ECF) contained within the integument of our bodies. Although this level of detail was not understood by the ancient Chinese, they did recognize the importance of body fluids. They understood that body water is derived from the dietary intake of food and water. Initially, it is absorbed from the gut into the venous blood supply to circulate throughout the body. Through various physiological activities, water is supplied to cells and interstitial spaces. Some water is formed in the body as a metabolic by-product of aerobic respiration in the mitochondria, where glucose is metabolized in the presence of oxygen to activate the high-energy phosphate compound ATP.

Blood plasma (fluid component) and cells make up the total blood volume.[1] The Chinese were not aware of the cellular component of circulation, which is mainly oxygen-carrying red blood cells and white blood cells. Control of total body water is mediated through the blood plasma. This is the fluid medium circulating in the vessel system that communicates with all the internal organs, tissues, and pores of the skin. The kidneys have the leading role in water metabolism, although the gut—and in particular the small intestine—also has an important role. A small quantity of water can also be gained or lost through the lungs. Water is lost through the skin by means of perspiration.

Body Fluids and Water

Body fluids, collectively known by the two Chinese characters, jin and ye, have a moistening and a nourishing function. The jin category of body fluid is more dilute, and flows easily in the pores, skin, and muscles. The ye part of body fluid is thick, and flows less easily in the joints, viscera, bowels, brain, and spinal cord. Because it is difficult to separate these two categories, body fluids are generally referred to in combination as jinye, and are equivalent to the intercellular and extracellular fluids of modern times.

The process of absorbing nutrients and water from the gut is noted in *NJSW 21* (*Distribution Vessel Pulse Differentiation*):

> When vital foods are ingested through the stomach, the refined substances are dispersed to the liver [via the portal vein], where the overflowing refined substances supply the muscles. Of the vital foods ingested by the stomach, the murky part is returned to the heart [lymphatics drain into the subclavian vein], and the refined substances overflow [are absorbed] into the blood vessels [mesenteric veins]. These refined substances of the blood vessels flow to the longitudinal distribution vessels [vena cava]. The distribution vessels, in turn, return the refined substances to the lungs [pulmonary arteries], and the lungs in turn send it out to all the vessels and transport the refined substances to the skin and body hair.
>
> Refined substances converge to bring about balance. When the balance is harmonious, the condition will be reflected at the radial pulse, from where the prospects for death or life can be determined.
>
> Liquids that enter the stomach slosh around, and their refined substances overflow [to the small intestine veins] to be directed upward by the spleen. The spleen's functional activity disperses the refined substances upward to converge at the lungs. The lungs regulate the water passages and transport liquids downward to the bladder.

Water is absorbed from the small intestine by the inferior mesenteric veins (small intestine vessels), which flow into the splenic vein (spleen vessel) and then on to the portal vein, the liver, the heart via the vena cava, and then the lungs (Figure 10.1). Since the lungs have a role in dispersing vital air (qi), they also direct water to the kidneys via the aorta and renal arteries (bladder vessels). Water is filtered in the kidneys and reabsorbed into the renal veins (kidney vessels), except for the small amount that forms as urine. The superior mesenteric arteries (heart vessels) direct water back to the small intestine to aid digestion.

Function of Body Fluids

The main function of body water is to provide the fluid medium through which all nutrients (ying), defensive substances (wei), organ vitalities (shenjing), and vital air (qi) are distributed throughout the body, and the products of their metabolic processes are eliminated from the body. Lymphatic fluid is derived from ECF and the function of the lymphatic vessels is to drain the interstitial spaces. Water is used to aid digestion of food, and to control body temperature through perspiration. Another important function of water is to moisten the body tissues and cavities—including the mucus membranes, oral and nasal cavities, lung tissues, joint capsules, and cerebral spinal cavities—to ensure proper function.

With respect to body water metabolism, the two most important substrates are nutrients (ying) and defensive substances (wei). Nutrients are transported via blood plasma to the interstitial fluid to be taken up by the intracellular fluid, where they are used for cell maintenance and fuel. Metabolic waste products are transported back to the blood plasma, where they are eliminated from the body in the urine formed in the kidneys. Defensive substances can flow from the capillaries (*sun*, 孙 vessels) into the interstitial fluid to mount a defensive reaction or normal warming function. In this situation they are absorbed back into the plasma by means of the lymphatic vessels. Defensive substances are also transported to the pores, where they have a role in perspiration.

It is now known that oxygen from vital air (qi) is absorbed into the blood plasma through the lungs, and carried by the hemoglobin contained in the red blood cells. Oxygen is given up through the interstitial fluid directly into the cells, where it is necessary for essential metabolism. Carbon dioxide (CO_2) produced as a by-product of cellular metabolism is transported back to the lungs for elimination from the body by the same red blood cells that deliver oxygen derived from vital air (qi).

Relationship between Vital Substances and Body Fluids

Vital substances differ from body fluids (jinye) both in nature and form. Nutrient and defensive components of vital substances are derived from food and water, just as body fluids are. There are similarities in their formation and circulation in the body. Formation, distribution, and excretion of body fluids depend on the circulation of vital substances, involving localized interrelationships as well as the function of the lungs, kidneys, bladder, internal membrane system associated with the gut (*sanjiao*, 三焦), and the liver. Impairment of these organs results in insufficient body fluids or the accumulation of fluids.

Deficiency in the function of these organs can impair their controlling function, resulting in loss of body fluid. Conversely, the accumulation of body fluids, to the extent that it impairs circulation of vital substances, affects the functional activity of many internal organs. Profound loss of body fluids leads to a significant loss of vital substances, and can result in death under conditions of high temperature exposure.

Relationship between Blood and Body Fluids

Both blood and body fluids are liquids that function to moisten and nourish the body. Body fluids are derived from the blood, and are produced when they leave the blood vessels to form sweat, tears, saliva, joint capsule fluid, water for digestion, and urine. Body fluids can be injured by recurrent or frequent blood loss, resulting in scanty urination, dry skin, and thirst. Severe loss of body fluids affects the blood volume, manifesting as exhaustion of both body fluids and blood.

For this reason, diaphoretic herbs or medications are avoided in cases of hemorrhage. Likewise, bloodletting treatments are avoided if there are symptoms of body fluid loss due to excessive sweating. Similarly, these strategies and other therapies involving reducing techniques are avoided in all cases where there is either blood or body fluid loss, including diarrhea, severe blood loss, emaciation, severe sweating, or loss of blood following childbirth.

Role and Function of Blood

All primitive societies have understood that blood is the life essence of humans and animals alike. It is no surprise that the ancient Chinese had a clear comprehension of the role of blood in circulating vital air, nutrients, defensive substances, and refined substances of vitality. Certain clinical conditions can manifest due to blood deficiencies, blood stagnation, and heat in the blood (Table 8.2). Some ideas about the role of blood are discussed in *NJLS 47* (*Root of the Viscera*), where the Yellow Emperor notes:

Table 8.2 Abnormal conditions in the blood and related syndromes.

Syndrome	*Etiology*	*Manifestations*
Blood deficiency	Blood deficiency failing to nourish the internal organs and vessels due to profuse bleeding, weak stomach and spleen function, mental strain, and consumption of body fluids.	Pallor or sallow completion, pale lips and nails, dizziness, blurring of vision, palpitations, insomnia, numbness of the hands and feet, pale menses, prolonged menstrual cycle, or menopause.
Blood stagnation	Sluggish blood flow, coagulation of extravasated blood, stagnation of cold, stagnation of vital substances, or trauma.	Localized cutting or stabbing pain that is worse on pressure or at night, mass tumors, hemorrhage, and ecchymoses or petechiae.
Heat in blood	Spontaneous bleeding resulting in extravasation of blood due to excess heat in the internal organs and its attack on the blood system.	Mental restlessness, or mania in severe cases, a dry mouth with no desire to drink, possible occurrence of various hemorrhagic syndromes, or profuse menstrual flow in women.

> A person's blood, vital air [qi], refined substances [ying and wei], and refined substances of vitality [shenjing] are necessary to respectfully support birth and growth, and circulate throughout the body to sustain life. The distribution vessels are required to circulate blood and vital air [qi], nourish body function [yin and yang], moisten the muscles and bones, and facilitate articulation of the joints. Defensive substances [wei] are necessary to warm the striated muscles, serve the skin—including the fat between the skin and flesh [adipose tissue], and manage the closing and opening of the pores...
>
> Therefore, when blood is in harmony it flows through the distribution vessels. Body function [yin and yang] is nourished. The muscles and bones are strong and powerful, and the joint articulations are completely functional. When defensive substances are harmonious, the striated muscles are smooth and functional, the skin is regulated and soft, and the pores are fine and dense.

The Chinese discerned that blood is dependent on the intake of nutrients and water. This is true with regard to the blood plasma. Discovery of the cellular portion of blood and its relationship to bone marrow was not possible during early times. Blood volume was thought to be related to intake of food under the control of the stomach and spleen. It is interesting to note that during fetal development, blood cells are generated not only in bone marrow, but also in the spleen, and some within the liver. Spleen production of blood cells can also occur under certain pathological conditions.

The dependence of blood on food and water intake, and the utilization of nutrients by oxygenation of blood in the lungs, is noted in *NJLS 18* (*The Meeting and Interaction of Nutrients and Defensive Substances*), where Qibo explains:

> The abdominal peritoneum [middle *jiao*] converges at the stomach, and issues forth after the thoracic membranes [upper jiao] from where the stomach receives food [via the esophagus]. From here [stomach] waste material gushes forth, from which the body fluids are evaporated, and from which digestion yields the minute refined substances [jing]. These [absorbed water and nutrients] travel upward [via the venous system] to pour into the lung vessels, and are then transformed and benefit blood to serve life and the body. For this reason there is nothing more precious circulating within the distribution vessels than that which are called nutrients [ying].

Blood contains a complex coagulation system mediated by certain proteins and zymogens. These circulate in the blood to maintain its free flow and protect against mechanical damage that could result in blood loss. In the Chinese view this coagulation system is controlled by the spleen and prevents blood extravasation, and also controls blood clotting. The blood coagulation system has an important interaction with the immune system, related to vasodilatory reactions, which are also thought to be under the influence of the spleen.

Role of Blood

The distribution of vital substances (ying, wei, shenjing, and qi) and body fluids (jinye) is the most critical role of blood. Vital substances and body fluids constitute the material basis of bodily function; consequently, there are important physiological and pathological relationships between blood, vital substances, and body function. Increased formation and circulation of blood can lead to increased levels of oxygen, nutrients, and functional activity. Similarly, an increase in the formation of these vital substances and body function has a corresponding effect on blood.

A deficiency (*xu*, 虛) of blood can lead to a deficiency of nutrients, oxygen, and body function. A deficiency of vital substances leads to a corresponding deficiency in blood. Stagnation of blood can cause a stagnation of vital substances, and similarly a stagnation of vital substances can cause a stagnation of blood. The importance of blood in the functioning of the body is noted in *NJSW 10* (*Development of the Five Viscera*):

> All the blood vessels relate to the eyes, neural tissue belongs to the brain, the muscles and tendons belong to the joints, blood belongs to the heart, vital air [qi] belongs to the lungs. These provide function to the four extremities and eight articulations [elbows, wrists, knees, and ankles] from morning to night.
>
> When a person sleeps, blood converges in the liver, and when the liver receives blood the eyes are able to see. When the feet receive blood they are able to walk, when the palms receive blood they are able to hold, and when the fingers receive blood they are able to grasp.

Blood and Internal Organs

Under normal conditions blood circulates in the vessels because of the mechanical motive forces of the heart (Chapter 10). The liver has an influence on the blood by acting as a storage area, however the liver's main task is that of dispersing the constructive substances and nutrients. The spleen keeps the blood within the vessels and dominates the digestive processes (pancreatic contribution), which result in the absorption of nutrients and water. These three organs (heart, liver, and spleen) provide coordinated activity to ensure adequate blood supply and volume, and to maintain continuous blood flow throughout the body.

Pathological conditions or dysfunction of the heart, spleen, or liver can result in blood system problems. Deficiency in heart function can lead to reduced blood circulation or blood stagnation. Inability of the spleen to control blood coagulation can result in bloody stools, uterine bleeding, subcutaneous bleeding, and ecchymoses. Insufficiency of liver blood can manifest in pale complexion, numbness of limbs, muscle spasms, eye dryness, blurred vision, dizziness and vertigo, and scanty menstrual flow.

Blood influences mental activities and the overall spirit or vitality of an individual. This is mainly due to the circulation of oxygen and nutrients, as well as organ vitalities (shenjing) (hormones and other substances), to the brain. Heart or liver blood deficiencies can result in mental disorders, including restlessness, insomnia, dream-disturbed sleep, and palpitations.

Similarity between Blood and Vital Substances

Blood and vital substances are considered to be similar in nature, and both have a critical role in life and vitality. This relationship is discussed in *NJLS 18*, where Qibo says:

> Just as nutrients [ying] and defensive substances [wei] belong to the same category of refined substances [jing], blood is the vitality of the spirit and this is why blood and vital substance [qi] have different names, but in this situation they are similar.

Blood dominates nourishment and moistening, while vital substances dominate warmth, metabolism, and motive force. Weak or deficient vital substances lead to a deficiency in blood. Furthermore, heart functional activity controls blood circulation. Lung function dominates the dispersion of vital substances by oxygenation of the blood. Liver functional activity is involved in metabolic processing, and therefore controls the free flow of nutrients throughout the body. These three organs (heart, lungs, and liver) are responsible for the circulation of vital substances, which are closely related to the circulation of blood.

Retarded circulation of vital substance or weakness in the heart to propel blood results in blood circulation problems and blood stasis. Weakness in vital substance in maintaining normal circulation within the vessels, preventing blood extravasation, leads to hemorrhage. If blood supply is not sufficient to provide proper nourishment, physiological functions are impaired. In cases of severe blood loss, there is an accompanying loss of vital substances. Exhaustion of blood is followed by exhaustion of vital function.

Key Metabolic Features

The early Chinese theoretical foundations of metabolism correlate closely with a modern understanding of these processes. One concept involves the idea that human life and genetic individuality start at conception—this is the person's original or source function (*yuanqi*, 元气). The other main idea concerns metabolic processes at the lowest tissue levels that convert nutrients (ying) and oxygen from vital air (qi) to useable energy for all bodily processes under the influence of source function. This process is called true or genuine function (zhenqi). Another significant theory considers that the heart is controlled by a primordial or ancestral function (zongqi), responsible for the heartbeat and also for dominating respiration. These three main components and other aspects of overall metabolism are noted in Table 8.3.

Original Vital Function

The original or source (*yuan*, 元) vital function (qi), called yuanqi, is formed at conception from the congenital essence that provides the primary motive force for life activities. Source function (yuanqi) defines a person's genetic disposition, and is considered to be fixed and cannot be improved upon. The best an individual can expect is to achieve their full genetic potential. Source function is operative at the lowest tissue levels and is thought to influence energy conversion at the cellular level by genetically determined factors. Source function is also thought to have a genetic influence at the visceral level, especially involving function of the lungs and stomach.

Once embryonic source function (yuanqi) is formed it is nurtured by acquired nutrients and oxygen supplied by the mother. The developing fetal viscera, particularly the heart, liver, and kidneys, have a vital role in circulating fetal blood and eliminating waste products. Once birth occurs the function of breathing is activated. The infant's own organs take over the role of the body's function and maintenance. From this point on, the individual obtains all nutrients from acquired sources to support life and to maintain source function.

A person's source function predisposes them to achieving a certain potential life span. However, environmental, emotional, and dietary stress, as well as substance abuse, inappropriate lifestyles, toxic exposure, and even excess sunlight can all have a negative impact on source function. In present times there are additional hazards that can damage source function, including X-rays, nuclear radiation, and electromagnetic radiation (emanations from radio,

Table 8.3 Correlation of Chinese concepts of metabolic processes in the human body with modern equivalents.

Item	*Name*	*Chinese Description*	*Modern Equivalent*
Yuanqi	Source vital breath or function	Inborn vital air and function established at conception.	Spark of life and genetic disposition.
Qingqi	Clear air	Fresh air.	Fresh air containing oxygen.
Guqi	Food vitality	Fundamental nutrients in food and water.	Fundamental nutrients in food and water.
Hou Tian Zhi Qi	Acquired nutrients	Sustaining substances derived from absorbed food, nutrients, water, and inhaled air.	Sustaining substances derived from absorbed food, nutrients, water, and inhaled air.
Zongqi	Pectoral or ancestral function	Function that provides basic rhythmic heartbeat, with a relationship to respiration.	Contractile and rhythmic nature of cardiac muscle tissue producing heartbeat, with a relationship to respiration.
Weiqi	Defensive substances	System that provides first line protection from environment and infections disease.	Immune cells and system, lymph fluid, and lymphatic system.
Yingqi	Nutrients	Absorbed nutrients flowing in blood vascular system.	Absorbed nutrients flowing in blood vascular system.
Jing	Refined substances	Refined substances including ying, wei, shenjing, reproductive substances, and other biologically active substances.	Refined substances, including all nutrients, immune cells, hormones, enzymes, neurochemicals, reproductive substances, etc.
Zhenqi	True or genuine function	Basic dynamic force of all vital function.	Energy production and use at cellular or mitochondrial level, adenosine triphosphate (ATP).

television, power lines, microwaves, magnets, and so on). One can work toward achieving one's own full potential life span by living a moderate life, obtaining adequate exercise, and reducing exposure to factors that are harmful to genetic processes.

True Function

The true or genuine function (zhenqi) of the body is an important concept that explains how the basic nutrients are used by the body and the influence of genetic determinants (source function, yuanqi) on energy production in the body. Genetic influence on metabolism is thought to be inherited from the mother (see reference to *NJLS 54* in Chapter 7). It has recently been shown that mitochondrial DNA, which controls the energy conversion process within the cells, is inherited exclusively from one's mother.

True or genuine function is recognized as the basic functional process responsible for all vital functions in the body. It operates at the lowest levels using nutrients (ying) and oxygen from vital air (qi) under the influence of the source function (yuanqi). True function is responsible for true energy production in the body, now known to occur at the mitochondrial level of each cell. Its principal reaction involves the use of glucose and oxygen to convert high-energy nucleotide adenosine diphosphate (ADP) to ATP, releasing CO_2 and water in the process. ATP is used in the cells as the energetic substrate for most biological functions.

Ancestral Function

The ancestral or primordial function (zongqi) is the process that controls heart contractions and respiration. The critical nature of the heart in maintaining life was understood by the early Chinese (Chapter 10); they recognized that heart tissue is different from striated muscles, and that therefore some unique processes must have been involved in keeping the heart beating. Undoubtedly, they also observed that animal hearts, such as those of turtles, continued to beat after being removed from the body. They rightly identified the unique contractile properties of cardiac muscle tissue as being a primordial characteristic.

Ancestral function is also referred to as pectoral function, and is specifically concentrated in the heart. It is responsible for the basic motive force of the heart, and causes the other vital substances (blood, oxygen, nutrients, and defensive substances) to circulate throughout the body. In addition, pectoral function also influences respiration and voice. A close regulatory function was noted between the heartbeat and respiratory rate, which is now known to be influenced by blood oxygen/CO_2 ratios.

Overall Metabolic Processes

The Chinese view of metabolism and energy production within the body is close to modern ideas. The overall scheme, depicted in Figure 8.1, is divided into two major branches. The first of these is the sky- or nature-given contribution to vital air. The second part involves the contribution from the intake of food and water.

Sky-Given Vital Air

The sky-given vital air (qi) consists of the spark of life that is created at conception (inborn vital breath) and the fresh air (*qingqi*, 清气) that is breathed in from the atmosphere (see Sky-Given Vital Air in Figure 8.1). The intake of clean air (qingqi) can be impaired by air pollution and other noxious elements (*zaqi*, 杂气) in the atmosphere.

Conception results from the reproductive material essence (sperm and ovum) supplied by the mother and father. This material is known as the "before heaven" or "inborn vital essence (*xian tian zhi jing*, 先天之精)." When the mother's egg and the father's sperm combine, a person's original or source function (yuanqi) is created.

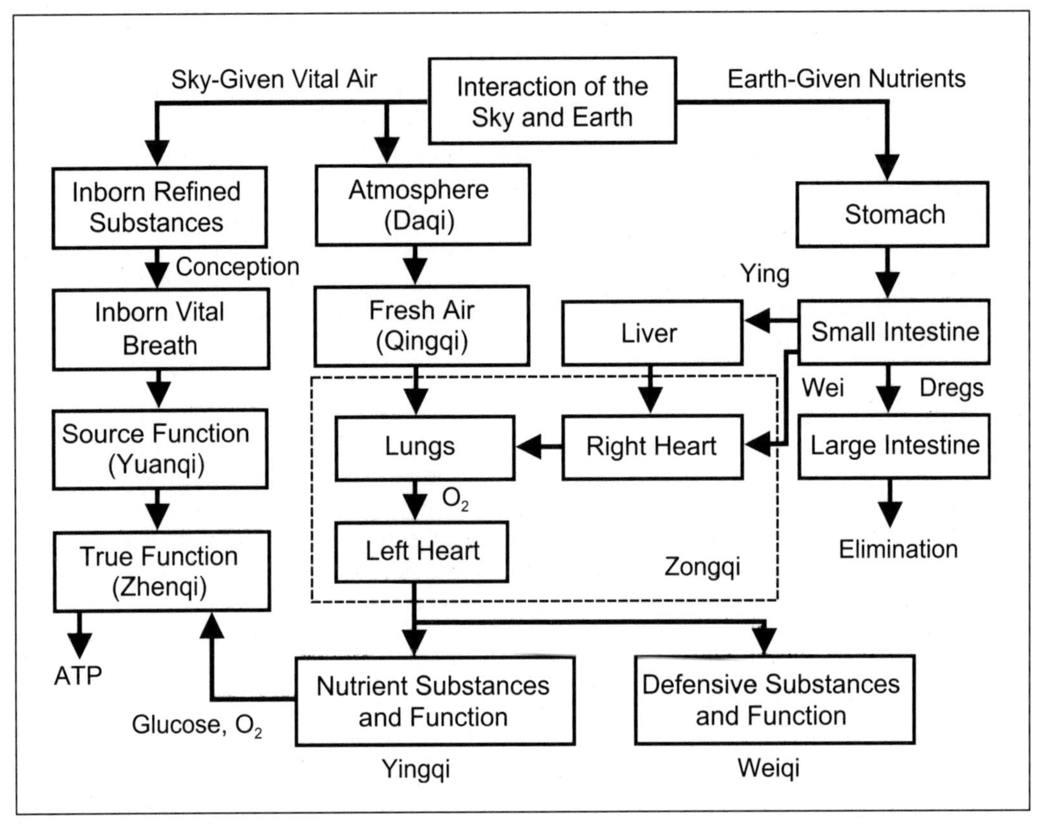

Figure 8.1 Principal interaction of the sky and earth in relation to traditional metabolic processes, including inhalation of vital air, intake of food and water, and genetic influence.

Source function (yuanqi) also has a role in the function of the lungs and stomach. In addition, source function has a major influence on the ancestral function (zongqi) responsible for the contractile nature of cardiac tissue, and the relationship between the heart and lungs in maintaining the heartbeat and respiration.

Earth-Given Nutrients

The contribution of food and water to metabolism involves the food and fluid intake that ultimately serves as the material substrate for energy production in the body (see Earth-Given Nutrients in Figure 8.1). Sometimes food is referred to as "water (*shui*, 水) and grains (*gu*, 谷)." After ingestion, food and water are first broken down in the stomach to form the initial material (*shuigu zhi qi*, 水谷之气). This initial material is passed along to the small intestine to complete the digestion processes. The usable part of the digestate (*guqi*, 谷气) is further broken down, and separated to provide the nutrients that are absorbed into the body by the small intestine veins. The dregs of digestion, or remaining solid and waste products (*zhuo*, 浊), are passed along to the large intestine for collection and elimination from the body.

The refined nutrients in food and water are sent on to the liver through the portal vein. From the liver the nutrients flow in the vena cava to the heart. The murky part of food (dietary fat and defensive substances) is absorbed into the deep lymphatics and along with lymph fluid is sent on to the heart.

The absorbed nutrients are sent on to the lungs, where they are distributed throughout the body along with oxygenated blood. This constitutes the acquired vital material (*hou tian zhi qi*, 后天之气) that is the fuel for all energetic processes in the body. Tissue level metabolism, represented by true function (zhenqi), converts refined nutrients, including glucose, protein, and fats. These nutrients, together with oxygen from vital air, work to convert ADP to ATP in the mitochondria, under the influence of source function (yuanqi). Nutrients are also needed for maintenance and repair.

The defensive substances of the immune system include lymph fluid, immune cells, and immune plasma proteins. Body fluids, including sweat and saliva, are also in this category. Initially defensive substances are circulated in the blood system, but they can leave the blood vessels to occupy the interstitial spaces that are drained by the lymphatic vessels. This occurs in response to immune reactions.

9
Vessels and Collaterals

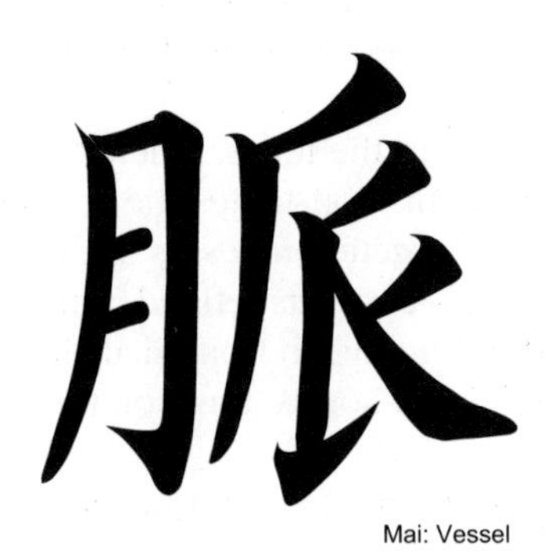

Mai: Vessel

> The vessels start to form in order to circulate nutrients, and the muscles and tendons form to make the body strong. The flesh develops to form the trunk of the body, the skin becomes firm, and the hair grows long. Food broken down in the mother's stomach supplies vital nutrients to the fetus. The vessel pathways then develop and open up, so that blood and vital substances can be circulated.
>
> Yellow Emperor, *NJLS 10 (Distribution Vessels)*

The study of therapeutic bloodletting led to early investigation of the vascular system. Much effort went into understanding vessel pathways, branching, and organization. All significant blood vessels of the body were identified, and many are named in relation to the anatomical region they serve, as well as to an associated internal organ. Twelve pairs of matched longitudinal arteries and veins (six pairs on each half of the body) comprise the organ-related main distribution vessels (*jingmai*, 经脉). The collateral branches (*luomai*, 络脉) of these main vessels supply tissues in the superficial and deep areas of the body. Collateral vessels divide further into fine vessels (*sunmai*, 孙脉), which comprise arterioles, capillaries, and venules. Fine vessels communicate between the outflowing arteries and the return flow venous supply, thus ensuring continuous blood circulation. Vessels, along with associated nerves, provide the anatomical means of communication between the internal and external body, a factor that is essential to health, disease processes, and treatment mechanisms.

Because there are more veins than arteries, the ancient Chinese identified five pairs of superficial venous networks that are not associated with the internal organs. These veins, plus two deep major veins, are classed as singular vessels (*jimai*, 奇脉). About 70 percent of blood is now known to be in the slow-flowing systemic veins, 11 to 12 percent is found in the fast-moving systemic arteries, and 5 to 6 percent is contained in the systemic capillaries. The remainder is in the lungs (8 percent) and heart (5 percent). Normally, the volumetric rate of flow in the veins and arteries is equal, even though the veins hold six times more blood than the arteries. The Chinese understood that veins are capacitance vessels, noting that they have additional capacity to control the relative blood volume between the arteries and veins.

Fine branching of vessels (sunmai) in the skin regions form networks called critical junctures, comprising neurovascular nodes (acupoints). All these sites involve vessels, with the main distribution vessels (jingmai) and their collaterals (luomai) giving rise to the greatest number of nodes (Chapter 11). Other locations, such as collateral (*luo*, 络), source (*yuan*, 原), and confluent or meeting sites are thought to influence the relative blood flow between specific vessels. Still other vessel locations have special communication (*shu*, 输) capabilities for specific purposes. Superficial fine vessels (sunmai) provide the initial means by which the influence of environmental factors transmit along the vessels to affect the internal organs (Figure 13.2).

Vessel Organization

For convenience, the names of the longitudinal distribution (*jing*, 经) and collateral (*luo*, 络) vessels are often combined to form the word *jingluo* (经络), which is used to describe the vascular system. This is especially true when discussing the distribution and collateral vessel pathways associated with nodal pathways (Chapter 11). The organization of the body's vessel system in terms of major longitudinal distribution and collateral vessels comprises the "theory of the jingluo." The structure and function of the vascular system in Chinese medical theory is identical to that in the modern Western view, except the Chinese place greater emphasis on branching in the superficial and deep body, and the relationship of vessels to each other. Attention to the branching nature of the vessels may not have been appreciated in the West, even in Willem ten Rhijne's time. He reports the Chinese and Japanese view of vessel branching being like a net:

> [The Chinese and Japanese structure of the vessels] is nonetheless netlike. The fibers in the leaf of any vegetable begin large, gradually decrease, and become very small in the fashion of a net, and finally end uniformly in pellicles. In the same way, when the anatomist's knife uncovers vessels, there are found to be lurking the previously concealed branches of blood.
>
> You may deduce the Chinese origin of the illustrations from the fact that they are not entirely in accord with correct anatomy, an art the Chinese do not value, except for the structure of the blood vessels and the circulation of the blood.

Vessels initially distribute blood to and from the heart through large deep vessels, which progressively branch into smaller vessels as they disseminate to the extremities (Figure 9.1). The left portion of the heart receives blood from the lungs via the pulmonary vein, which pumps blood into the thoroughfare vessel (*chong*, 冲 aorta). This artery, classed as a singular vessel (jimai), directs blood to the internal organs and slightly smaller communication or transporting vessels (*shumai*, 输脉). The arterial communication vessels (shumai) consist of the brachiocephalic, subclavian, external iliac, and femoral arteries, which then supply six slightly smaller distribution (jingmai) arteries on each side of the body, which in turn distribute blood longitudinally to the extremities, head, face, and neck, and to the superficial regions of the trunk. Distribution vessels branch further into collateral vessels (luomai), which then branch into finer vessels (sunmai), correlating with arterioles, capillaries, and venules.

Venous return from the extremities and internal organs follows the reverse process, starting with the venules (sunmai) that supply venous collateral vessels (luomai), which then flow into the six main distribution veins (jingmai) and five superficial singular venous networks (jimai) on each side of the body. These vessels then supply the venous communication vessels (brachiocephalic and external iliac veins), which in turn return venous blood to two additional deep singular vessels; the allowance (*ren*, 任) vessel (vena cava), and the governing (*du*, 督) vessel (azygos, hemiazygos, and ascending lumbar veins). The allowance (ren) vessel

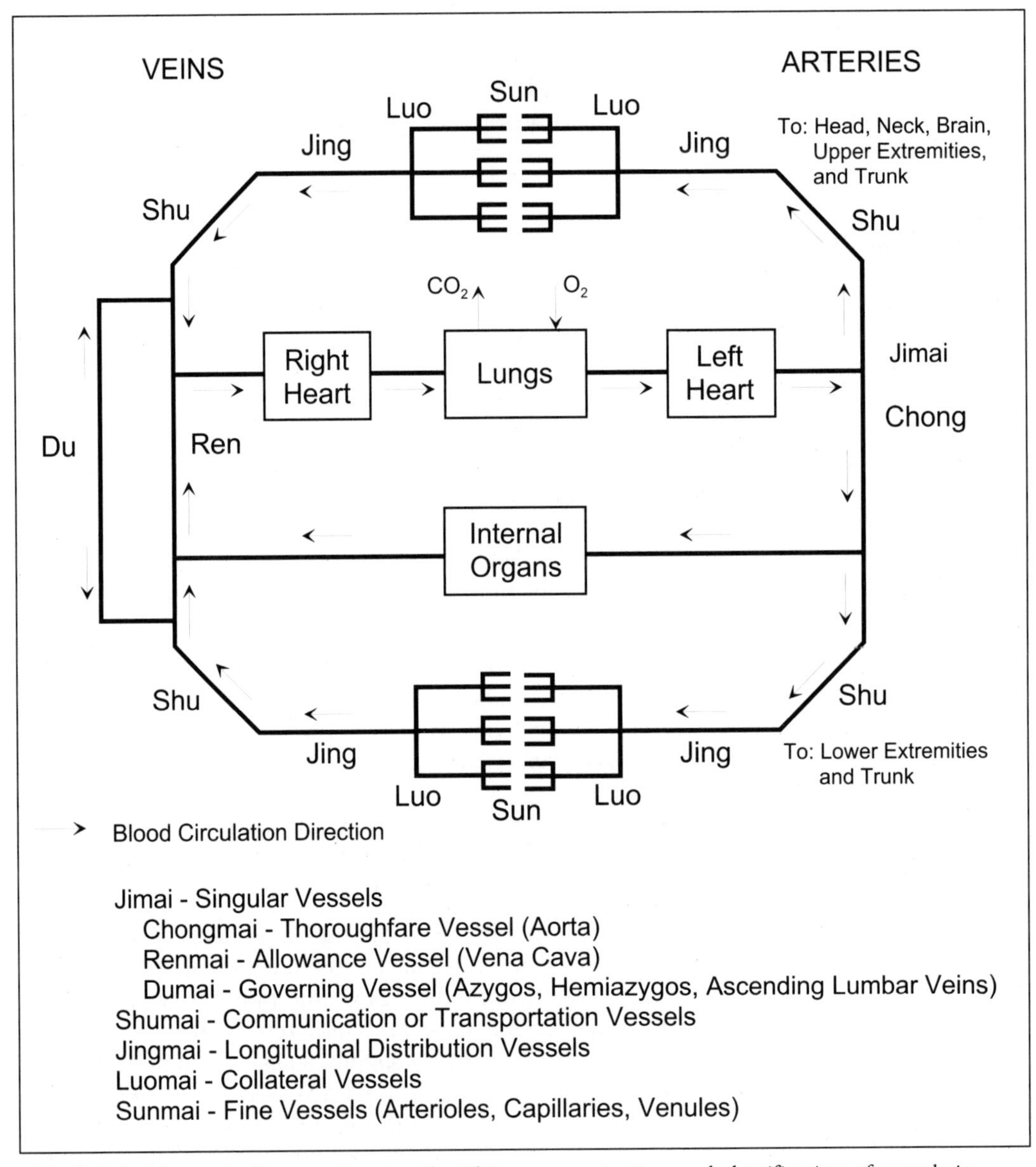

Figure 9.1 Schematic diagram showing the Chinese organization and classification of vessels in terms of branching from larger to smaller arterial vessels, and the reverse for veins.

connects directly with the right portion of the heart, which subsequently directs the venous blood to the lungs via the pulmonary arteries.

Because the circulatory system is one continuous network of outflowing arteries and returning veins, the names of specific vessels actually apply only to a portion of a vascular route. In describing pathways related to internal organs, portions of the deeper vessels are included in each route, along with the superficial course of the particular distribution vessel.

In total, some sixty-five major vessel pathways were identified, and include twelve pairs of distribution, thirteen pairs of collateral, two unpaired collateral, five pairs of superficial singular, and three unpaired deep singular vessels (Table 9.1). The twelve pairs of main distribution vessels have identified nodal sites. Two of the singular vessels, the governing (du) and allowance (ren), also give rise to nodes, while the thoroughfare vessel (chong aorta) shares locations on the lower abdomen with the kidney vessels. All eight of the singular vessels have confluent and communication sites.

Branching of Rivers and Vessels

One of the more auspicious Chinese characters, *yong* (永)—originally derived from the character for water (*shui*, 水)—describes the convergence of small rivulets and streams to form larger water flows and main rivers (Figure 9.2). From this, the character took on the meaning of perpetual, eternal, long, or far-reaching to describe the nature of a major river. A mirror image of the original form of yong was used to create the character component *pai* that describes the branching typical of veins and arteries. The character for blood (*xue*, 血) was added to pai, forming the word *mai* (脉), which means blood vessel, as applied to veins and arteries. The radical for flesh, *rou* (肉), used to indicate that something is related to the human body, later replaced the radical for blood. The character yong has also been used to replace the pai component. Mainland China now uses this latter character form for vessel in the simplified character set (Figure 9.2). The corollary of veins and arteries being like large streams and rivers formed from the joining of smaller creeks and rivulets is conveyed in the Chinese character mai, and provides a comprehensive overview of the physical branching of blood vessels. In addition to meaning vessel, the character mai is used to mean pulse.

Vessels are differentiated into outflowing arteries and returning veins. Outflowing and returning vessels are also differentiated by the presence of a pulse. Outflowing vessels are arteries, and as such are located between the heart and the fine vessels (sunmai). At certain locations along these vessels, the pulse generated by heart contractions can be felt as a peripheral pulse. Because this pulse is not transmitted past the sun vessels, no pulse is detected in the returning vessels, which are veins. When specifically referring to arteries, the Chinese use the term *dongmai* (动脉) to indicate the presence of a pulse. Here, *dong* (动) means to move or to act. The term *jingmai* (静脉)—this character *jing* (静) not being the same as the one for distribution—is used when referring specifically to veins, and means quiet or peaceful, with no pulse present.

Superficial Branching at Nodal Sites

A significant aspect of the traditional view of vessels is the importance accorded to superficial branching. This arrangement of vessels is described in *NJLS 17* (*Length of the Vessels*):

> The main longitudinal distribution [jing] vessels are deeper and branch into horizontal or collateral [luo] vessels. The collateral [luo] vessels are further differentiated into the fine [sun] vessels [arterioles, capillaries, and venules].

The collateral (luo) vessels branch into the very fine (sun) vessels that distribute to the skin (Figure 9.3). This arrangement of collateral (luo) branching is also present in the arrangement of vessels supplying the internal organs. The concentration of fine vessels creates

Table 9.1 Summary of the major superficial and deep vessels, along with the number of related nodal sites.

	Type	*Location (Chinese anatomical orientation)*	*Class*	*Nodes*
Twelve Distribution				
Lung	Artery	Upper chest, anterior medial arm, and hand	Yin	11
Large Intestine	Vein	Anterior lateral hand and arm, and face	Yang	20
Stomach	Artery	Face, trunk, anterior lateral leg, and foot	Yang	45
Spleen	Vein	Anterior medial foot, leg, and anterior lateral trunk	Yin	21
Heart	Artery	Posterior medial arm and hand	Yin	9
Small Intestine	Vein	Posterior lateral hand and arm, shoulder and face	Yang	19
Bladder	Artery	Forehead, head, back, posterior lateral leg and foot	Yang	67
Kidney	Vein	Bottom of foot, posterior medial leg, and anterior trunk	Yin	27
Pericardium	Artery	Upper chest, medial arm and hand	Yin	9
Internal Membrane	Vein	Lateral hand and arm, shoulder, and ear	Yang	23
Gallbladder	Artery	Lateral head, body and leg, and anterior lateral foot	Yang	44
Liver	Vein	Foot, medial leg, lower abdomen, and thorax	Yin	14
Eight Singular				
Thoroughfare	Artery	Aorta, and surface of lower abdomen		(14)
Allowance	Vein	Vena cava, and anterior body center line	Yin	24
Governing	Vein	Azygos, hemiazygos, and ascending lumbar v.v., and the posterior body centerline	Yang	28
Belt	Vein	Around waist from back to lower abdomen		
Medial Lifting	Vein	Medial leg, anterior medial trunk, neck, and face	Yin	
Lateral Lifting	Vein	Lateral leg, trunk, shoulder, face, and head	Yang	
Medial Holding	Vein	Medial leg, ant. med. trunk, and anterior neck	Yin	
Lateral Holding	Vein	Lateral foot, leg, trunk, shoulder, and head	Yang	
Fifteen Collateral				
Lung, Heart, Pericardium	Arteries	Hand	Yin	
Large and Small Intestine, Internal Membrane	Veins	Hand	Yang	
Stomach, Bladder, Gallbladder	Arteries	Foot	Yang	
Spleen, Kidney, Liver	Veins	Foot	Yin	
Great Spleen	Vein	Lateral thorax	Yin	
Governing	Vein	Posterior trunk, head, and face	Yang	
Allowance	Vein	Mouth, thorax, and lower abdomen	Yin	

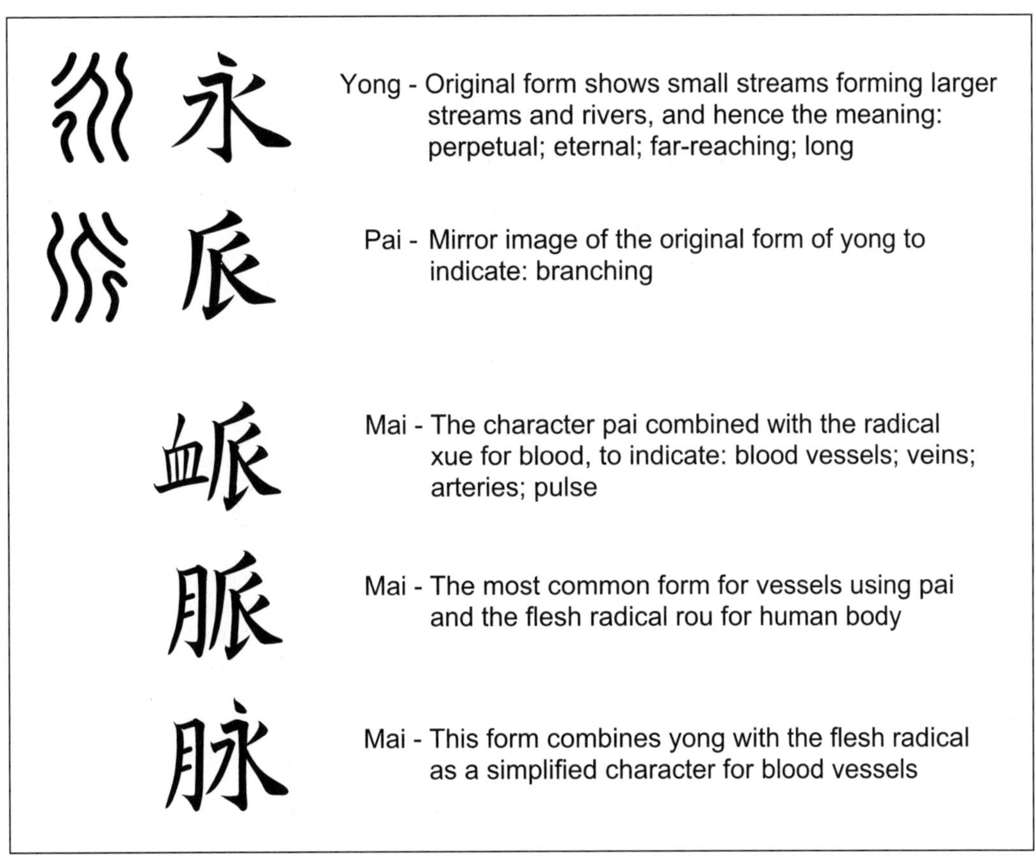

Figure 9.2 Derivation of the Chinese character *mai* for vessel, from the original character forms—before brushstroke calligraphy—for *yong* and *pai.*

small superficial areas where a compact arrangement of fine blood vessels and nerves are found. These regions are called critical junctures (*jie*, 节) or nodes. The arrangement of fine branching of collateral (luo) vessels is common to all nodal sites, as noted in *NJLS 3* (*Understanding the Fine Needle*):

> The critical junctures or vital nodes consist of 365 specific locations. The collateral [luo] vessels nourish all of these sites.

Singular Distribution Vessels: Jimai

The singular distribution vessels consist of three major deep vessels of the body, including one arterial vessel and two venous vessels, in addition to five pairs of superficial distribution veins (Table 9.2). Called jimai in Chinese, these vessels are considered singular because they are not assigned to any particular internal organ. Here, the character *ji* (奇)[1] means singular, but is also identical in form to the character *qi* (奇), typically used to mean strange. This character qi can also be interpreted as extraordinary, which is commonly contracted to mean

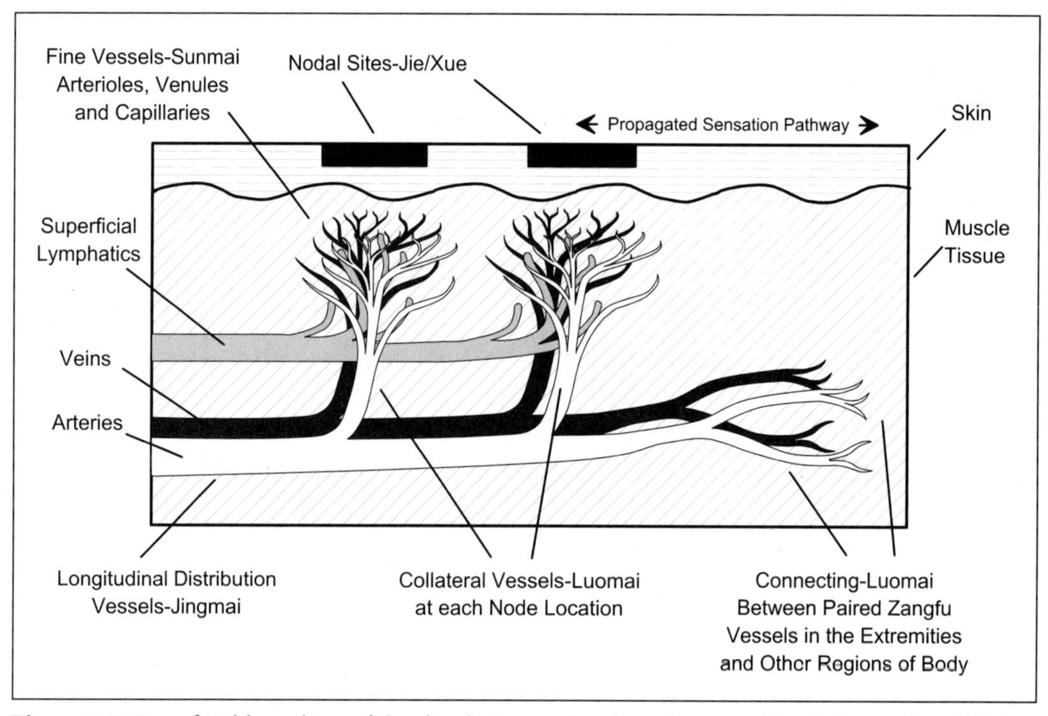

Figure 9.3 Superficial branching of the distribution and collateral vessels (*jingluo*) at each nodal site (acupoint), and the internal-external relationship in collateral terminals of the main distribution vessels in the extremities.

extra, resulting in the singular distribution vessels being referred to as the "eight extra vessels." Being a critical part of the circulatory network, the singular vessels have regulatory functions over particular main distribution (jing) vessels. Certain nodes on those regulated distribution vessels represent confluent locations (called master and couple nodes) that are applied in the treatment of particular clinical indications (Table 9.3).

The eight singular vessels are in a different category from the twelve main distribution vessels: the latter are responsible for the basic distribution of blood and vital substances to the internal organs and superficial parts of the body; the eight singular vessels (except the thoroughfare vessel, or chong aorta) are responsible for providing the necessary volumetric capacity to handle the runoff when the main distribution vessels are excessive. Physiologically, three of the eight singular vessels are represented by the large deep vessels of the body, while the other five were identified to account for the body's greater number of venous networks, compared to arteries. The reduced velocity of blood flow in the veins requires a greater number of venous structures. Also, veins are usually slightly larger than their corresponding arteries.

Veins are considered capacitance vessels, and help regulate the volume of venous and arterial blood. With the exception of the thoroughfare vessel (chong aorta), the singular vessels are all veins. Consequently, seven of the eight singular distribution vessels provide venous mechanisms to regulate the main distribution vessels. The one arterial singular vessel, the thoroughfare vessel (chong aorta), helps regulate arterial flow. The capacitance and

Table 9.2 Indications for the eight singular (*ji*) distribution vessels.

Ji *Vessels*	*Indications*
Thoroughfare (*Chong*)	An upsurge in flow causing internal (abdominal) disturbances and contraction of the genital organs (one of seven kinds of impairment in males); pain, panting, and shaking of hands due to internal cold.
Allowance (*Ren*)	Internal pain and congestion, and in men it will cause the seven types of hernia; in women there will be gynecological disorders and accumulated coagulation (abdominal mass).
Governing (*Du*)	Stiffness along the back that can lead to fainting; curvature of the spine.
Belt (*Dai*)	Abdominal fullness, with the lumbar region feeling like water flowing down, as if sitting in water.
Lateral Lifting (*Yangqiao*)	Relaxation of yin and excitation of yang.
Medial Lifting (*Yinqiao*)	Relaxation of yang and excitation of yin.
Lateral Holding (*Yangwei*)	When yin and yang are not able to hold each other together, this causes upset and disappointment with loss of will (*zhi*) and drive, and a significant inability to control and grasp (loss of physical strength); pain with cold and hot sensations.
Medial Holding (*Yinwei*)	When yin and yang are not able to hold each other together, this will cause upset and disappointment with loss of will (*zhi*) and drive, and a significant inability to control and grasp (loss of physical strength); pain and cardiac pain.

Table 9.3 Confluent nodes of the eight singular vessels and indications for regional areas.

Singular Vessel	*Regulated Vessel*	*Confluent Nodes*	*Regional Indications*
Governing Lateral Lifting	Small Intestine Bladder	Houxi (SI 3) Shenmai (BL 62)	Inner canthus, ear, neck, shoulder, and back.
Allowance Medial Lifting	Lungs Kidneys	Lieque (LU 7) Zhaohai (KD 6)	Throat, chest, lungs, and diaphragm.
Thoroughfare Medial Holding	Spleen Pericardium	Gongsun (SP 4) Neiguan (PC 6)	Heart, chest, and stomach.
Belt Lateral Holding	Gallbladder Internal Membrane	Zulinqi (GB 41) Waiguan (SJ 5)	Outer canthus, retroauricle, cheek, and diaphragm.

regulatory nature of the singular vessels is described in the *Nanjing* (*Difficulty 27: Content and Meaning of the Singular Distribution Vessels*), which uses the analogy of the main distribution vessels being regular irrigation canals, while the eight singular vessels are for emergency runoff:

> There are the lateral holding [*yangwei*, 阳维], medial holding [*yinwei*, 阴维], lateral lifting [*yangqiao*, 阳跷], medial lifting [*yinqiao*, 阴跷], thoroughfare [chong], governing [du], allowance [ren], and the belt [*dai*, 带] vessels. Normally they are not constrained by the twelve main distribution vessels. Therefore, they are called the eight singular distribution vessels... When the Sage drew up the design for the main irrigation ditches and canals to facilitate the passage of water and prepare for emergencies in case of heavy rains, he had no choice but to design the singular vessels to accommodate the extra amount of water which might overflow from the regular vessels. This is why the eight singular vessels are not restricted to the main distribution vessels in the body.

Much the same idea is presented in the *Nanjing* (*Difficulty 28: The Eight Singular Distribution Vessels*), along with a description of singular vessel pathways:

> By analogy, the eight singular vessels are like a plan drawn up by the Sage of irrigation ditches and canals. When these irrigation ditches and canals are filled to overflow capacity, they pour into deep lakes. Therefore, using the Sage's analogy, when there is an inability to constrain the distribution of blood and vital substances, the vessels in the human body will swell and bulge to excess. Blood then flows into the eight singular vessels so as not to circulate throughout the periphery and therefore relieve the twelve main distribution vessels when they cannot constrain the flow.

Deep Singular Vessels

The three deep singular vessels consist of the thoroughfare (chong aorta), the allowance (ren), and the governing (du) vessels. The internal pathways of the chong vessel and the ren vessel both originate in the uterus (uterine artery and vein, respectively) and travel up alongside the spine (aorta and vena cava, respectively). The thoroughfare (chong aorta) and allowance (ren) vessels connect directly to the left ventricle and right atrium of the heart, respectively. The thoroughfare vessel is the aorta, and the allowance is the vena cava. The governing vessel is represented by the paired azygos and hemiazygos and the ascending lumbar veins (Figure 10.1).

All three of the deep singular vessels have related superficial vessel pathways that give rise to associated nodes. The nodal pathways of the allowance (ren) and governing (du) vessels traverse the anterior and posterior centerlines of the head and trunk (Chapter 11), and represent a total of fifty-one nodal site locations. The thoroughfare (chong aorta) has superficial collateral vessels (arteries) and related nodes as well, located on the lower abdomen. These nodal locations are shared with a portion of the kidney (vein) superficial distribution vessel. These nodes have their own unique indications and functions.

Since the thoroughfare vessel directs blood oxygenated by inhaled vital air from the left ventricle of the heart to all the arterial distribution vessels, which return as venous blood, the thoroughfare vessel is called the "sea of the twelve vessels." The thoroughfare vessel (chong aorta) regulates the flow of blood and vital substances to the twelve main *zangfu* (脏腑)

distribution vessels. The allowance (ren) vessel (vena cava) controls the internal vessels. The thoroughfare and allowance vessels also distribute to the face, where they coincide with parts of the main distribution vessel pathways. A description of the internal and superficial vessel pathways, including those to the lips and mouth, is included in *NJLS 65* (*Five Sounds and Five Flavors*):

> The thoroughfare vessel [chong aorta] and the allowance [ren] vessel both originate from the uterus [uterine arteries and veins] and travel up alongside the spine [aorta and vena cava], and are the sea of the distribution and collateral vessels. Their superficial branches travel upward along the abdominal region and both pathways meet at the throat [carotid artery and jugular vein, respectively]. Separate collateral branches then distribute to the lips and mouth [superior and inferior labial arteries and veins].

Thoroughfare Distribution Vessel

The thoroughfare distribution vessel (chong aorta)[2] functions as the thoroughfare of blood, nutrients, defensive substances, organ vitality substances, and vital air. This vessel is characterized by always having a pulse beat. The thoroughfare vessel has an important communication node in the upper region at Dazhu (BL 11), and in the lower regions at the upper and lower Juxu nodes (Shangjuxu, ST 37 and Xiajuxu, ST 39). Because the thoroughfare vessel (and stomach distribution vessel) includes the superior and inferior labial arteries, it communicates with the sites Renzhong (DU 26, also known as Shuigou) and Chengjiang (RN 24). The thoroughfare vessel also communicates with Huiyin (RN 1). The thoroughfare vessel regulates the spleen distribution vessel, and its master nodal site (Gongsun, SP 4) is on that distribution vessel (Table 9.3). The thoroughfare vessel is coupled with the medial holding (yinwei) vessel, which regulates the pericardium distribution vessel. Its couple node is Neiguan (PC 6). One description of the thoroughfare vessel is provided in the *Nanjing* (*Difficulty 28*):

> The thoroughfare vessel [chong aorta] arises at Qichong [ST 30] where it merges with the stomach–foot *yangming* [阳明] distribution vessel. It travels upward along each side of the navel to reach the thorax where it disperses.

The superficial pathway of the thoroughfare vessel, where it shares nodal sites with the kidney distribution vessel, is also described in *NJSW 60* (*Bone Cavities*):

> The thoroughfare superficial vessel starts at the vital substance street [Qichong, ST 30], where it travels with the superficial *shaoyin* [少阴] kidney vessel. From here [Qichong, ST 30] it distributes up along each side of the umbilicus to the thorax where it disperses.

Distribution through the thoroughfare vessel to the lower extremities is described by Qibo in *NJLS 62* (*Pulsating Transport*), cited in Chapter 10. Here, the pulse beat of the posterior tibial artery (a branch of the thoroughfare vessel) is detected below and posterior to the medial anklebone. Since this location is near kidney distribution vessels nodal sites, some considered the kidney vessel to be an artery instead of a vein. The *NJLS 38* (*Upstream and Downstream Flow in Treating Fat and Thin People*) resolves this issue where the Yellow Emperor asks:

> The shaoyin [kidney] vessels only circulate [flow] downward, what about that?
>
> Qibo replies: That's not true. The thoroughfare vessel [chong aorta] is the sea of the five viscera and the six bowels, and they all receive nourishment from here. It [thoroughfare

> vessel] travels upward [carotid artery] and moves outward to distribute to the forehead, where it nourishes all the yang vessels and irrigates [supplies] all refined substances. The thoroughfare vessel also travels downward where it pours into the shaoyin [kidney] major collateral [renal artery], exits at the vital substance street [Qichong, ST 30] [external iliac artery], follows along the medial aspect of the thigh and enters the popliteal fossa at a slant, and goes down to circulate along the tibia [posterior tibial artery] down to below the medial malleolus where it divides; it then moves down to travel with the shaoyin vessel [kidney] and nourishes [supplies] the three yin vessels [kidney, spleen, and liver distribution veins].

Reference to the thoroughfare vessel supplying the yang vessels of the head and neck involves the three arterial routes of the stomach, gallbladder, and bladder distribution vessels. The thoroughfare vessel also supplies the stomach distribution vessels of the legs, which in turn supply the muscles. This information, along with other vascular details, is presented in *NJSW 44* (*Paralysis*):

> The yangming [stomach] vessel is the sea of the five viscera [*zang*, 藏] and the six bowels [*fu*, 府]. It is responsible for lubricating the ancestral muscle, and the ancestral muscle is responsible for binding the bones and muscles of the lumbar region. The thoroughfare vessel [chong aorta] is the sea of the main distribution vessels, responsible for irrigating the streams and valleys [referring to the skeletal muscles], and it joins the yangming [stomach] vessel at the ancestral muscle [meeting of external iliac and inferior epigastric arteries]. The yin and yang vessels meet to empty the ancestral muscle. Their meeting is at the vital substance street [external iliac artery and vein], and the yangming [stomach] vessel is the chief of the vital substance street [Qichong, ST 30]. All these vessels depend upon the belt [dai] vessels [subcostal veins], which are collateral branches of the governing [du] vessel. Therefore, when the yangming [stomach] vessel is in deficiency the ancestral muscle will be relaxed. The belt [dai] vessels will not pull the other vessels together, and therefore, the person will suffer paralysis of the legs and not be able to walk.

Allowance Vessel

The allowance (ren)[3] distribution vessel meets all the yin (inflowing) vessels and therefore is referred to as the "sea of yin." It bears the vital substances of the yin vessels, and the yin substance and function of the internal organs (zangfu). The allowance (ren) vessel regulates the lung distribution vessel with Lieque (LU 7) as a master node, and is coupled with the medial lifting (yinqiao) vessel, with Zhaohai (KD 6) as its couple node (Table 9.3). From the *Nanjing* (*Difficulty 28*), the allowance (ren) vessel starts at Zhongji (RN 3) and travels up below it through the pubic hair following along the interior aspect of the abdomen, up through the node Guanyuan (RN 4) and continuing upward until it reaches the throat. This pathway description is close to that noted in *NJSW 60*:

> The allowance [ren] vessel [vena cava] starts below the node Zhongji [RN 3] and travels up through the border of the pubic hair to follow along the interior aspect of the abdomen [medial branches of the superior and inferior epigastric veins], past Guanyuan [RN 4] and up to the throat. It then continues up the cheek, following along the face, to enter the eyes [Chengqi, ST 1].

Additional information on the allowance (ren) vessel is provided in *NJLS 2 (Origin of Communication Sites)*, where Qibo describes the major veins draining the head, face, and brain as secondary branches of the superior vena cava. Three major venous branches of the superior vena cava include the internal jugular vein that drains the brain and portions of the face, the vertebral veins (including the ascending and deep cervical vein branches), which drain the brain and neck, and the external jugular vein, which drains the head and face. Seven secondary branching pathways involving these three vessels are discussed. Each secondary branch is assigned either to a particular main distribution vessel or a related arterial counterpart, and has an associated communication (shu) node as follows:

> The allowance [ren] vessel [vena cava] travels between the centers of the supraclavicular fossi where the node Tiantu [RN 22] is located. The first of the secondary branches [internal jugular vein] of the allowance [ren] vessel travels beside the external carotid artery that belongs to the stomach–foot yangming distribution vessel where the node Renying [ST 9] is located. The second secondary branch [internal jugular, facial, inferior alveolar, superior labial, and superior labial veins] of the allowance [ren] vessel belongs to the large intestine–hand yangming distribution vessel, where the node Futu [LI 18] is located. The third secondary branch [external jugular, retromandibular, and middle temporal vein] of the allowance [ren] vessel corresponds with the small intestine–hand *taiyang* (太阳) distribution vessel, where the node Tianchuang [SI 16] is located. The fourth secondary branch [external jugular, retromandibular, and superficial temporal veins] of the allowance [ren] vessel travels with the gallbladder–foot *shaoyang* (少阳) distribution vessel, where the node called Tianrong [SI 17] is located. The fifth secondary branch [external jugular and posterior auricular veins] of the allowance [ren] vessel corresponds with the internal membrane [*sanjiao*, 三焦]–hand shaoyang distribution vessel, where the node Tianyou [SJ 16] is located. The sixth secondary branch [external jugular and occipital vein] of the allowance [ren] vessel travels with the urinary bladder–foot taiyang distribution vessel, where the node Tianzhu [BL 10] is located. The seventh secondary branch [vertebral vein] of the allowance [ren] vessel is the vessel located in the middle of the neck, and corresponds with the governing [du] vessel, where the node Fengfu [DU 16] is located.

Another portion of the allowance (ren) vessel is noted in *NJLS 69 (Loss of Voice due to Grief and Rage)*, where Qibo describes treating loss of voice:

> The kidney–foot shaoyin distribution vessel has fine branches above that supply the tongue, which are collaterals from the region of the hyoid bone, and terminate in the epiglottis. The blood vessels on both sides can be drained off [reduced] to eliminate the turbid condition. The vessels that meet at the epiglottis are upper branches of the allowance [ren] vessel. Select the node Tiantu [RN 22] to restore the condition of the epiglottis [restore voice function, since the epiglottis is door of the voice].

Governing Vessel

The superficial pathway of the governing (du)[4] vessel starts below the coccyx and runs up the posterior midline of the body, traversing over the head to terminate at the upper lip and gums. The deep pathway is given in the *Nanjing (Difficulty 28)*:

> The governing [du] distribution vessel begins in front of the lowest part of the perineum, and from this area travels side-by-side up the interior part of the back [azygos and hemiazygos, and the ascending lumbar veins] to enter the node Fengfu [DU 16], where it connects with the brain.

The governing (du) vessel meets all the yang (superficial back) vessels at Dazhui (DU 14) and is therefore referred to as the "sea of yang." It functions to govern the vital substances of the yang vessels and the yang function of the internal organs (zangfu). It regulates the small intestine distribution vessel with Houxi (SI 3) as a master node (Table 9.3). Shenmai (BL 62) is the couple node for the lateral lifting (yangqiao) vessel and the governing (du) vessel.

Superficial Singular Vessels

Superficial singular vessels consist of four pairs of longitudinal venous network routes (yinqiao, yangqiao, yinwei, and yangwei), plus one additional set of vessels (*daimai*, 带脉 or belt vessel) that distribute from each side of the back around to the abdomen. These venous pathways do not include those assigned to the paired distribution arteries and veins related to the internal organs—these matched organ pairs only account for six of the main distribution veins. Consequently, the remaining superficial veins are classified as singular vessels. For the most part, the four longitudinal pairs flow lengthwise along the body forming complex networks, which is typical of the superficial veins. The Chinese named these vessels for their numerous interconnections in draining the superficial regions, but the English translations for these terms fail to convey an equivalent understanding. Unlike the twelve organ-related main distribution vessels, these five superficial singular vessels do not give rise to nodes (acupoints). However, nodes related to other vessels are found along their pathways. The superficial singular vessels are considered similar in nature to the main distribution (jing) vessels, and are not considered to be collateral (luo) vessels, noted in *NJLS 17* where the Yellow Emperor asks:

> The lifting [*qiao*, 蹻] vessel is designated as both yin and yang, which vessel belongs to the correct category?
>
> Qibo answers: In males the lifting [qiao] vessel belongs to yang, in females it belongs to yin. This category correctly applies to the distribution vessels, but does not correctly apply to the collateral [luo] vessels.

Belt Vessel

The pathway of the belt (dai) vessels is noted in the *Nanjing* (*Difficulty 28*):

> The belt [dai] vessel starts at the last rib and circles once [right and left subcostal veins] around the circumference of the body. The belt [dai] vessel branches from the governing [du] vessel [ascending lumbar veins] at the level of the second lumbar vertebra. It goes around the waist and functions to bind all the other vessel together.

The belt vessel regulates the gallbladder distribution vessel, with corresponding superficial communication nodes located on the gallbladder distribution vessel, including Daimai (GB 26), Wushu (GB 27), and Weidao (GB 28). The master node of the belt vessel is Zulinqi (GB 41), with Waiguan (SJ 5) as its couple location (Table 9.3).

Medial Lifting Vessel
The pathway of the medial lifting (yinqiao)[5] vessel is provided in the *Nanjing* (*Difficulty 28*):

> The medial lifting [yinqiao] vessel also starts at the heel and follows along the medial malleolus, travels up to the throat, where it crosses the thoroughfare vessel [chong aorta], and is then linked with the thoroughfare vessel.

The medial lifting (yinqiao) vessel regulates the kidney distribution vessel, and its master node is Zhaohai (KD 6), with Lieque (LU 7) as its couple node (Table 9.3). A detailed description of the medial lifting (yinqiao) vessel superficial pathway is given in *NJLS 17*, where the Yellow Emperor asks:

> What is the origin of the medial lifting [yinqiao] vessel and where does it terminate? What is its vital substance flow vessel?
>
> Qibo answers: The medial lifting [yinqiao] vessel is another vessel of the kidney–shaoyin vessel and it starts behind Rangu [KD 2, navicular prominence] to travel in front of the medial malleolus, continuing in a straight upward path along the medial aspect of the thigh to enter the inguinal region, and then up to the chest to enter the supraclavicular fossa [Quepen, ST 12]. From here it travels up to and in front of Renying [ST 9], entering the cheekbone and then joining the eye at the inner canthus [Jingming, BL 1]. Here it joins the bladder–taiyang vessel and the lateral lifting [yangqiao] vessel, and travels with the lateral lifting vessel in the upper regions [of the head], where their vital substances merge with each other and normally moisten the eyes. When vital substances are deficient in the medial and lateral lifting vessels, the eyes cannot close.

Lateral Lifting Vessel
The pathway of the lateral lifting (yangqiao) vessel is given in the *Nanjing* (*Difficulty 28*):

> The lateral lifting [yangqiao] vessel starts at the heel and follows along the lateral malleolus to travel upward to enter Fengchi [GB 20].

The lateral lifting (yangqiao) vessel regulates the bladder distribution vessel with Shenmai (BL 62) as its master node, and Houxi (SI 3) as its couple node (Table 9.3).

Medial Holding Vessel
The lateral holding (yangwei) and medial holding (yinwei)[6] vessels are described in the *Nanjing* (*Difficulty 28*):

> The lateral holding [yangwei] and medial holding [yinwei] vessels tie collateral vessels together [venous networks] to handle overflow of blood and vital substances. These vessels are stimulated to drain off the excess from all the main distribution vessels. The medial holding vessel begins where all the medial [yin] vessels of the leg cross.

The medial holding (yinwei) vessel regulates the pericardium distribution vessel with Neiguan (PC 6) as its master node, and is coupled with the spleen distribution vessel with Gongsun (SP 4) as its couple node (Table 9.3).

Lateral Holding Vessel
The lateral holding (yangwei) distribution vessel starts where all the lateral [yang] vessels of the leg meet (*Nanjing, Difficulty 28*). The lateral holding (yangwei) vessel regulates the

internal membrane (sanjiao) vessel with Waiguan (SJ 5) as its master node, and is coupled with the gallbladder vessel with Zulinqi (GB 41) as its couple node (Table 9.3).

Disease Manifestations of the Eight Singular Vessels

The eight singular distribution vessels function to strengthen the relationship between the twelve main distribution vessels, and regulate their vital substances and blood. They are closely related to the liver and kidneys, as well as the extraordinary organs such as the uterus, brain, and spinal cord. Pathological indications for the eight singular distribution vessels are based on their physiological functions and the areas they traverse (Table 9.2). These are derived from specific references in the *Neijing* and the *Nanjing*.

Communication Vessels: Shumai

Shumai can be translated as "communication" or "transportation" vessels. They serve as the transitional structures from the large deep singular vessels to the distribution vessels (jingmai) of the extremities, head, face, neck, and trunk. In terms of arterial flow they consist of the brachiocephalic artery and then the subclavian artery in the upper trunk, and the external iliac artery and then the femoral artery in the lower trunk. These arterial communication vessels are extensions of the aorta (chong) and serve to direct circulation out of the body core. For venous return circulation to the body core, the communication vessels are transitions between the distribution vessels and the vena cava (ren), and consist of the subclavian vein and then the brachiocephalic vein in the upper region, and the femoral vein and then the external iliac vein in the lower region of the trunk. Communication vessels also supply other important vessels to the head, brain, and trunk that are part of the distribution pathways. For outward flow, these include the common carotid, vertebral, internal thoracic, and inferior epigastric arteries. For return flow they consist of the jugular, vertebral, internal thoracic, and inferior epigastric veins. The jugulars, vertebral veins, and other major veins of the neck are also referred to as secondary vessels of the vena cava. In addition, the intercostal arteries and veins are sometimes referred to as communication vessels.

Main Distribution Vessels: Jingmai

Longitudinal vessels distributing to the extremities, head, face, and trunk derive from the communication or transportation vessels (shumai). A central feature of the distribution vessels concerns their unique pathways, their relationship to internal organs, and the fact that these vessels give rise to most nodal sites (see Chapter 11 for a detailed description of the twelve main distribution vessels and their nodal pathways). The role of the distribution vessels is to supply blood, nutrients, defensive substances, refined substances of vitality, and vital air to all parts of the body, while providing collateral vessels to form nodal sites along their superficial courses. These arteries and return veins are identifiable, and the pathways of some of the veins are visible. Collateral vessels, such as the veins on the back of the hand, are visible. The *NJLS 10* (*Distribution Vessels*) discusses the visibility of the vessels, as follows:

> The twelve distribution vessels are hidden to circulate within the striated muscles, and since they are deeper vessels they are not visible to the naked eye. The only possible exception to this is the spleen–foot *taiyin* (太阴) distribution vessel, which travels above the lateral malleolus and has no place to hide. All the vessels that are often visible to the eye are superficial, and they are all collateral [luo] vessels. Of the six distribution vessels and collaterals of the hand, the large intestine [yangming], internal membrane [sanjiao], and small intestine [shaoyang] are the largest [and most visible] collateral vessels. They arise in the region between the five fingers, and also meet each other in the center of the elbow.

Some of the distribution vessels travel over portions of the body trunk. The three yang distribution vessels of the feet (stomach, gallbladder, and urinary bladder) travel from the face, cross the entire trunk, and then course down the legs to terminate in the toes. In the head region these vessels are supplied by branches from the thoroughfare vessel (chong aorta). In the leg region they are supplied by communication branches (shumai) of the aorta. On the body trunk the yang vessels of the feet are supplied by the superficial vessels of the trunk. Superficial trunk vessels of the stomach and gallbladder distribution vessels are supplied by branches with either the aorta or communication vessels (shumai) in both the upper and lower part of the trunk. Superficial trunk vessels for the bladder distribution vessel are supplied by the aorta by means of intercostal arteries. The trunk portion of the distribution vessels supplies collateral vessels that penetrate the muscle fascia where arteries, veins, and nerves are distributed to the superficial regions. Many of the nodes on the trunk of the body are located at these sites.

Confluence of the Main Distribution Vessels

Early teachers and practitioners of Chinese medicine were challenged by the task of explaining the complete circulatory system involving distribution vessels with related collateral vessels that supply critical nodes along specific anatomical regions, and the internal vascular routes. Examination of the superficial nodal pathways on the body, as depicted on acupuncture charts, gives little idea of the internal vascular routes. Nodal sites of arterial and venous matched yin-yang distribution vessels lie in close proximity to their respective main vessels in the extremities. Above the knee or elbow the distribution vessels start to diverge from their superficial nodal pathways. Eventually, the vessels connect to the internal organs, and later along the vessel routes the yin-yang matched arteries and veins converge at other appropriate anatomical sites. These superficial and deep relationships are discussed in terms of "parting and gathering," referred to as the six confluences of the yin-yang matched distribution vessel pairs in *NJLS 11* (*Parting of Distribution Vessels*), where the Yellow Emperor asks:

> The twelve distribution vessels are not only involved in life and birth for a person, and the attack of disease, but also in the treatment and cause of human disease. This must be studied by the beginner practitioner and mastered by the skilled physicians. Only a negligent or unskilled practitioner would consider this topic to be easy. A highly skilled practitioner will appreciate the difficulties involved. Can you please explain how the twelve distribution vessels part and gather, and describe their exiting and entering locations?

Qibo bows his head again in great respect and replies: These are indeed bright questions. These are the same questions that are ignored by negligent practitioners, but are the ones considered by skilled physicians. Please let me explain:

First Confluence

The bladder–foot taiyang distribution vessel parts from its main pathway at the popliteal fossa. It then travels as a single pathway to 5 *cun* [寸] [1 cun, or Chinese inch, is equal to 0.902 inches or 2.30 centimeters] below the buttocks and branches into the anus [internal pudendal arteries]; it then joins the urinary bladder [superior and inferior vesicle arteries] and disperses into the kidneys [renal arteries]. It follows along the spine [aorta] to disperse into the heart, and in a straight path continues upward to the spine to reach the nape of the neck [vertebral arteries] where it rejoins its main [superficial] pathway. This is the first distribution vessel.

The kidney–foot shaoyin distribution vessel parts from its regular pathway at the popliteal fossa where it [internal pudendal veins, vesicle veins] travels along with the bladder-taiyang vessel. It travels up [inferior vena cava] to the kidneys [renal veins] at the fourteenth vertebra [L2] where it crosses the belt vessel [subcostal vein]. It travels straight up [superior vena cava and internal jugular vein] to the root of the tongue [lingual vein], and turns back to the nape of the neck [vertebral veins] to join the bladder-taiyang vessel. This is the first gathering [confluence] between the six yin and six yang distribution vessels. The parting [vessel] pathways to the various internal organs serve each main distribution vessel superficial and peripheral course.

Second Confluence

The gallbladder–foot shaoyang distribution vessel main pathway travels to the buttocks where it winds around to enter the border of the pubic hair [external pudendal arteries, dorsal arteries of penis] where it joins the liver-*jueyin* [厥阴] vessel [external pudendal veins, dorsal vein of penis]. From here it separates from its regular pathway to enter among the lower ribs [abdominal aorta], following up the hypochondriac region to join the gallbladder [cystic artery] and disperse up into the liver [hepatic arteries], following in a continuous line to the heart [aorta]. It continues upward following the esophagus and exiting at the lower jawbone, dispersing in the face and then relating to the eye connections [optic nerve and related blood vessels]. It rejoins the gallbladder-shaoyang vessel at the outer canthus of the eye.

The liver–foot jueyin distribution vessel separates from its main pathway at the dorsum of the foot, traveling upward to the border of the pubic hair [external pudendal veins, dorsal vein of penis]. Here it joins the gallbladder-shaoyang vessel and travels along its route [cystic vein, hepatic veins, superior vena cava]. This is the second confluence.

Third Confluence

The stomach–foot yangming distribution vessel travels up to the thigh [femoral and iliac arteries] to enter the abdominal cavity [abdominal aorta], there joining the stomach [gastric artery] and dispersing to the spleen [splenic artery]. Then it travels up to the heart [aorta] and following along the esophagus [throat] [external carotid artery] it reaches the mouth [facial artery, superior and inferior labial arteries]. It continues to travel upward beside the nose [dorsal nasal artery] and infraorbital bone [zygomaticoorbital artery] to make connection with the eye [angular artery], and then rejoins the yangming distribution vessel.

The spleen–foot taiyin distribution vessel travels up to the thigh [external iliac] to join the yangming [stomach] vessel, and it separates [from its superficial route] to follow completely along the course of the stomach vessel [inferior vena cava, and gastric, splenic, and portal veins]. It continues to travel upward [superior vena cava] to join at the throat [external jugular and superior thyroid veins], linking together with the tongue [hypoglossal and sublingual veins]. This is the third confluence between the yin and yang distribution vessels.

Fourth Confluence

The small intestine–hand taiyang distribution vessel starts at the small finger and branches at the division of the shoulder [shoulder joint], entering the axilla [axillary vein] and traveling to the heart [subclavian vein, superior vena cava, and coronary veins], and making connections with the small intestines [vena cava, portal vein, and inferior and superior mesenteric veins supplying the small intestines].

The heart–hand shaoyin distribution vessel branches at the axilla [axillary artery] between the two muscles. It joins the heart [brachiocephalic, subclavian, aorta, and coronary arteries] and then travels upward to the larynx [internal carotid artery], stemming from the face to join the eye [anterior cerebral and ophthalmic arteries, and then the ethmoidal, supraorbital, and lacrimal arteries] at the inner canthus. This is the fourth confluence of yin and yang distribution vessels.

Fifth Confluence

The internal membrane–hand shaoyang distribution vessel, deriving from the fourth finger, parts from its regular pathway at the shoulder to enter the supraclavicular fossa [subclavian vein]. It descends [vena cava and pericardiacophrenic veins] to travel to the internal membrane system [sanjiao], dispersing in the thorax region.

The heart protector [pericardium] distribution vessel parts from its main pathway 3 cun below the axilla [Yuanye, GB 22] [lateral thoracic artery] and enters the thorax region [subclavian artery, aorta, and pericardiacophrenic arteries], and then divides to join the internal membrane system [sanjiao]. It then travels up along the larynx to the throat [external carotid artery], reaching behind the ear [posterior auricular artery] to join with the internal membrane distribution vessel [posterior auricular vein] at the mastoid process [Wangu, GB 12]. This is the fifth confluence.

Sixth Confluence

The large intestine–hand yangming distribution vessel travels from the hand [cephalic vein] to the breast region [subclavian vein], and parts from this pathway at the top of the shoulder [transverse cervical vein] at Jianyu [LI 15] to reach the vertebrae [superficial cervical vein]. Below [vena cava, portal vein], it travels to the large intestine [inferior and superior mesenteric veins]. It makes connections with the lungs [bronchial veins], traveling up along the larynx and throat to reach the supraclavicular fossa [subclavian vein], where it joins the regular large intestine–hand yangming distribution vessel.

The lung–hand taiyin distribution vessel parts from its main pathway [radial artery] at the axilla [axillary artery], anterior to the heart–hand shaoyin distribution vessel, and travels to the lungs [aorta, bronchial arteries], and then disperses in the large intestine [aorta, inferior and superior mesenteric arteries]. Above, it reaches the supraclavicular fossa [subclavian artery] traveling along the larynx and throat, converging with the hand yangming vessels. This is the sixth confluence of the yin and yang distribution vessels.

Collateral Vessels: Luomai

Longitudinal distribution vessels form many collateral branches in order to serve all areas of the body. Collateral vessels branch further into fine vessels (sunmai) to directly communicate with body tissues, organs, and the superficial body regions. Collateral vessels also supply each nodal site (acupoint), as well as other areas of the body. Important collateral vessels occur between major distribution vessel arteries and veins in the distal and peripheral regions. In each of these pairings, if the visceral vessel is an artery, its matching bowel vessel is the vein related to the area, and vice versa. These comprise twelve major internal organ–external body related collateral (luo) vessels and one major spleen collateral on each side of the body. In addition, the allowance (ren) and governing (du) vessels have collateral vessels, resulting in a total of twenty-eight of these vessels (Table 9.1).

The internal-external related collateral vessels have symptomatic indications (Table 9.4). Furthermore, special nodes exist on the distribution vessel pathways that are called source (yuan) and collateral (luo) locations (Table 9.5). These sites are used to adjust blood flow between vessels of matched internal organ (zangfu) pairs. Internal-external related collateral vessels are described in *NJLS 10*, as follows:

Lungs and Large Intestine Collateral Vessels

The collateral of the lung–hand taiyin vessel branches from its distribution vessel [radial artery] at the region called Lieque [LU 7]. It arises above the wrist crease within the muscles and travels side-by-side with a straight branch of the distribution vessel to enter the palm of the hand [deep palmar arch]. It also disperses or spreads along the border of the thenar eminence [superficial palmar branch of radial artery and palmar digital arteries]... Another collateral branch of the lung vessel [proper palmar digital arteries] travels to meet the large intestine–hand yangming distribution vessel.

The collateral of the large intestine–hand yangming vessel branches from its distribution vessel [cephalic vein] at the region called Pianli [LI 6], which is located 3 cun above the wrist crease. From here it [digital veins of thumb and index finger] reaches the lung–hand taiyin distribution vessel. Another collateral branch travels up along the arm, ascending the shoulder at Jianyu [LI 15] [transverse cervical vein] and above this [subclavian and external jugular veins] it bends at the cheek [facial vein] to travel at a slant to the teeth [superior and inferior labial veins]. Another branch [retromandibular vein] enters the ear and joins with the prime artery [superficial temporal artery].

Stomach and Spleen Collateral Vessels

The collateral of the stomach–foot yangming vessel branches from its distribution vessel at the node called Fenglong [ST 40], located 8 cun above the ankle. This branch travels

Table 9.4 Indications for the fifteen collateral (*luo*) vessels.

Collateral	*Condition*	*Indications*	*Nodes*
Lung	Solid Hollow	Heat sensation in wrist and palm. Shortness of breath, enuresis, frequent urination.	Lieque (LU 7)
Heart	Solid Hollow	Chest and diaphragm fullness. Loss of speech (aphasia).	Tongli (HT 5)
Pericardium	Solid Hollow	Cardiac pain. Irritability and mental vexations.	Neiguan (PC 6)
Large Intestine	Solid Hollow	Toothache, deafness. Coldness in teeth, blockage of the ear diaphragm.	Pianli (LI 6)
Small Intestine	Solid Hollow	Joint weakness, atrophy and motor impairment of the elbow. Scabs, scabies, or warts on skin.	Zhizheng (SI 7)
Internal Membrane	Solid Hollow	Spasms and contractions of elbow. Dysfunction of elbow joint.	Waiguan (SJ 5)
Stomach	Inverse Solid Hollow	Blockage of larynx, fatigue, and dumbness. Madness. Foot dysfunction, withering of tibia.	Fenglong (ST 40)
Bladder	Solid Hollow	Allergic rhinitis, blocked stuffy nose, headache, and back pain. Allergic rhinitis with nosebleed.	Feiyang (BL 58)
Gallbladder	Solid Hollow	Cold feet. Allergic rhinitis and nosebleed.	Guangming (GB 37)
Spleen	Inverse Solid Hollow	Acute gastroenteritis or cholera. Cutting intestinal pain. Abdominal swelling and distension.	Gongsun (SP 4)
Kidney	Inverse Solid Hollow	Irritability and unhappiness. Difficult urination and retention of urine. Low back pain.	Dazhong (KD 4)
Liver	Inverse Solid Hollow	Swelling of testicles and unexpected acute disease of external genitalia, testis, and scrotum. Abnormal erection (priapism). Itching in region of genitalia	Ligou (LV 5)
Great Spleen	Solid Hollow	Pain through extent of body Weak/loosened joints throughout extent of body.	Dabao (SP 21)
Allowance (*Ren*)	Solid Hollow	Pain in skin over abdomen. Itching and scratching in abdominal region.	Jiuwei (RN 15)
Governing (*Du*)	Solid Hollow	Spinal stiffness. Heavy sensation of head.	Changqiang (DU 1)

Table 9.5 Collateral, source, and accumulation nodes for the *zangfu* main distribution vessels and singular vessels.

	Collateral (Luo)	*Source* (Yuan)	*Accumulation* (Xi)
Vessel			
Lung	Lieque (LU 7)	Taiyuan (LU 9)	Kongzui (LU 6)
Large Intestine	Pianli (LI 6)	Hegu (LI 4)	Wenliu (LI 7)
Stomach	Fenglong (ST 40)	Chongyang (ST 42)	Liangqiu (ST 34)
Spleen	Gongsun (SP 4)	Taibai (SP 3)	Diji (SP 8)
Heart	Tongli (HT 5)	Shenmen (HT 7)	Yinxi (HT 6)
Small Intestine	Zhizheng (SI 7)	Wangu (SI 4)	Yanglao (SI 6)
Bladder	Feiyang (BL 58)	Jinggu (BL 64)	Jinmen (BL 63)
Kidney	Dazhong (KD 4)	Taixi (KD 3)	Shuiquan (KD 5)
Pericardium	Neiguan (PC 6)	Daling (PC 7)	Ximen (PC 4)
Internal Membrane	Waiguan (SJ 5)	Yangchi (SJ 4)	Huizong (SJ 7)
Gallbladder	Guangming (GB 37)	Qiuxu (GB 40)	Waiqiu (GB 36)
Liver	Ligou (LV 5)	Taichong (LV 3)	Zhongdu (LV 6)
Great Spleen	Dabao (SP 21)		
Singular Vessels			
Allowance	Jiuwei (RN 15)		
Governing	Changqiang (DU 1)		
Lateral Lifting			Fuyang (BL 59)
Medial Lifting			Jiaoxin (KD 8)
Lateral Holding			Yangqiao (GB 35)
Medial Holding			Zhubin (KD 9)

to the taiyin [spleen] vessel. It travels down along the outer aspect of the tibia. In the upper regions of the body there are collateral branches to the head and nape of the neck where they join all the distribution vessels in respect to vital substance circulation. Below this area collateral branches distribute to the larynx and throat.

The collateral of the spleen–foot taiyin vessel branches from its distribution vessel at the region called Gongsun [SP 4], which is located 1 cun behind the first metatarsophalangeal joint. This branch travels down to the yangming [stomach] distribution vessel. Branches of this vessel also form collateral connections to the intestines and stomach. A disruption and inverse flow in the upper region [abdominal] will cause acute gastroenteritis or cholera.

Heart and Small Intestine Collateral Vessels

The collateral of the heart–hand shaoyin vessel branches from its distribution vessel at the region called Tongli [HT 5], which is located 1 cun above the wrist crease. Another branch travels upward to follow along with the distribution vessel to the heart, and also connects with the root of the tongue [lingual artery] and joins connections with the eye [internal carotid artery]... Another branch travels to the small intestine–hand taiyang vessel.

The collateral of the small intestine–hand taiyang vessel branches from its distribution vessel at the region called Zhizheng [SI 7], which is located 5 cun above the wrist crease. Internally it connects with the heart shaoyin vessel. Another branch travels up to the elbow and has a collateral branch to the shoulder at the extremity of the acromiun [Jianyu LI 15].

Bladder and Kidney Collateral Vessels

The collateral of the bladder–foot taiyang vessel branches from its distribution vessel at the region called Feiyang [BL 58], located 7 cun above the ankle [lateral malleolus]. This branch travels to the kidney–foot shaoyin distribution vessel.

The collateral of the kidney–foot shaoyin vessel branches from its distribution vessel at the region called Dazhong [KD 4]. From here it passes behind the medial malleolus, and winds around the heel. One branch travels to the bladder distribution vessel; one branch merges with its regular distribution vessel to travel upward to below the level of the pericardium, where it is linked externally with the lumbar spine.

Pericardium and Internal Membrane Collateral Vessels

The collateral of the pericardium–hand jueyin vessel branches from its distribution vessel at the region called Neiguan [PC 6], which is located 2 cun above the wrist crease. It disperses between the two tendons [flexor carpi radialis tendon and palmaris longus tendon], and another branch travels to the internal membrane–hand shaoyang vessel. It also travels upward with the distribution vessel to join the external membrane of the heart [pericardiacophrenic arteries], and then makes connections with the heart.

The collateral of the internal membrane–hand shaoyang vessel branches from its distribution vessel at the region called Waiguan [SJ 5], which is located 2 cun above the wrist crease. It winds around the outer aspect of the arm and flows into the chest [pericardiacophrenic veins] to join the pericardium vessel.

Gallbladder and Liver Collateral Vessels

The collateral of the gallbladder–foot shaoyang vessel branches from its distribution vessel at the region called Guangming [GB 37], which is located 5 cun above the ankle [lateral malleolus]. This branch travels to the liver–foot jueyin vessel, with a collateral below to the instep of the foot.

The collateral of the liver–foot jueyin vessel branches from its distribution vessel at the region called Ligou [LV 5], which is located 5 cun above the medial malleolus. This branch travels to the gallbladder shaoyang vessel. A branch travels along the tibia upward to the testicles [external pudendal veins]; a collateral branch distributes to the penis [dorsal vein of penis].

Great Collateral of the Spleen Vessel

The great collateral [*daluo*, 大络] of the spleen–foot taiyin vessel branches from its distribution vessel at the region called Dabao [SP 21], which is located 3 cun below the axilla where it spreads across the upper part of the side of the thorax [thoracoepigastric vein].

Allowance Collateral Vessel

The collateral of the allowance [ren] vessel branches from its distribution vessel at the region called Weiyi [RN 15, now called Jiuwei], which is located below the xiphoid process [turtledove tail], where it disperses in the abdominal region.

Governing Collateral Vessel

The collateral of the governing [du] vessel branches from its distribution vessel at the region called Changqiang [DU 1], travels up each side of the backbone [azygos, hemiazygos, and ascending lumbar veins] to the nape of the neck, where it disperses over the top of the head. Below this region it sends branches to the left and right sides of the scapula. It also branches to the bladder–taiyang vessel, entering the vertebral foramen [vertebral veins].

Fine Vessels: Sunmai

The fine branches of the collateral vessels directly serve all body tissues. They represent arterioles, capillaries, and venules that provide a connection between arteries and veins (Figure 9.3). One of the more important roles of the fine vessels is their function in the superficial skin. Here, they have an important temperature control and defensive task. Sunmai are also found concentrated at nodal locations. Because of the extent of the fine vessels concentrated in the skin area, environmental exposure can impact the body via fine branching vessels, collaterals, and distribution vessels. Since these vessels communicate with the internal organs, superficial environmental influences can penetrate into deeper regions to cause illness (Chapter 13).

10
Blood Circulation

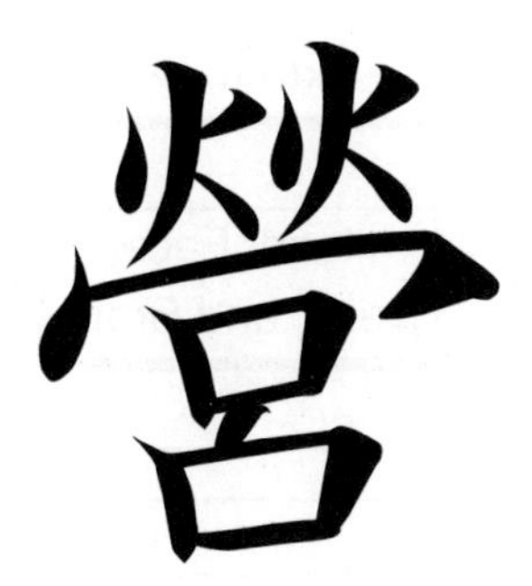

Ying: Nutrients

> [Absorbed water and nutrients] travel upward [via the venous system] to pour into the lung vessels, which are then transformed for the benefit of blood to serve life and the body. For this reason there is nothing more precious circulating in the distribution vessel tunnels than that which is called nutrients [ying].
>
> Qibo, *NJLS 18 (The Meeting and Interaction of Nutrients and Defensive Substances)*

In the Chinese view, the key relevance of the blood circulatory system is the continuous supply of nutrients (*ying*, 营), defensive substances (*wei*, 卫), organ vitality substances (*shenjing*, 神精), vital air (*qi*, 气), and fluids (*jinye*, 津液) to the superficial and internal body tissues. All regions need a constant distribution of these essential materials to maintain health, vigor, and life. Even a slight impairment in blood circulation, either in the arterial or venous flow, leads to dysfunction and pain. The heart provides the motive force for circulating blood through all the vessels in the body in an endless circuit. In addition to discovering blood circulation, the Chinese also determined that defensive substances (wei) can leave the arterial circulation to mount a defensive response. Products of this function are then reabsorbed back into the blood supply through what is now known as the lymphatic system. The description of these processes by the ancient Chinese was the first attempt to describe the immune and lymphatic systems. In the Chinese view, both nutrients and defensive substances make fifty circulation cycles daily through the linear pathway of the body vessels. One cycle is completed in 2 *ke* (刻),[1] where 1 ke is one-hundredth of a day (14.4 minutes), and 2 ke is 28.8 minutes. When viewed in its entirety, the Chinese model of the circulatory system (*jingluo*, 经络) is consistent with Western understanding (Figure 10.1).

The reason for viewing blood circulation through the linear pathway of the vessels is related to the Chinese emphasis on the outflowing arteries and returning venous supply in the yin-yang superficial body regions and assigned organ-related distribution vessel pairs (Table 4.3). Tracing a linear pathway to and from the extremities and internal regions to sequentially include all the distribution vessels results in a long, tortuous route. The 28.8 minutes calculated for such a long, looping circuit is probably just under double the true value—not unimpressive, especially considering the methodology employed and the period in history when this calculation was made. Despite evidence that the Chinese realized blood

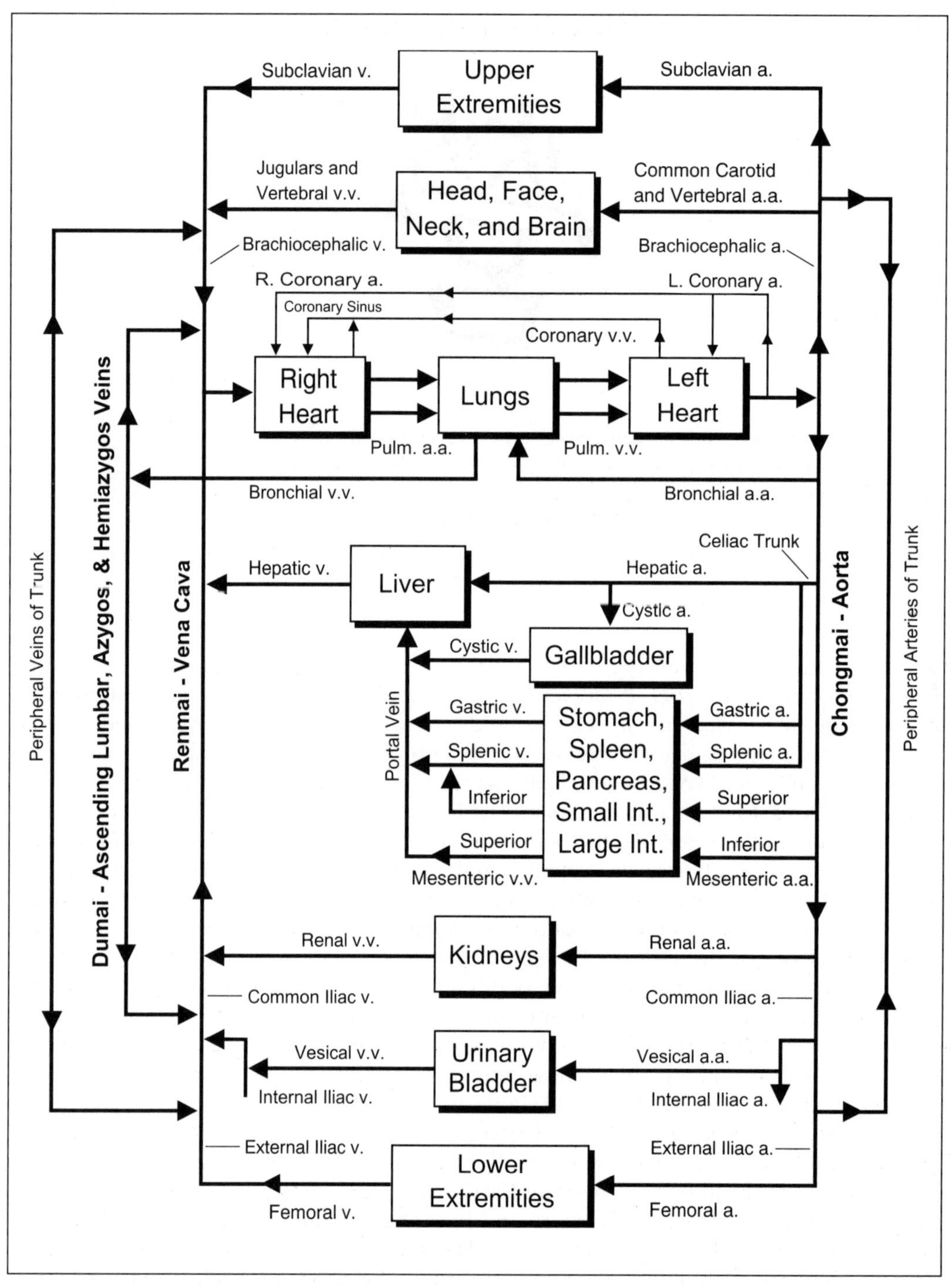

Figure 10.1 Schematic diagram of blood circulation through the body and internal organs, indicating deep relationship of the singular vessels (*chong*, *ren*, and *du*), and peripheral vessels of the trunk and extremities.

is simultaneously circulated out to all the main arteries and returned via the veins in a continuous fashion, no calculation of time for this simultaneous recirculation of total blood volume is given. Modern measurements indicate that in an average person it takes less than a minute to turn over the total volume of blood.

The detailed study, identification, and organization of all the main vessels (Chapters 9 and 11), in addition to their knowledge of the pulses being generated by the heart, demonstrates that the Chinese had an understanding of simultaneous circulation throughout the body. They identified the outward flow from the heart in the arteries, and the return flow to the heart in the veins. Further, they noted that the heartbeat is only detected in arteries because the pulse wave cannot transmit through the capillaries. A slight delay in the radial pulse, which is further from the heart compared to the carotid pulse, shows that the pulse is a wave phenomenon. The Chinese described the pulse characteristics as a wave crashing on a shore.

Role of the Heart in Circulation

Blood is oxygenated by vital air breathed into the lungs, and is then directed to the left side of the heart (Figure 10.1). From here, blood is forced into circulation by the contraction of the heart's left ventricle. This contraction results in the pulse beat, which is detected only in the arteries. Knowledge of these physiological processes led to a realization by the Chinese that all oxygenated blood, containing nutrients and defensive substances, comes directly from the lungs. From this the Chinese put the peripheral distribution vessels assigned to the lungs first in their linear circulation order. Although blood is simultaneously circulated through all the vessels, it was viewed in terms of circulation patterns consistent with the yin-yang divisions of the body supplied by the main organ-related distribution vessels. There is a close relationship between pulsation and respiration cycles of the lungs.

Heart Produces Pulse

The heart is the monarch from which vitality is derived (*NJSW 8*: *Canon of Precious Secrets*), and is considered master of all the viscera and bowels (*NJLS 29*: *Commentaries of the Masters*). The heart is in charge of blood circulation, while the lungs are in charge of inhaling vital air (*NJSW 10*: *Development of the Five Viscera*). The lungs are considered to be the prime minister with respect to the other organs. Further proof of the heart's role in circulating blood and nutrients is provided in *NJSW 21* (*Distribution Vessel Pulse Differentiation*). Here, a discussion on the effects of one's home life, emotions, and certain activities on the heart pulse leads to a general review of the circulation process. The role of the heart in providing the pulse function to circulate blood and nutrients is noted as follows:

> Refined substances from food broken down in the stomach are dispersed to the liver [via mesenteric and portal veins], from where the overflowing nutrients supply the muscles and tendons. Of the vital foods broken down in the stomach, the murky nutrients are returned to the heart [via deep lymphatic drainage into subclavian vein], which in turn overflows the refined substances into the pulse. The functional activity of the pulse circulates blood and nutrients through the distribution vessels.

Additional comments that confirm the understanding that the heart circulates blood are provided in *NJLS 54* (*Natural Life Span*). Here the discussion focuses on the normal decline in organ functional capability as a result of aging:

> At the age of sixty the functional capability of the heart declines, causing the circulation of blood and vital substances [nutrients, defensive materials, and vital air] to be slowed.

Chinese physicians of ancient times understood the close relationship between the heart and lungs. Oxygen demand has a direct influence on the heart rate. In a wide range of different situations, the heart normally beats four times during each complete breathing cycle (inhaling and exhaling). If this ratio either increases or decreases, it indicates an abnormal condition. Problems of the lungs or a decline in the functional capability of the lungs only affects the process of respiration. The main effect is on the intake and utilization of vital air containing oxygen, which has a direct impact on overall strength and vigor. The *NJLS 54* notes:

> At the age of eighty the lungs decline in function resulting in the loss of vigor, with the individual starting to make frequent errors in speech.[2]

The heart corresponds to the blood vessels (*NJLS 47*: *Root of the Viscera*), since they all emanate from and return to the heart. As a consequence, the heart is considered to be in tune with the vessels and the condition of the heart is reflected in the facial complexion (*NJSW 10*). This is due to the rich superficial blood supply to the face. Observation of facial coloration, such as pale white or blue, indicates possible problems with the heart and circulation.

Pulse Only Detected in Arteries

The recognition that the pulse is only observed in arteries confirms the role of the heart in blood circulation. Easily detected pulse beats are palpated on the radial and carotid arteries, and their individual condition and relative strength are used for diagnosis. The heartbeat is also detected in certain other regions of the legs and face (Table 10.1). One interesting discussion on blood circulation, including the role of the heart, is provided in *NJLS 62* (*Pulsating Transport*), where the Yellow Emperor asks:

> Of the twelve main distribution vessels, only the lung–hand *taiyin* (太阴), kidney–foot *shaoyin* (少阴), and the stomach–foot *yangming* (阳明) have areas that pulsate without ceasing, why is that?
>
> Qibo replies: It is understood that the stomach [role in fluid absorption and blood formation] is related to the pulse. The stomach is the sea of the five viscera and the six bowels, and its clear substances travel upward [in the vessels] to concentrate in the lungs. From there, lung vital substances [including oxygen from vital air] enter the lung taiyin vessel to circulate throughout the body. The coming and going of its circulation relies on respiration, so that each time a person exhales the pulse beats and then beats another time [two beats], on each inhalation the pulse beats and also repeats [two beats]. Since breathing continues without stop, the pulsation does not stop.
>
> The Yellow Emperor asks: The vital substances travel to the radial pulse location [Taiyuan, LU 9] in ten beats, where it discontinues [capillaries and venules] and bends around [large intestine vessel] to return in eight beats. What are the originating and return pathways? This is not fully understood.

Table 10.1 Nine pulse indications in the three regions, along with the carotid (ST 9) artery pulse.

Node Site	*Pulse Location*	*Indications*
Taiyang (Extra)	Zygomaticoorbital and deep temporal arteries on both sides of forehead at depression 1 cun posterior to midpoint between the lateral tip of eyebrow and the angulus oculi lateralis.	Conditions related to forehead
Ermen (SJ 21)	Superficial temporal artery at anterior border of ear at level of the superior tragic notch.	Conditions related to eyes and ears
Daying (ST 5)	Facial artery at lower border of mandible.	Conditions related to mouth and teeth
Taiyuan (LU 9)[1]	Radial artery at wrist crease distal to styloid process.	Internal conditions, state of distribution vessels, and conditions of the lungs
Shenmen (HT 7)	Ulnar artery at wrist crease.	Condition of heart
Hegu (LI 4)	Princeps pollicus artery lying below the highest spot on first m. interosseous at midpoint of 2nd metacarpal bone.	Conditions of chest and lungs
Zuwuli (LV 10)[2]	Superficial branches of medial circumflex femoral artery 3 cun directly below inguinal grove and Qichong (ST 30).	Condition of liver
	Or Taichong (LV 3): First metatarsal artery on dorsum in depression distal to junction of 1st and 2nd metatarsal bones.	Condition of liver
Jimen (SP 11)[2]	Lateral side of femoral artery 6 cun above Xuehai (SP 10) on line between Xuehai (SP 10) and Chongmen (SP 12).	Condition of spleen and stomach, or complete digestive system
	Or Chongyang (ST 42): Dorsal pedis artery at highest spot on dorsum of foot in depression between 2nd and 3rd metatarsal and cuneiform bones (pedipulse).	Condition of spleen and stomach, or complete digestive system
Taixi (KD 3)	Posterior tibial artery anterior to tendocalcaneous at level of medial malleolus, pulse is best felt slightly below and anterior to Taixi.	Condition of the kidneys, bladder, and reproductive organs
Renying (ST 9)[1]	Carotid artery on both sides of neck at level of laryngeal prominence on anterior border of m. sternocleidomastoideus.	External conditions, state of distribution vessels, and conditions of stomach

1. Differential diagnosis between relative magnitude of wrist (Taiyuan, LU 9) and neck (Renying, ST 9) pulses provides information on diseased area of the body.
2. As the *Neijing* did not indicate specific nodal sites, two possible pulses that can be used for these regions are provided.

Qibo replies: Vital substances depart from the heart [left ventricle] suddenly, like shooting a crossbow or like a wave hitting the shore. When it reaches the thenar eminence it starts to reverse and decline. The remaining vital substances disperse while traveling upward, which is why no pulsation is perceptible in the return [venous] circulation.

The Yellow Emperor asks: How do you account for the stomach–foot yangming having a pulsating location?

Qibo replies: Stomach vital substances travel upward to concentrate in the lungs, its intense force flows up alongside the pharynx [carotid artery] upward through cavities and apertures [of head and face], providing branches to the eyes, joining major collateral vessels to the brain, and reaching the forehead. Below, it distributes to Kezhuren [Shangguan, GB 3] to follow the mandible where it joins with the yangming vessel and simultaneously descends to Renying [ST 9]. This is how the stomach vital substances travel separately to the yangming vessel. Therefore, the yin [lung] and yang [stomach] pulses in the upper [Renying, ST 9] and lower [Taiyuan, LU 9] regions correspond with each other [seem to be as one]. Therefore, a yang disorder with a small yang pulse is a contrary condition, a yin disorder with a large yin pulse is a contrary condition. When the yin and yang pulses both appear to be calm or forceful, like a cord being stretched which is about to break or fail, this is a sign of disorder.

The Yellow Emperor asks: How do you account for the pulse on the foot shaoyin [vessel]?

Qibo replies: The thoroughfare vessel [*chong*, 冲 aorta] is the sea of the twelve main distribution vessels. It has a major collateral branch to the shaoyin that starts at the kidneys [renal artery] and then travels downward [common iliac artery] and outward [external iliac artery] at the vital substance street [Qichong, ST 30] to follow along the medial aspect of the thigh [femoral artery], internally slanting to enter the popliteal fossa [popliteal artery]. It then follows the medial side of the tibia [posterior tibial artery] to travel with the shaoyin [kidney] distribution vessel [posterior tibial vein], moving downward to enter behind the medial anklebone and to the underside of the foot [medial plantar artery]. A branch is diverted into the ankle and moves out at the instep [lateral plantar artery] to enter the joint of the big toe, concentrating vital substances in all the distribution vessels in order to warm up the feet and tibial region. This vessel always has a pulse that beats constantly [located slightly below and posterior to the medial anklebone on a line between Zhaohai, KD 6 and Taixi, KD 3].

Importance of Blood Flow to Specific Regions

Disrupted or impaired blood distribution in the peripheral regions can manifest in pain and dysfunction in the affected area, and can also be symptomatic of visceral problems. Appreciating the subtleties of arterial (outward) and venous (return) blood flow allows identification of possible symptoms in each body region. Circulation to the upper, middle, and lower regions of the body is examined in terms of these regions being further subdivided into three. Divisions are named sky, earth, and human, depending on their relative position or relative organ position in the body; sky is above, earth is below, human stands between the two. Each of the nine divisions on each side of the body manifest conditions that are indicative or symptomatic of organ pathology. These regions, including their corresponding nine pulses, are examined for diagnostic purposes (Table 10.1). This unique attention to the effects of blood flow in specific regions is presented in *NJSW 20* (*The Three Regions and Nine Subdivisions*).

Comprehending the importance of arterial and venous flow in the various regions of the body and how to restore disruption by therapeutic means is discussed throughout the *Neijing*. One key reference is provided in *NJSW 27* (*Departing and Combining of True Function and Pathogenic Forces*), as follows:

> Those who know nothing about the three regions cannot differentiate between internal [yin] and external [yang], and cannot understand the divisions of sky and earth. The earth represents the earth subdivisions, sky represents the sky subdivisions, and the human represents the human subdivisions. These are regulated by the internal bowels in order to stabilize the three regions.
>
> Therefore, it is said that to apply needle therapy without understanding the three regions and the nine subdivisions, as well as symptomatic vessel indications and locations, although they are excessive only for a moment, such a practitioner will not be able to contain the disorder. To practice in this manner is to punish those without fault [the patients]. This is called the grand delusion. This contrary treatment causes disorder of the large distribution vessels, and true or genuine function [*zhenqi*, 真气] cannot be sustained. Such practitioners take solidness [excess] for hollowness [deficiency], and pathogenic forces for true function. This practice of needling is meaningless. Instead, this practice is like a thief of vital substances and competes for the patient's physiological balance [*zhengqi*, 正气]. These practitioners take direct [arterial] flow for indirect [venous] flow, causing a dispersion of nutrients and defensive substances. This results in a loss of true function with only the pathogenic forces residing in the body. This cuts short the person's long life, which is a heavenly calamity. A practitioner without the understanding of the three regions and nine subdivisions [and their symptoms] therefore cannot stay in practice for long.

Nutrient Circulation Cycles

The ancient attempt to calculate the time it takes nutrients to be circulated in the linear pathway of the vessels of the body is probably the first recorded attempt to conduct such an analysis. It is a true scientific effort, albeit primitive science, but for its time it demonstrated a sound logical approach. The twelve organ-related distribution vessels on each side of the body were included in the circulation route, as were the governing (*du*, 督), allowance (*ren*, 任), and two medial lifting (*yinqiao*, 阴蹺) singular vessels. This results in twenty-eight vessel pathways, equal in number to the constellations in the Chinese celestial sphere. A water clock was used to measure ke periods (14.4 minutes), while a device similar to a sun dial was used to measure *fen* (分), each being one-thirty-sixths of the distance between the constellations, or 1.43 minutes. An average blood perfusion flow rate was calculated using pulse beats and respiration cycles. One cycle of nutrients being circulated throughout the linear route of all vessels was calculated at 28.8 minutes. The same information provided in the *Neijing* can also be recalculated to arrive at a fairly accurate rate of total simultaneous blood volume turnover.

Linear Order of Circulation

The order of circulation of nutrients in the vascular system is presented in *NJLS 16* (*Nutrients*), starting with the following:

> Nutrients are the precious components of consumed grains. After grains enter the stomach [and are digested] they are sent to the lungs and overflow into the middle region [heart] from where they are dispersed to the external [body] regions. The food essence then travels through the distribution tunnels [distribution vessels], supplying nutrients continuously. After coming to an end the circulation sequence starts again to repeat the process. This is called the patterns of sky and earth... These are the traveling routes of nutrients, which indicate the common state of upstream [venous] and downstream [arterial] flow.

Due to the critical role of the lungs in breathing in vital air, the lung vessel is first in the sequential order. The lung (artery) distribution vessel supplies the hand with return circulation by the large intestine (vein) vessels. The large intestine vessels communicate with the stomach distribution vessel (artery) on the face, which distributes down to the feet, where the spleen distribution vessel (vein) is the return vessel. This view of linear circulation continues on one side of the body until all twelve distribution vessels (*jingmai*, 经脉) have participated (Figure 10.2). After the liver distribution vessel (vein), the sequence moves on to the governing (du), allowance (ren), and the two medial lifting (yinqiao) vessels. After this, the linear circulation continues with the lung distribution vessels on the other side of the body.

Length of Vessel Linear Pathway

The *NJLS 17* (*Length of the Vessels*) provides measurements for the length of the distribution vessels, based on an average height of 75 *cun* (寸) or Chinese inch (1 cun is equal to 0.902 inches or 2.30 centimeters). The length of the foot yang distribution vessels (arteries) are 80 cun each, while the foot yin vessels (veins) are 65 cun each, since the latter do not travel to the face. Hand yang distribution vessels (veins) are all 50 cun, while hand yin vessels (arteries) are each 35 cun in length, since the yin hand vessels do not travel to the face. Both the governing (du) and the allowance (ren) vessels (both veins) are measured at 45 cun each. Each of the two medial lifting (yinqiao) veins are measured at 75 cun, since they travel from the foot up to the face. Altogether, the linear pathway of these vessels combined totals 1,620 cun. Note that the thoroughfare vessel (chong aorta) is not included in the linear calculation, since it is considered the blood source for the distribution vessels. The superficial singular vessels, other than the medial lifting, are not included in the primary circulation route.

Average Blood Perfusion Rate

The *NJLS 15* (*Fifty Nutrient Circulations*) provides the speed at which the nutrients (ying) are distributed through the blood system. This value is taken as the average perfusion rate through a typical distribution vessel, its corresponding collateral vessels, and the finer vessels that supply the superficial regions and nodes (acupoints), supplying all the muscle, skeletal, neural, and superficial tissues supplied by the vessel. Nutrients are described as traveling 3 cun in two heartbeats, or 6 cun in one respiration cycle (four heartbeats in one respiration cycle). No clues are provided to how the ancients derived this figure. While the rate of blood flow is

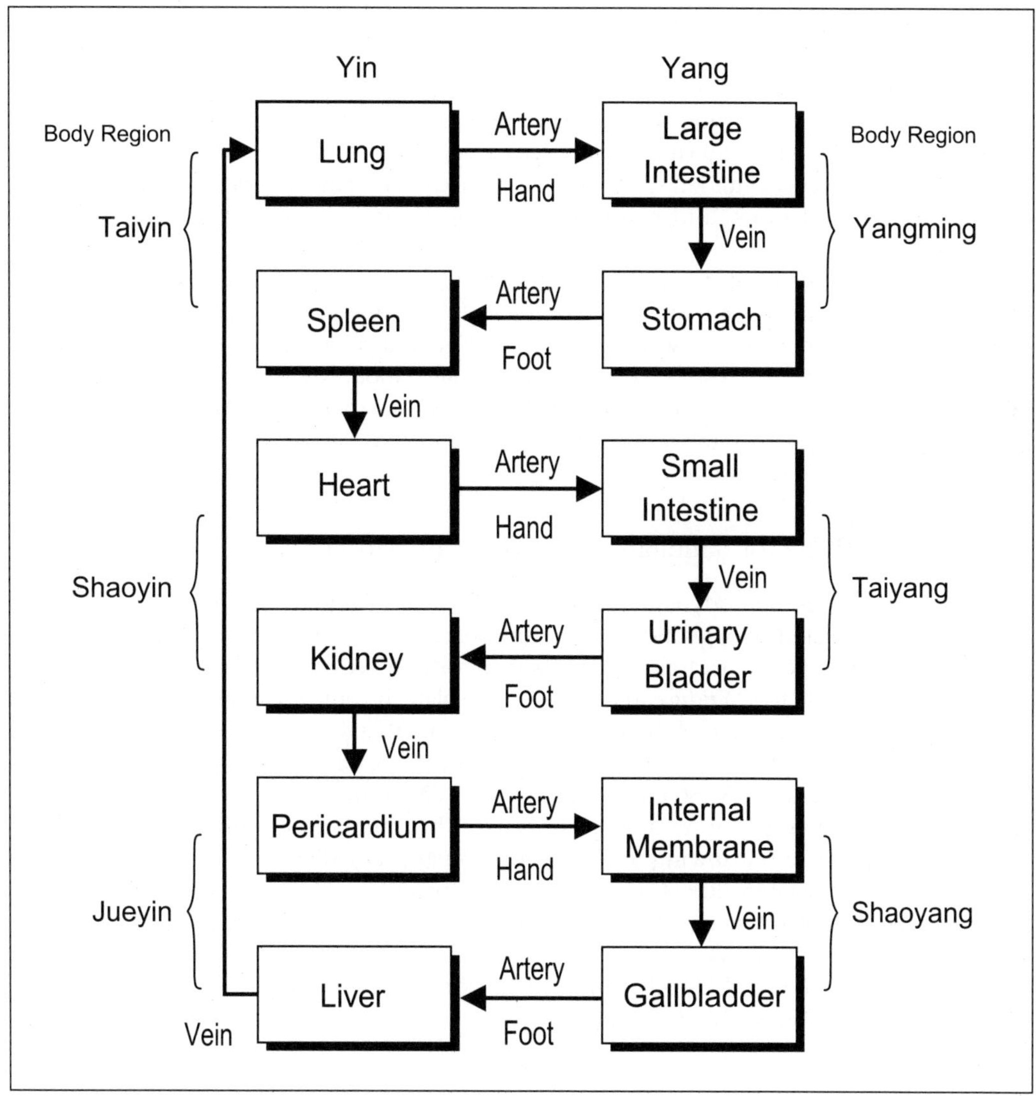

Figure 10.2 Circulation order of nutrients (*ying*) through the superficial distribution vessel pathways of the twelve internal organs (circulation through the *du*, *ren*, and *yinqiao* vessels is not shown).

now known to be considerably faster in the arteries than in the veins, the Chinese value of nutrients traveling 6 cun per respiration cycle is nevertheless useful in understanding the ancient view of hemodynamics.

Fifty Nutrient Circulations a Day

Using the value of nutrients traveling 6 cun per respiration cycle, *NJLS 15* notes that blood can circulate through the 1,620-cun linear pathway of the main distribution vessels in 270 respiration cycles (length of linear pathway divided by distance traveled by nutrients per respiration cycle). The time taken for 270 respirations, and hence one nutrient circulation, was measured using a twenty-four-hour water-drip clock as 2 ke (28.8 minutes). A total of 13,500 respiration cycles were noted to occur in a typical day, therefore fifty complete linear circulations of nutrients take place each day (respiration cycles per day divided by number of respiration cycles needed to circulate nutrients)—twenty-five cycles during the day along with the passage of fourteen constellations, and twenty-five during the night, through another fourteen constellations.

The value of 28.8 minutes for a typical nutrient circulation cycle may be in error by a factor of two, since the number of daily respiration cycles presented in the *Neijing* appears to be only half of what is normally observed today—dividing the value of 270 respiration cycles by 28.8 minutes gives only 9.3 respiration cycles per minute, about half the average. This suggests that the individual being measured was at rest or even meditating. Doubling the figure of 9.3 respiration cycles per minute results in a linear circulation cycle of only 1 ke (14.4 minutes), which is closer to the real value.

Calculation of Time for Simultaneous Blood Circulation

The Western view of hemodynamics considers how long it takes the body's total blood volume to be circulated through the heart. In an average-sized person at rest, it takes less than one minute. This works out to 1,440 daily blood circulation cycles, the number of minutes per day. Data presented in the *Neijing* can be used to calculate the time for simultaneous circulation to determine the turnover rate of the total blood volume. By taking the Chinese measurement of 1,620 cun for the total length of the twenty-eight major distribution arteries and return veins, an average value of 57.86 cun is obtained for either an arterial or venous route (total length of vessels divided by number of vessels). This number is doubled (115.7 cun) to represent the average outflowing and return pathways. Dividing this last number by the blood perfusion flow rate value of 6 cun per respiration cycle yields 19.3 respiration cycles to recirculate the total blood volume through the heart. An average person requires about twenty respiration cycles per minute. Dividing 19.3 by twenty gives a number of 58 seconds for the time to recirculate the total blood volume. This compares well with the Western value of 60 seconds for the average blood turnover rate.

Circulation of Defensive Substances

The circulation of defensive substances (wei) is also considered critical. The ancient Chinese described outflowing circulation in the arteries and drainage back to the venous supply via the lymphatic vessels. Defensive substances also make fifty linear cycles each day. The early Chinese analysis of the circulation of defensive substances in the superficial and deep regions does not correlate precisely with present understanding, but this was the first discussion in history of these concepts. The mathematical model used to calculate the period of defensive substance circulation used common fractions, which when rounded off results in a slight error compared with the calculation for nutrient circulation. An elaborate explanation was constructed in the *Neijing* to explain why there is a slight difference between the times of nutrient and defensive substance circulation; it seems that the ancient Chinese physicians had not realized this was simply a mathematical problem.

One of the complications undoubtedly faced by early Chinese researchers is that lymphatic vessels are more difficult to follow in the body than blood vessels. Despite this limitation, the fundamental ideas they developed are for the most part correct. Lymphatic structures are terminal vessels that do not form a continuous ring, as with blood vessels. They drain the interstitial spaces in the deep and superficial regions, draining back to the subclavian vein. Here the lymph fluid drains back into the blood plasma. The defensive substances and lymph fluid are transported out to the superficial regions in the arteries. The ancient Chinese lymphatic model is based on defensive substances being circulated by the arteries to the superficial yang regions and drained back to the subclavian vein by the lymphatic vessels in the superficial yin regions. Modern anatomy shows there are indeed more lymphatic structures in the superficial yin regions than in the yang regions.

The most important of the early concepts was that defensive substance circulation to the superficial regions and deep circulation involving the internal organs is drastically different from blood circulation. Defensive substances circulate through both superficial and deep regions with some degree of independence. The functional activity of the internal organs, especially the kidneys and the liver, depends on critical processes involving the lymphatics. Also, the absorption of dietary fat from the small intestine is accomplished by means of the deep lymphatics. These activities play more of a functional than a defensive role, although there are important defensive roles for the deep system involving both the spleen and its related thymus gland.

Defensive Substances Leave Blood Circulation

The Chinese appreciated the fact that defensive substances can easily flow out of the blood circulation via the fine vessels, such as capillaries, to mount a reaction. The way these materials leave the circulation is discussed in *NJLS 18* (*The Meeting and Interaction of Nutrients and Defensive Substances*):

> The nature of defensive [wei] function is so fierce, smooth, and quick that it leaves [the vessels] through any opening and diverts from its normal distribution route. This is called oozing or leaked excretion.

The fifty daily defensive substance circulation cycles through the body and internal organs involve being distributed by the arterial supply and then drained back into the venous system by what are now known as lymphatics vessels. This is summarized in *NJLS 71* (*Invasion of Pathogenic Forces*):

> With respect to defensive substances, they flow out fiercely and are high spirited and fast moving. Initially they circulate to the four extremities and the spaces between the striated muscles and the skin without stopping. During the day, defensive substances circulate in the yang phase, and during the night they circulate in the yin phase, constantly traveling between the yang regions [of the body] and the kidney–foot shaoyin superficial regions, and the five viscera and six bowels.

Lymphatics at Critical Nodes

Lymphatic or defensive (wei) vessels have similar branching arrangements in the superficial regions to the distribution and collateral vessels (Figure 9.3). However, these are terminal vessels originating in the more superficial levels, which function to drain the tissue spaces. The circulation route for the Chinese defensive system is illustrated in Figure 10.3. Defensive substances (immune cells and related materials) are transported to the superficial regions by the arterial blood supply. Defensive substances can leave the blood circulation through the walls of the capillaries to fight off an external assault, or respond to tissue damage resulting from trauma. By-products of this reaction are then drained back into the circulation by the lymphatic vessels.

The defensive interaction takes place due to an interplay between nutrients (ying), which include blood coagulation system proteins, and defensive substances (wei), which include immune cells and complement proteins (Chapter 14). In the case of needle insertion, this reaction is critical to stimulate restorative processes, which also involve afferent and efferent nerves. In the case of trauma, this reaction results in swelling and edema in the region that has been assaulted. This is explained in *NJLS 35* (*Swelling*):

> When nutrients [ying] travel along the [arterial] vessels and encounter defensive substances [wei] traveling inversely [normal direction of flow for lymphatics], it causes swelling of the vessels. When defensive substances converge with the vessels traveling between the dividing muscles, it causes swelling of the skin.

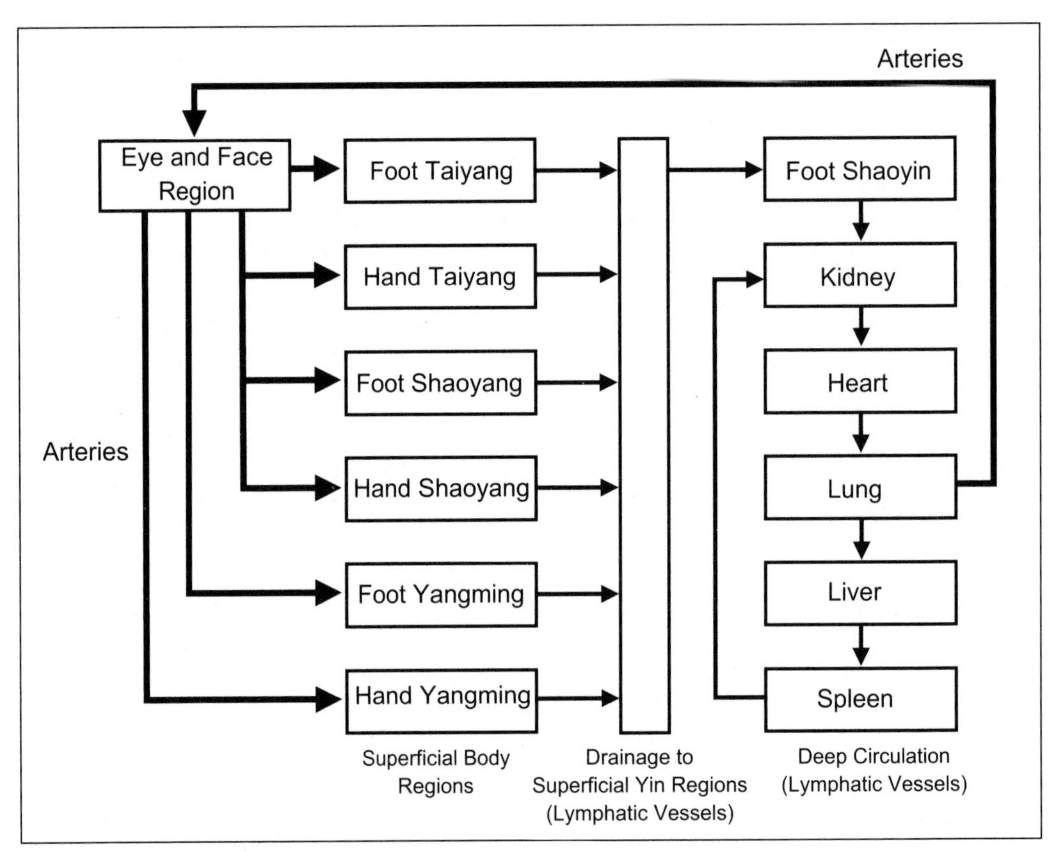

Figure 10.3 Circulation pathway for defensive substances (*wei*) through the blood vessels, superficial lymphatics, and deep lymphatic vessels of the body.

Superficial and Deep Circulation

Defensive substances are circulated simultaneously to all the superficial and deep regions of the body by means of the arteries. When these substances leave the blood circulation in response to protective needs, immune reaction, or response to needling they are drained back into the lymphatic vessels. In the superficial regions, lymphatic vessels lie between the skin and muscles, and drain the interstitial spaces in the superficial body. Deep lymphatics drain the areas related to the internal organs, and also transport the murky defensive material derived from dietary intake from the gut to the venous blood supply. The early Chinese noted that defensive substances circulate simultaneously to all superficial yang areas of the body by means of the arteries. They are then drained back through the yin regions via the lymphatic vessels to recirculate back to the superficial areas, thus completing one typical cycle. Meanwhile the defensive substances also circulate through the internal organs (Figure 10.3).

The order of defensive substance circulation starts at the eyes and face, where all yang regions communicate with the face. The first circulation cycle is taken to start at daybreak, when a person awakes and opens their eyes. In calculating the circulation cycles, the twenty-eight minor constellations were used as a time reference. As with nutrient circulation, twenty-five circulation cycles occur during the yang phase (day) of the earth's rotation, and twenty-five during the yin phase (night). Hence each defensive substance cycle should take exactly 2 ke (28.8 minutes). Using the position of the constellations to measure defensive substance circulation results in about one-and-eight-tenths of a cycle[3] for each constellation segment. Decimal fractions were not in general use at the time the *Neijing* was compiled—the use of common fractions results in a rounding error causing a slight discrepancy between circulation cycle times for nutrients and for defensive substances; had decimal fractions been employed, these two would be identical. Another drawback with using constellation periods is that circulation during the yin and yang phases of the day can be confused with circulation within the yin and yang regions of the body. The distribution pathways are described in *NJLS 76* (*Circulation of Defensive Substances*):

> The period from *fang* [房, fourth constellation] to *bi* [毕, nineteenth constellation, Hyades] belongs to yang, while the period from *mao* [昴, eighteenth constellation] to *xin* [心, fifth constellation] belongs to yin. The yang phase [of the constellations] is in charge of day, while the yin phase is in charge of night. Thus, in one day and one night, defensive substances circulate to make fifty circuits through the body. During the day, defensive substances travel to complete twenty-five circulations during the yang phase. At night, defensive substances travel to complete twenty-five circulations during the yin phase. The defensive substances also circulate through the five viscera.
>
> Thus, the yin phase ends at dawn, and the yang phase begins with defensive substances flowing from the region of the eye [medial angle]. From the eye the defensive substance route extends upward over the head and follows along the back of the neck down the bladder–foot *taiyang* [太阳] superficial regions. It continues to follow along the back down to the extremity of the small toe. As the defensive substances continue to disperse, another path from the lateral angle of the eye travels down the small intestine–hand taiyang regions to terminate at the lateral aspect of the small finger.
>
> Another branch disperses from the lateral angle of the eye traveling down the gallbladder–foot *shaoyang* [少阳] superficial region, flowing to the area between the fourth and fifth toe. Another branch above travels down along the internal membrane

[*sanjiao*, 三焦]–hand shaoyang superficial regions, to the area between the fourth and fifth finger.

Another path at the frontal area of the eye meets with the chin artery [facial artery] and travels down the stomach–foot yangming superficial regions to the dorsum of the foot, entering the region of the fifth toe. The defensive substances also disperse from the region below the ear, traveling down the large intestine–hand yangming superficial regions, entering the area of the thumb and palm of the hand. The pathway traveling down the stomach–foot yangming region also enters the sole of the foot and travels outward below the medial malleolus. Defensive substances then travel in the yin divisions and return [in the arterial system] to meet at the eye, thus completing one circulation cycle [28.8 minutes].

Defensive substances normally enter the internal regions [yin] from the kidney–foot shaoyin superficial region to flow into the kidneys. From the kidneys they flow to the heart and from the heart they flow to the lungs. From the lungs they flow to the liver and from the liver they flow to the spleen. From the spleen they return to flow back to the kidneys, making one internal circulation.

Pattern of Circulation

Defensive substances that leave the arterial blood supply in the yang regions are drained back to the yin regions by the superficial lymphatic vessels. Internally, the deep lymphatics drain the internal organs and gut, meeting the superficial lymphatic return at the subclavian vein. From here, defensive substances return to the heart. This is an endless process with defensive substances being continuously circulated in the superficial and deep regions. While this is not explicit in the preceding quote from *NJLS 76*, it is clarified by Bogao later in the same treatise:

> The *Great Essentials* says: Generally, when the day rotates at the start of each additional constellation, defensive substances are present in the taiyang regions. Therefore, when the day rotates the angular distance of one full constellation, defensive substances travel[4] through all three yang regions, as well as the yin divisions [including internal]. This process is repeated without stopping, consistent with the periods of sky and earth, one after another in succession. After defensive substances complete one cycle the process starts again, after one day and one night, and is measured as 100 ke [1,440 minutes], without end.

The outflow drains from the yang superficial regions back to the yin regions because most of the superficial lymph nodes are located within these regions. Draining back to the deep regions via the lesser yin superficial regions (related to the kidneys) follows because this is the superficial area of the body that overlies the main deep lymphatic pathways and the lymphatic trunks that drain into the venous blood supply. The ancient Chinese probably considered defensive substance flow to be constant. Lymphatic circulation relies on muscle and body motion to stimulate defensive substance flow. Consequently, the flow rate is higher during the active daylight periods. While sleeping, the flow rate diminishes and reaches its lowest level in the early morning hours before awaking.

Correlating Treatment with Defensive Function

Defensive substances are thought to dominate specific superficial regions during certain times of the day, which will influence the response to disease involving the defensive or immune function and needling. When viewing the circulation through the superficial regions it seems to take 4 ke for one cycle in this area. The timing starts when a person awakes in the morning. As previously discussed, the day is divided into one hundred divisions called ke, each being 14.4 minutes long. The following information is given in *NJLS 76*:

> During the measurement of the first ke, defensive substances are in the taiyang superficial regions, and during the second ke they are in the shaoyang regions. During the third ke they are in the yangming superficial regions, and during the fourth ke defensive substances are in the yin [superficial] regions.

This repeats over and over. Therefore, needling a disease in a certain part of the body in ancient times had to be timed for when defensive function was dominant in that region. Presently these guidelines are given little attention, but as a general rule strong stimulation and short duration of needle insertion is used in clearing heat associated with an active infection (a solid condition). On the other hand, false heat due to a yin deficiency (a hollow condition) is treated with mild stimulation and longer duration of needle retention. The *NJLS 76* provides the following explanation:

> The practitioner must cautiously wait for the proper time since disease conditions have their own periods. To lose this timing, contrary to waiting for the proper time, the one hundred [all] diseases cannot be controlled. Therefore it is said that to treat a solid condition, needling is applied when the defensive reaction is coming on, and to treat a hollow condition, needling is applied when the defensive reaction is departing. This means that the defensive function is either present or gone at specific times, and so it is necessary to wait for the proper time when treating either a hollow or solid condition.

11

Distribution Vessels and Nodal Pathways

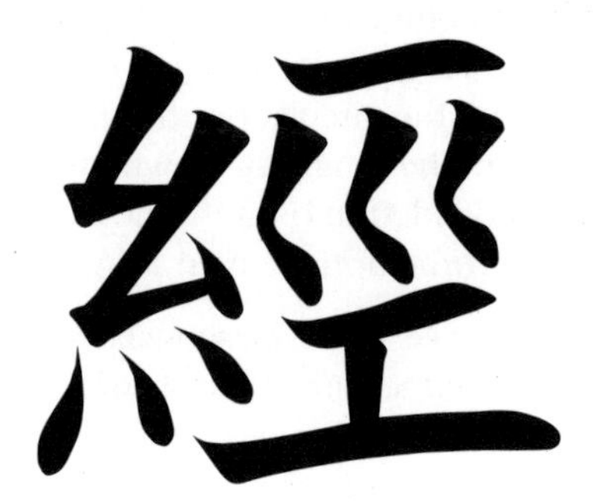

Jing: Distribution Vessel

> The distribution vessels are most important since they are capable of determining the fate of life, as well as regulating the balance between hollowness [deficiency] and solidness [excess]. To understand this is essential.
>
> Yellow Emperor, *NJLS 10 (Distribution Vessels)*

The account of the Chinese vascular system presented in Chapter 9 is completed in this chapter with a description of the longitudinal distribution vessels (*jingmai*, 经脉). These organ-related distribution blood vessels are neurovascular systems, and are critical both because they give rise to the collateral vessels (*luomai*, 络脉) and because they distribute nutrients, defensive substances, substances of vitality, and oxygen from vital air to all the internal organs, glands, muscular tissue, tendons, bones, the brain, neural tissue, sensory system, and skin, and transport metabolic waste products for disposal, including carbon dioxide, back to the lungs for exhalation. All processes and functions of the body depend on these vessels. The collateral vessels they form give rise to small receptive areas on the skin that provide added sensitivity for protective reasons. These small regions on the skin are the neurovascular nodes (acupoints) that can be stimulated to bring about profound restorative processes (Chapter 14).

Detailed information on the distribution vessels is presented in this chapter directly from *NJLS 10* (*Distribution Vessels*), which constitutes a comprehensive discussion on the distribution vessel superficial and deep pathways. The Western names given to the vessels along the distribution route are included to provide a correlation with the Chinese descriptions. Nodal locations (acupoints) and pathways associated with these vessels are provided separately in *NJSW 58* (*Vital Nodes*), *NJSW 59* (*On the Storehouses of Vital Substances*), and other sources for location, indications, and pathways. The nodal routes of the main distribution vessels are presented in Figures 11.1 to 11.14—the nodal sites in these diagrams are connected by a line that generally represents the stimulation-induced propagated sensation (PS) pathway, and is not meant to be an accurate depiction of the deeper distribution vessels. Information on pathology as a result of the vessels being adversely affected by external factors, as well as other problems related to each associated internal organ, dominant tissue, or responsibility, is summarized in Tables 11.1 through 11.6.

Clinically, nodal sites are important simply because they are used to influence circulation and induce restorative physiological reactions. These regions represent a compact arrangement of fine blood vessels, lymphatic vessels, and nerves (Figure 9.3), and have relationships to known anatomical features. Nodes on the arm and leg lie on lines that follow blood vessel, lymphatic, and neural pathways. On the trunk of the body, nodes are organized in relation to segmental innervation levels, where nerves and blood vessels penetrate muscle fascia. On the face and head they lie in proximity to cranial nerves and upper cervical nerves, once again alongside blood and lymphatic vessels. In the auricle, the same relationship between blood vessels and nerves (sprigs from cranial nerves) is also observed. The importance of the nodes is noted by the Yellow Emperor in *NJLS 1* (*Nine Needles and Twelve Sources*):

> The critical junctures [nodes] consist of 365 specific locations. If one understands their importance, one sentence can cover the whole topic. However, if one does not understand their significance, this knowledge will deteriorate and be endlessly dispersed.

Presently a total of 309 specifically identified nodes are known to be distributed along each side of the body in the well-defined pathways that represent the *zangfu* (脏腑), or twelve organ-related distribution vessels. The two major singular distribution vessels that traverse the anterior and posterior central body lines have an additional fifty-two sites: the governing (*du*, 督) vessel has twenty-eight, the allowance (*ren*, 任) vessel has twenty-four. Taking into account the nodes distributed on one side of the body along with those on the body centerline gives a total of 361 unique locations. The *Neijing* frequently refers to 365 such locations on the body, noted to be equal to the number of days in a year. However, more than 520 actual locations are noted in the *Neijing*, with only about 150 specifically mentioned by name or reference. A total of 670 sites is arrived at by adding all sites of the governing and allowance vessels to those of the twelve organ vessels that are distributed symmetrically on each side of the body.

Six of the singular vessel pathways do not have nodal sites of their own, so they utilize locations on the organ distribution vessels. Also, there are many additional nodes, perhaps one hundred or more, that are not located on one of the regular vessels, and there are additional sites found on the auricle.

The distribution vessel pathways in *NJLS 10* are presented by anterior, posterior, and medial and lateral regions of the body in the established circulation order. Western names of the vessels are included where possible, but it should be noted that the ancient Chinese described the vessels in their yin-yang anatomical reference system. Discussion of the distribution vessels in *NJLS 10* is preceded by introductory remarks by the Yellow Emperor:

> Life for the human first starts when refined substances combine [father's sperm and mother's egg]. As a result of this conception the brain and spinal medulla start to form, and the bones develop to provide a framework [structure] for the body. The vessels form in order to circulate nutrients [*ying*, 营]; the muscles and tendons develop to make the body strong. The flesh develops to form the trunk [walls] of the body, the skin becomes firm, and the hair can grow long. Food broken down in the mother's stomach supplies the fetus, and the vessel pathways then develop so that blood and vital substances can be circulated... The distribution vessels are most important since they are capable of determining the fate of life or death, and are essential in the treatment and cause of all disease ["one hundred diseases"], as well as mediating the balance between hollowness [deficiency] and solidness [excess]. To understand this is essential.

The treatment approach noted in *NJLS 10* for addressing specific pathological conditions is identical for each distribution vessel; the only variation being that nodes are selected along the affected vessel. The information that follows is therefore relevant for each distribution vessel:

> With respect to all diseases [of a particular distribution vessel], when they are abundant or flourishing [excess], they should be treated by the application of reducing [draining off] techniques. When disorders are hollow [deficient], they should be treated by reinforcing [mending] techniques. If they are hot [fever] diseases, they should be treated by needle insertion of a short duration. If they are cold disorders, they should be treated by retaining the needle [for a longer period]. If the distribution vessels are depressed, they should only be treated by the application of moxibustion. If the diseases are neither flourishing nor hollow disorders, they should be treated by selecting nodes along the [specifically indicated] distribution vessel.

Anterior Vessel and Nodal Pathways

The anterior aspect in the Chinese anatomical orientation of the arms, legs, face, and portions of the trunk are supplied by four major distribution vessels that serve the lungs, large intestine, stomach, and spleen, and give rise to nodal pathways that traverse this region of the body. The distribution pathways are discussed below individually for these vessels, along with pathology affecting the vessels themselves or along the vessel pathway, in addition to problems of the organs or their related tissues or functions. Table 11.1 summarizes this information for the vessels of the lungs and large intestine; Table 11.2 for the stomach and spleen.

The hand and arm are supplied by the yin-yang paired lung and large intestine distribution vessels. Referred to as the hand–anterior medial aspect (great yin) vessel, the lung vessel is an outflowing artery that supplies the anterior aspect of the arms (radial artery). Internally the lung distribution vessel includes the bronchial arteries and the superior and inferior mesenteric arteries that supply the large intestine. The hand–anterior lateral aspect large intestine vessel is a return-flowing venous network that drains the areas supplied by the lung vessels. Internally it includes the bronchial veins of the lungs, and the inferior and superior mesenteric veins that drain the large intestine.

Superficial nodes associated with the lung distribution vessel begin on the thorax. There are eleven sites starting with Zhongfu (LU 1), located lateral to the first intercostal space, 6 Chinese inches, or *cun* (寸), from the centerline of the chest and terminating at the thumb extremity with Shaoshang (LU 11) (Figure 11.1).

The distribution pathway of the large intestine distribution vessel has twenty nodes, beginning at the extremity of the index finger at Shangyang (LI 1). From here the superficial tract passes over the hand, traveling up to the elbow and to the shoulder, terminating next to the nasal ala on the face at Yingxiang (LI 20) (Figure 11.2).

The stomach distribution vessel consists of outflowing arteries distributing to the face, anterior trunk, and anterior lateral aspects of the lower extremities. Internally the vessels of the stomach consist of the gastric and splenic arteries. The spleen vessel is a return-flowing vein supplying the anterior medial aspects of the lower extremities, and drains the areas supplied by the stomach vessel, except for the head region. In the abdominal and thorax regions the spleen vessel is represented by the internal thoracic and the superior and inferior

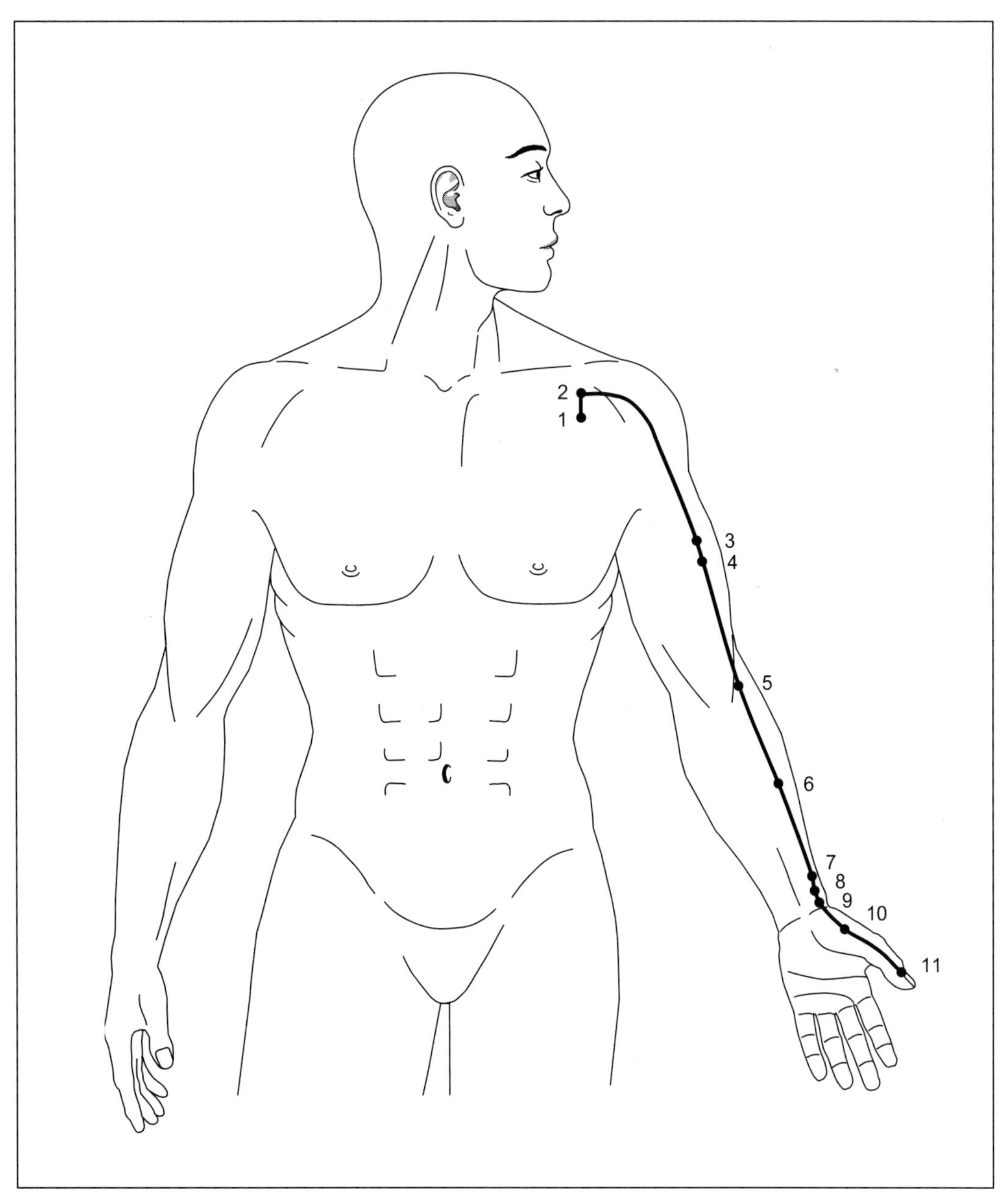

Figure 11.1 Nodal pathway associated with the anterior medial distribution and collateral vessels of the upper extremity (hand *taiyin*), related to the lungs.

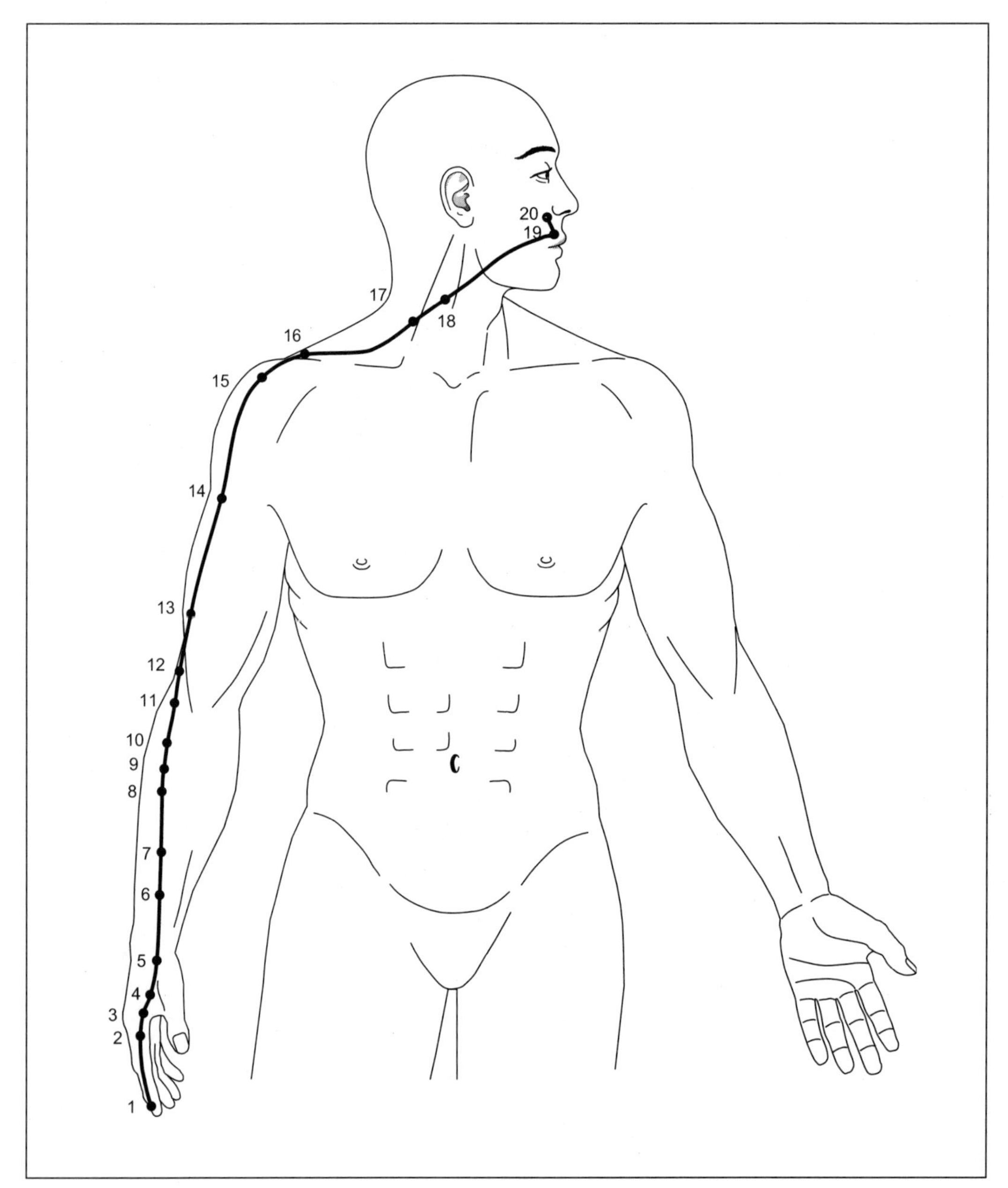

Figure 11.2 Nodal pathway associated with the anterior lateral distribution and collateral vessels of the upper extremity (hand *yangming*), related to the large intestine.

epigastric veins that travel along with the stomach superficial arteries. Internally the vessels of the spleen consist of the gastric and splenic veins.

There are forty-five nodes associated with the stomach distribution vessel, beginning with Chengqi (ST 1), located between the eyeball and the infraorbital ridge directly below the pupil. This pathway distributes down the face, chest, abdomen, and anterior legs, ending with Lidui (ST 45) on the lateral side of the second toe (Figure 11.3).

The spleen vessel distribution pathway has twenty-one associated superficial nodes. The first is Dabai (SP 1), located at the medial corner of the nail of the large toe. From here it travels up the medial side of the foot anterior to the malleolus, traveling up the anterior medial aspect of the leg, reaching the abdominal region and then traveling up to the lateral aspect of the thorax to terminate at Dabao (SP 21) (Figure 11.4).

Vessels of Anterior Medial Hand: Lungs

> The distribution vessel of the anterior medial aspect of the upper extremity[1] [lungs] arises in the upper abdominal cavity [middle *jiao*, or abdominal aorta] with collateral branches [inferior and superior mesenteric arteries] traveling below to the large intestine. Here it travels back up along the cardiac orifice of the stomach to join the lungs [bronchial arteries].
>
> From the lung connections it moves transversely [brachiocephalic, subclavian, and axillary arteries] to reach the region [on the arm] below the axilla, where it travels downward along the medial aspect of the humerus [brachial artery]. It reaches the cubital fossa below, traveling in front of the lesser yin [heart] and pericardium [*xinzhu*, 心主] distribution vessels. It follows along the inner aspect of the forearm and lower aspect of the radius bone [radial artery], entering the region where the radial pulse is detected. It then distributes to the thenar [superficial palmar branch of radial artery], and follows along the border of the thenar eminence [Yuji, LU 10] to reach the extremity of the thumb [proper palmar digital arteries]. From behind the wrist a branch of the lung distribution vessel [radial artery] travels along the inner aspect [radial side] of the index finger to reach its extremity [proper palmar digital arteries].

Disorders due to circulation in the lung distribution vessel, the lungs themselves, and excess and deficient conditions are noted in Table 11.1.

> When the above diseases are abundant [excess] disorders, the patient's pulse at Taiyuan [LU 9] will be four times as great as at the neck pulse at Renying [ST 9]. If the diseases are hollow [deficient] disorders, the patient's pulse at Taiyuan [LU 9] will conversely be smaller than the neck pulse at Renying [ST 9].

Vessels of Anterior Lateral Hand: Large Intestine

> The distribution vessel of the anterior lateral aspect of the upper extremity [large intestine] arises in the extremity of the thumb [digital veins] and index finger [digital veins]. This vessel follows along the upper margin of the finger passing through the region of Hegu [LI 4], located between the first and second metacarpal bones [cephalic vein]. Continuing upward it enters the region between the two tendons [extensor pollicis longus and extensor

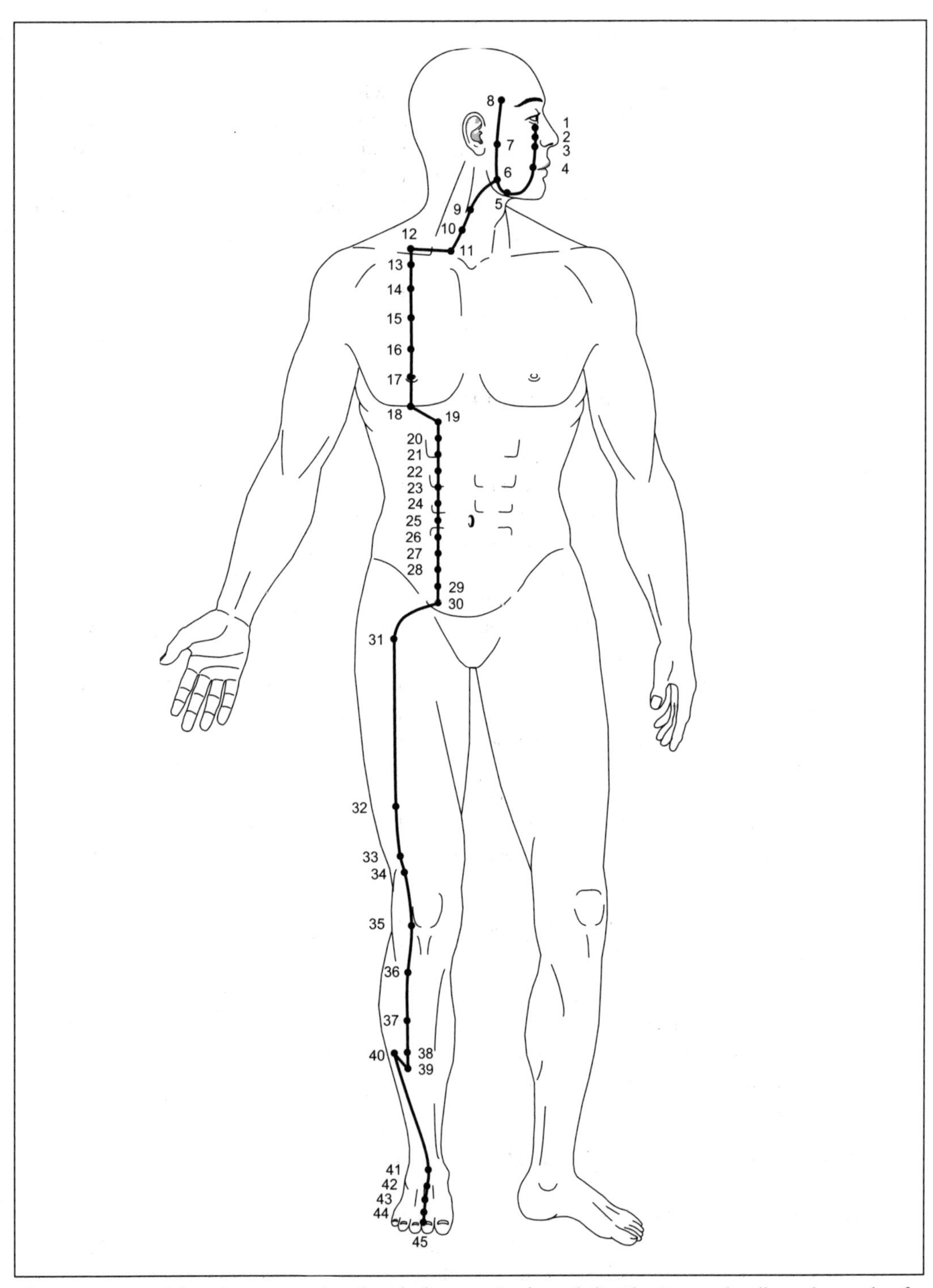

Figure 11.3 Nodal pathway associated with the anterior lateral distribution and collateral vessels of the lower extremity (foot *yangming*), related to the stomach.

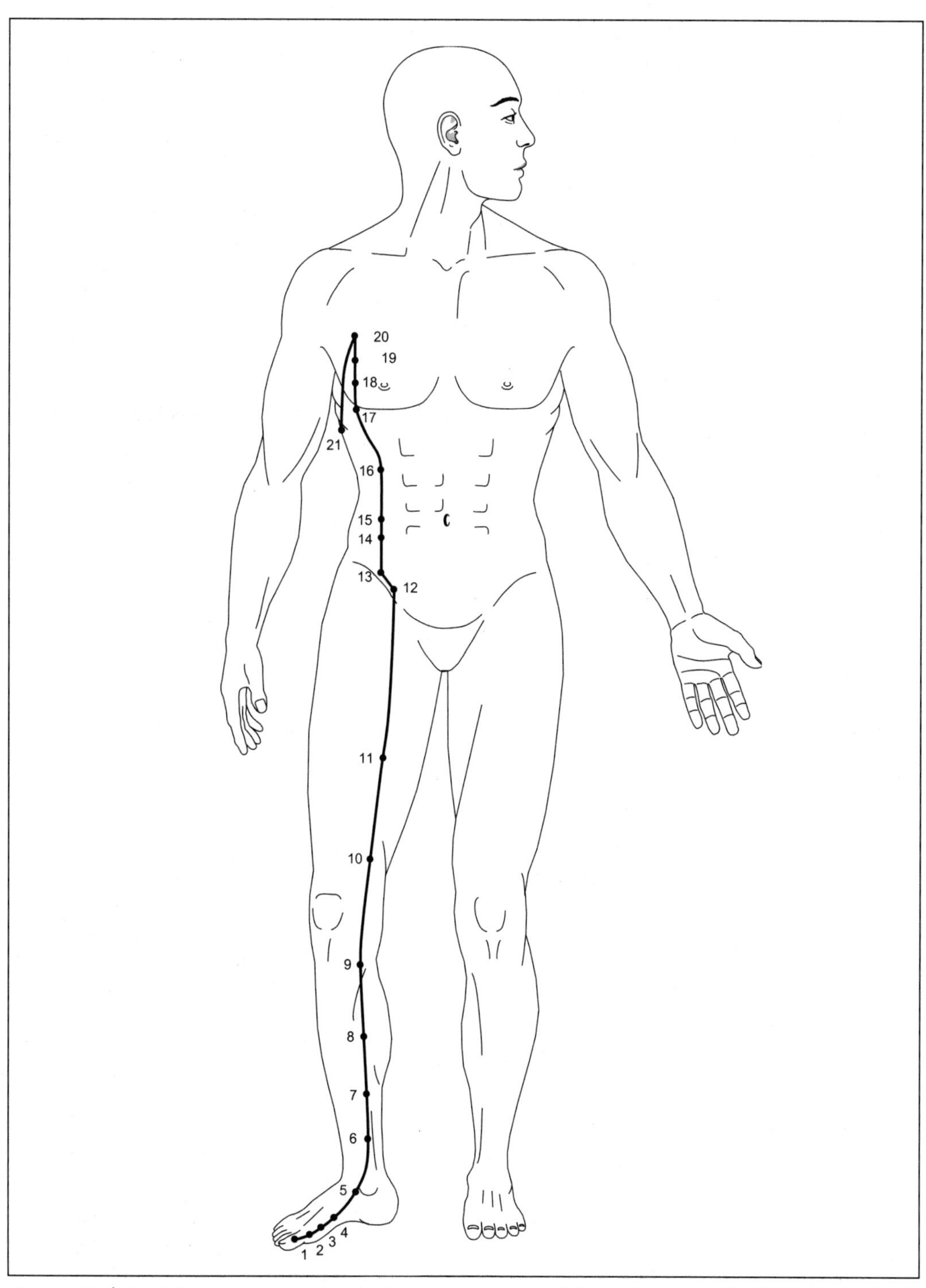

Figure 11.4 Nodal pathway associated with the anterior medial distribution and collateral vessels of the lower extremity (foot *taiyin*), related to the spleen.

Table 11.1 Indications for the two main distribution (*jing*) vessels of the upper extremity, supplying the anterior body superficial area (lungs and large intestine).

Jing *Vessel*	*Indications*
Lung	Anterior Medial Upper Extremity (Hand *Taiyin*)
Vessel	Swelling and congestion of lungs; expanded chest associated with asthma and cough; pain in supraclavicular fossa; and serious condition with arms folded across chest, associated with blurred vision.
Lung Organ	Cough; adverse rising of lung respiratory gases marked by long expiration, short inspiration, and dyspnea (could include asthma), accompanied by thirst; mental vexations (depression) with congested chest; pain and cold in medial anterior region of arm and forearm; and feverish palms.
Surplus (Excess)	Pain in shoulders and back due to wind-cold syndrome; abnormal perspiration due to attack of wind; and frequent urination with scanty urine.
Hollow (Deficient)	Pain and cold in shoulders and back; shortness of breath due to sighing; and change in the color of urine.
Large Intestine	Anterior Lateral Upper Extremity (Hand *Yangming*)
Vessel	Toothache and swelling in the neck.
Body Fluid	Yellowish eyes; dry mouth and allergic rhinitis, including chronic sinusitis; nosebleed; congested throat; pain in the anterior shoulder and upper arm; pain and dysfunction of the thumb and index finger.
Surplus (Excess)	Heat (fever, burning sensation) along the course of the vessels.
Hollow (Deficient)	Relentless cold feelings and shivering.

pollicis brevis], and follows along the forearm [cephalic vein] to reach the lateral aspect of the elbow. It then travels up the lateral anterior aspect of the upper arm to the shoulder [cephalic vein] and the anterior aspect of the acromion [transverse cervical vein]. Above this area it travels to the back [superficial cervical vein] where it meets with vessels above [external jugular vein].

Below this it enters the supraclavicular fossa region [meeting of subclavian and jugular veins], sending collateral branches [bronchial vein] to the lungs. It continues downward [inferior vena cava] through the diaphragm to form connections [inferior and superior mesenteric veins] with the large intestine [colic, ileocolic, and sigmoid veins].

A branch of the large intestine distribution vessel from the supraclavicular fossa region travels up the neck [external jugular vein] to pass through the cheek [facial vein], entering the lower teeth and continuing onward to distribute around the mouth [superior and inferior labial veins], reaching the philtrum [Renzhong, DU 26]. The branch on the left side distributes toward the right, and the branch on the right distributes toward the left,[2] then moves upward [angular vein, also infraorbital vein] to clasp each side of the nasal ala [Yingxiang, LI 20].

Disorders due to circulation in the large intestine distribution vessel, body fluids controlled by the large intestine, and excess and deficient conditions are noted in Table 11.1.

> When the above diseases are abundant [excess] disorders, the patient's neck pulse at Renying [ST 9] will be four times as great as at Taiyuan [LU 9]. If the diseases are hollow [deficient] disorders, the patient's pulse at Renying [ST 9] will conversely be smaller than the pulse at Taiyuan [LU 9].

Vessels of Anterior Lateral Foot: Stomach

> The distribution vessel of the anterior lateral aspect of the lower extremity[1] [stomach] arises at the nose [angular artery], reaching the junction of the nose and forehead [brow], where on each side it communicates [dorsal nasal artery] with the great yang [bladder] distribution vessel [supratrochlear artery], below which it follows along the lateral aspect of the nose to enter the upper teeth. It then returns to clasp the mouth by circling the lips [superior and inferior labial arteries]; the lower branch reaches to the node Chengjiang [RN 24].
>
> The stomach distribution vessel then declines to follow along behind the lower angle of the jaw [facial artery], passing over the jaw at Daying [ST 5], and traveling to the region of the masseter muscle [Jiache, ST 6], then traveling upward in front of the ear [superficial temporal artery], where a branch [zygomaticoorbital artery] distributes over to Kezhuren [Shangguan, GB 3], and continues upward [superficial temporal artery] to the hairline and brow of the skull [frontal branch of superficial temporal artery and then finer branches].
>
> A branch located in front of the node Daying [ST 5] [lingual or submental artery] travels to the external carotid artery at Renying [ST 9], which in turn travels down along the throat and larynx to enter the region of the supraclavicular fossa [Quepen, ST 12] [junction of the right common carotid and brachiocephalic arteries, or left common carotid and aorta]. It then continues below [the aorta], passing through the diaphragm and making connections to the stomach [celiac artery, and then left and right gastric arteries] with a collateral branch to the spleen [splenic artery].
>
> Another branch from the supraclavicular fossa region travels down the inside aspect of the thorax [internal thoracic artery], continuing down along each side of the umbilicus [superior and inferior epigastric arteries] to enter the vital substance street [Qichong, ST 30] [external iliac artery]. Another branch of this vessel [superior and inferior epigastric arteries] travels downward from the level of the cardia, along the inside of the abdominal wall to rejoin the former vessel at the vital substance street [Qichong, ST 30] [external iliac artery].
>
> It then continues down the anterior portion of the thigh [Biguan, ST 31] [femoral artery] to reach the rectus femoris muscle [Futu, ST 32]. Traveling below it reaches the knee and distributes to the patella [lateral superior and lateral inferior arteries], and continues downward following along the lateral aspect of the tibia [anterior tibial artery] to the dorsum of the foot [dorsalis pedis artery] and then [dorsal metatarsal artery] enters the medial aspect of the middle toe [dorsal digital artery of medial aspect of the third toe and lateral side of the second toe].

Another branch at the lower aspect of this vessel separates 3 cun from the dorsum [arcuate artery] to enter [dorsal metatarsal artery] the lateral margins of the middle toe [dorsal digital artery of lateral aspect of the third toe and medial side of the fourth toe]. Another branch of this vessel distributes from the dorsum of the foot, reaching the extremity of the big toe [lateral and medial dorsal digital arteries of the first toe and medial aspect of the second toe].

Disorders due to circulation in the stomach distribution vessel, blood controlled by the stomach, stomach surplus, and excess and deficient conditions are noted in Table 11.2.

When the above diseases are abundant [excess] disorders, the patient's neck pulse at Renying [ST 9] will be four times as great as at Taiyuan [LU 9]. If the diseases are hollow

Table 11.2 Indications for the two main distribution (*jing*) vessels of the lower extremity, supplying the anterior body superficial area (stomach and spleen).

Jing *Vessel*	*Indications*
Stomach	Anterior Lateral Lower Extremity (Foot *Yangming*)
Vessel	Continuous shaking due to cold; tendency to groan; frequent yawning; and a black coloration of the face, or black coloration in the area between the eyes and the eyebrows. Also includes behavioral problems[1] and intestinal noises ("running-pig" disorder) with abdominal distention due to an upsurge in activity along the tibia.
Blood	Mania and madness; malaria; warm disease with excessive perspiration; rhinitis and nosebleed; deviated mouth-canker (fever blister) on lips; swollen neck; congested throat; abdominal distension and edema; painful and swollen knees; pain along the chest, breast, groin (vital substance street), thigh, rectus femoris, lateral aspect of the tibia, and dorsum of the foot; and stiffness and dysfunction of the middle toe.
Surplus (Excess)	Anterior portion of body feels hot.
Stomach Surplus	Quick digestion with continual hunger and yellow urine.
Hollow (Deficient)	Anterior portion of body feels cold and shivering with a cold sensation in the stomach, along with abdominal distension and fullness.
Spleen	Anterior Medial Lower Extremity (Foot *Taiyin*)
Vessel	Stiffness in the root of the tongue; vomiting after eating; pain in epigastrium; abdominal distension; and frequent belching.
Spleen Organ	Pain in root of tongue; inability of body to move (body stiffness); inability to eat (swallow food); mental vexations (depression); acute pain below heart; loose stools; passage of abdominal mass (dysentery); oliguria; jaundice; inability to lie down; stubborn (chronic) swelling and coldness of medial aspect of thigh and knee when standing; and stiffness and dysfunction of big toe.

1. Includes aversion to angry people; watchful but yet startled or frightened when hearing sounds made on a wooden instrument; heart on verge of palpitations; and a desire to dwell shut up in a house with the windows covered. In extremely serious cases the person will have a longing to sing from high places (mountain, hill, etc.); discarding their clothes and walking around nude.

[deficient] disorders, the patient's neck pulse at Renying [ST 9] will conversely be smaller than the pulse at Taiyuan [LU 9].

Vessels of Anterior Medial Foot: Spleen

The distribution vessel of the anterior medial aspect of the lower extremity [spleen] begins at the extremity of the big toe [dorsal digital veins]. It follows along the medial side at the border of the white flesh and continues past the medial aspect of the first metatarsophalangeal joint. It then travels upward in front of the medial malleolus, and then up along the medial aspect of the gastrocnemius muscle [great saphenous vein]. It travels along the posterior aspect of the tibia, crossing in front of the transitional yin [liver] distribution vessel.

Continuing above the knee, it travels along the medial and anterior aspect of the upper thigh, where it enters the abdomen [external iliac vein] to form connections with the spleen [splenic vein], with collateral branches to the stomach [gastric vein]. Above the diaphragm this vessel [superior vena cava] clasps the pharynx [throat] [jugular vein, then superior thyroid vein] and links with the root of the tongue [hypoglossal vein], dispersing along the underside of the tongue [sublingual vein].

From the stomach this vessel travels up through the diaphragm to pour into the heart [gastric vein to portal vein and then vena cava].

Disorders due to circulation in the spleen distribution vessel and in the spleen itself are noted in Table 11.2.

When the above diseases are abundant [excess] disorders, the patient's pulse at Taiyuan [LU 9] will be four times as great as at the neck pulse at Renying [ST 9]. If the diseases are hollow [deficient] disorders, the patient's pulse at Taiyuan [LU 9] will conversely be smaller than the neck pulse at Renying [ST 9].

Posterior Vessel and Nodal Pathways

The posterior aspect in the Chinese anatomical orientation of the arms, legs, back of the head, and trunk are supplied by four major distribution vessels that serve the heart, small intestine, bladder, and kidneys, and give rise to nodal pathways that traverse this region of the body. The distribution pathways are discussed below individually for these vessels, along with pathology affecting the vessels themselves or along the vessel pathway, in addition to problems of the organs or their related tissues or functions. Table 11.3 summarizes this information for the vessels of the heart and small intestine; Table 11.4 for the bladder and kidneys.

The heart vessel is an outflowing artery supplying the posterior medial aspect of the upper extremity, and internally it consists of the coronary arteries and the superior mesenteric arteries that supply the small intestines. The small intestine vessel supplies the posterior lateral aspect of the upper extremity, and is a return-flowing vein that drains the region supplied by the heart vessel and regions of the scapula, neck, and face. Internally it consists of the coronary veins and the superior mesenteric veins that drain the small intestines.

The bladder vessel distribution is an outflowing artery that supplies the head, scalp, back, posterior lateral legs, and lateral foot regions, and includes the vertebral and intercostal arteries.

Internally it includes the renal arteries and the superior vesical arteries supplying the bladder. The kidney distribution vessel is a return-flowing vein supplying the posterior medial aspects of the lower extremities, and it drains the area supplied by the bladder distribution vessel, except for some regions of the face. On the trunk of the body the kidney distribution vessel is represented by the intercostal veins that match the intercostal arteries of the bladder, and includes the vertebral veins. Internally it includes the renal veins and the superior vesical veins that drain the bladder.

The heart vessel distribution pathway has a total of nine nodes, and starts at the axilla center at Jiquan (HT 1). From here it courses down the anterior medial arm and travels across the palm of the hand to end on the radial side of the extremity of the little finger at Shaochong (HT 9) (Figure 11.5).

The small intestine vessel distribution pathway contains nineteen nodes, and begins at the extremity of the little finger at Shaoze (SI 1). From here it courses up along the medial aspect of the hand and then travels up the posterior regions of the arm to continue over to the scapula. Then it travels up the neck to end at Tinggong (SI 19), located anterior to the auricle at the level of the tragus (Figure 11.6).

The bladder vessel distribution pathway has sixty-five nodes, beginning at the medial canthus of the eye at the node Jingming (BL 1). From here it distributes up over the head and courses down each side of the neck and back. It continues down the posterior aspect of the leg, passing under the lateral malleolus and ending on the lateral side of the extremity of the small toe at Zhiyin (BL 67) (Figure 11.7).

The kidney vessel distribution pathway has twenty-seven nodes, and starts on the bottom of the foot at the junction between the anterior third and posterior two-thirds of the sole at Yongquan (KD 1). It then continues to the medial aspect of the foot, passing under the malleolus and up the medial posterior aspect of the leg and thigh. From here it continues up on the anterior trunk of the body, passing on each side of the central body line and ending at the lower border of the clavicle, 2 cun from the chest center at Shufu (KD 27) (Figure 11.8).

Vessels of Posterior Medial Hand: Heart

> The distribution vessel of the posterior medial aspect of the upper extremity [heart] arises at the heart to form connections with the heart system [coronary arteries]. Below, it passes through the diaphragm [abdominal aorta] to make collateral branches with the small intestine [superior mesenteric arteries].
>
> A branch of this distribution vessel from the heart connections travels up along each side of the throat [internal carotid arteries] to form a system of connections [internal to brain] with the eyes [anterior cerebral artery, ophthalmic artery, then the ethmoidal, supraorbital, and lacrimal arteries].
>
> Direct branches from the heart connections drive back over the top of the lungs [brachiocephalic, subclavian, and then axillary artery] to reach the region below the axilla. This then travels down the medial posterior aspect of the humerus, traveling behind the great yin [lung] and xinzhu [pericardium] distribution vessels to reach the medial aspect of the elbow below. It continues down along the medial posterior aspect of the forearm [ulnar artery], arriving at the beginning of the palm, passing behind [radial side] the pisiform bone. It continues along the medial aspect of the palm [common

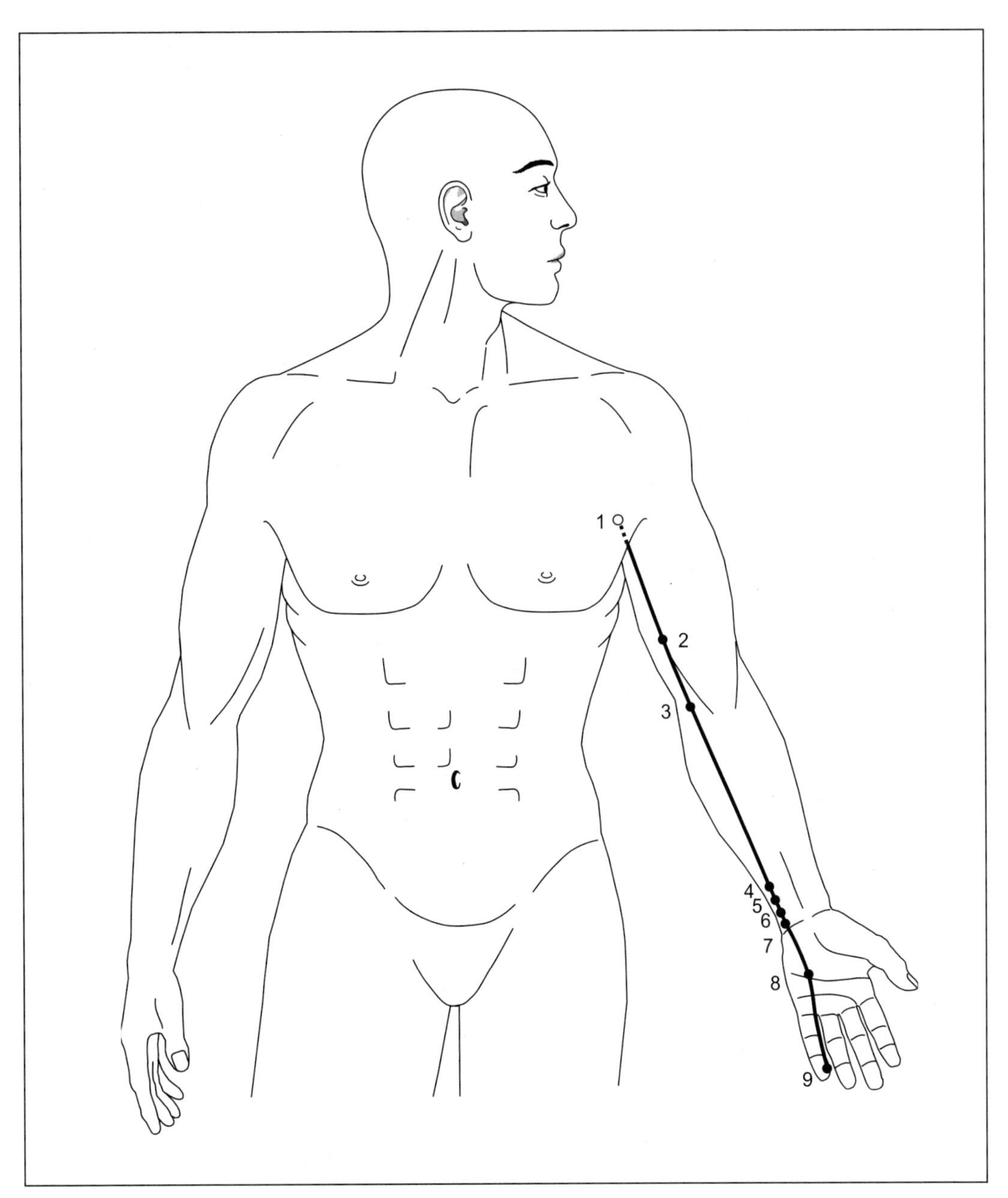

Figure 11.5 Nodal pathway associated with the posterior medial distribution and collateral vessels of the upper extremity (hand *shaoyin*), related to the heart.

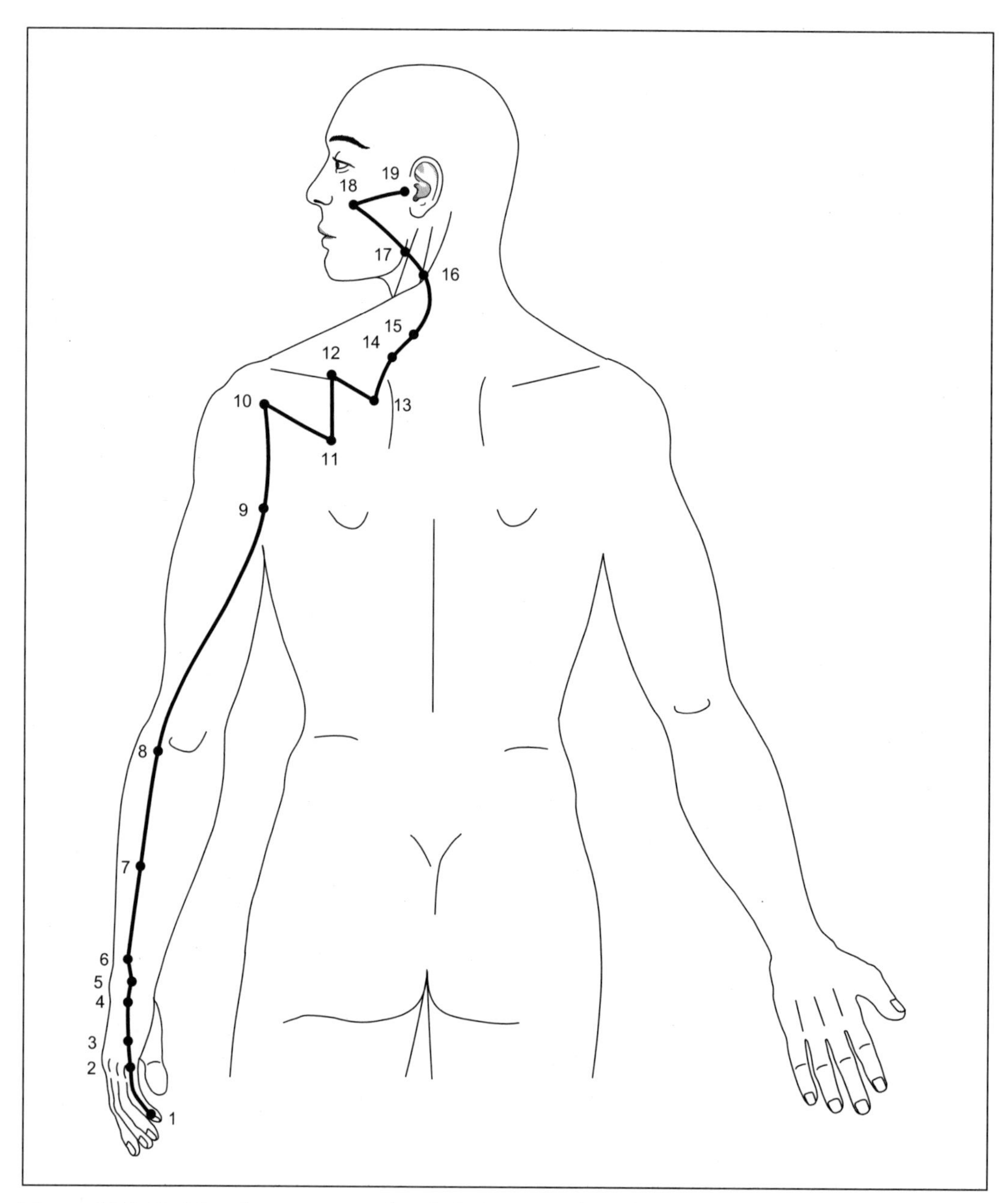

Figure 11.6 Nodal pathway associated with the posterior lateral distribution and collateral vessels of the upper extremity (hand *taiyang*), related to the small intestine.

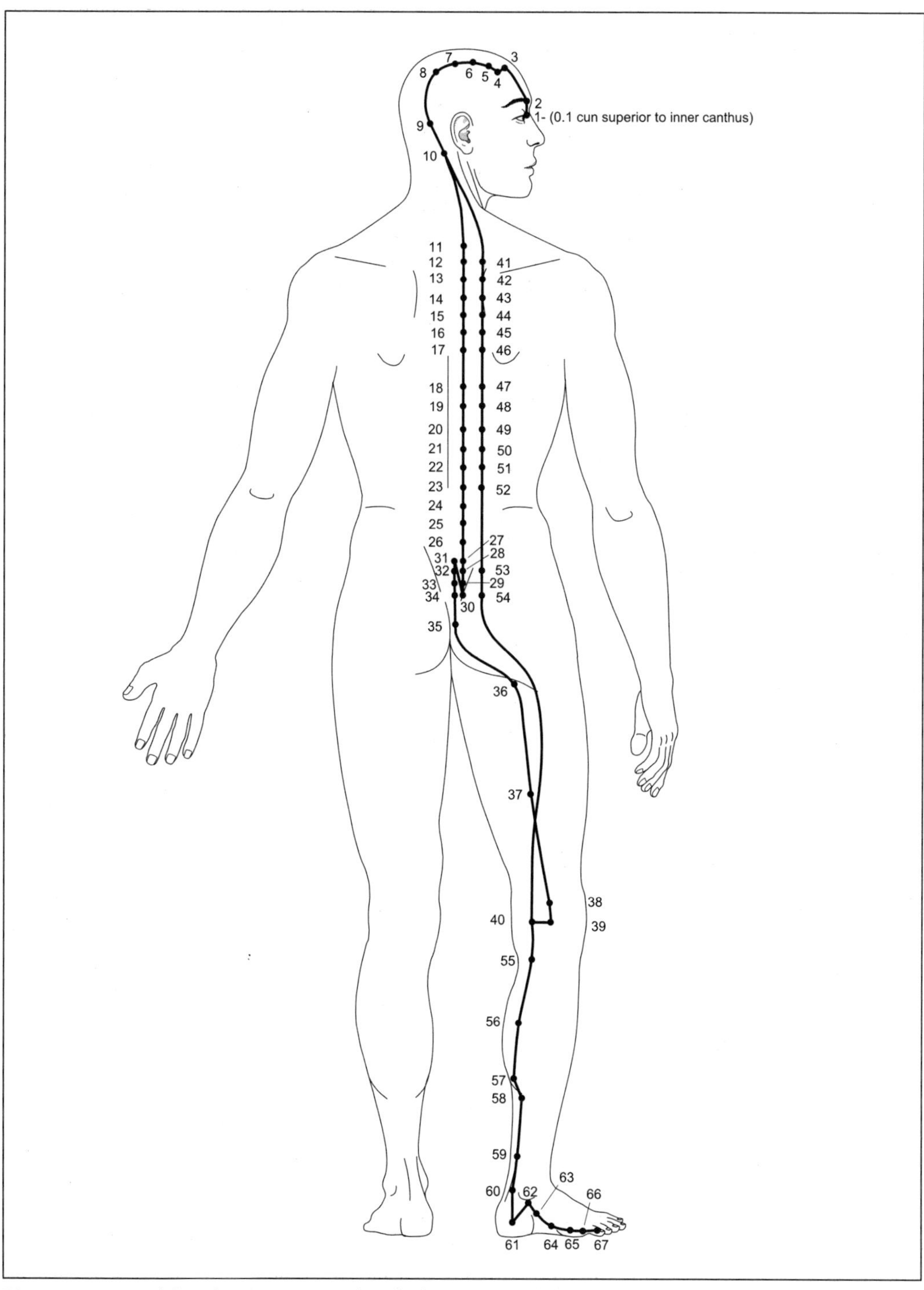

Figure 11.7 Nodal pathway associated with the posterior lateral distribution and collateral vessels of the lower extremity (foot *taiyang*), related to the bladder.

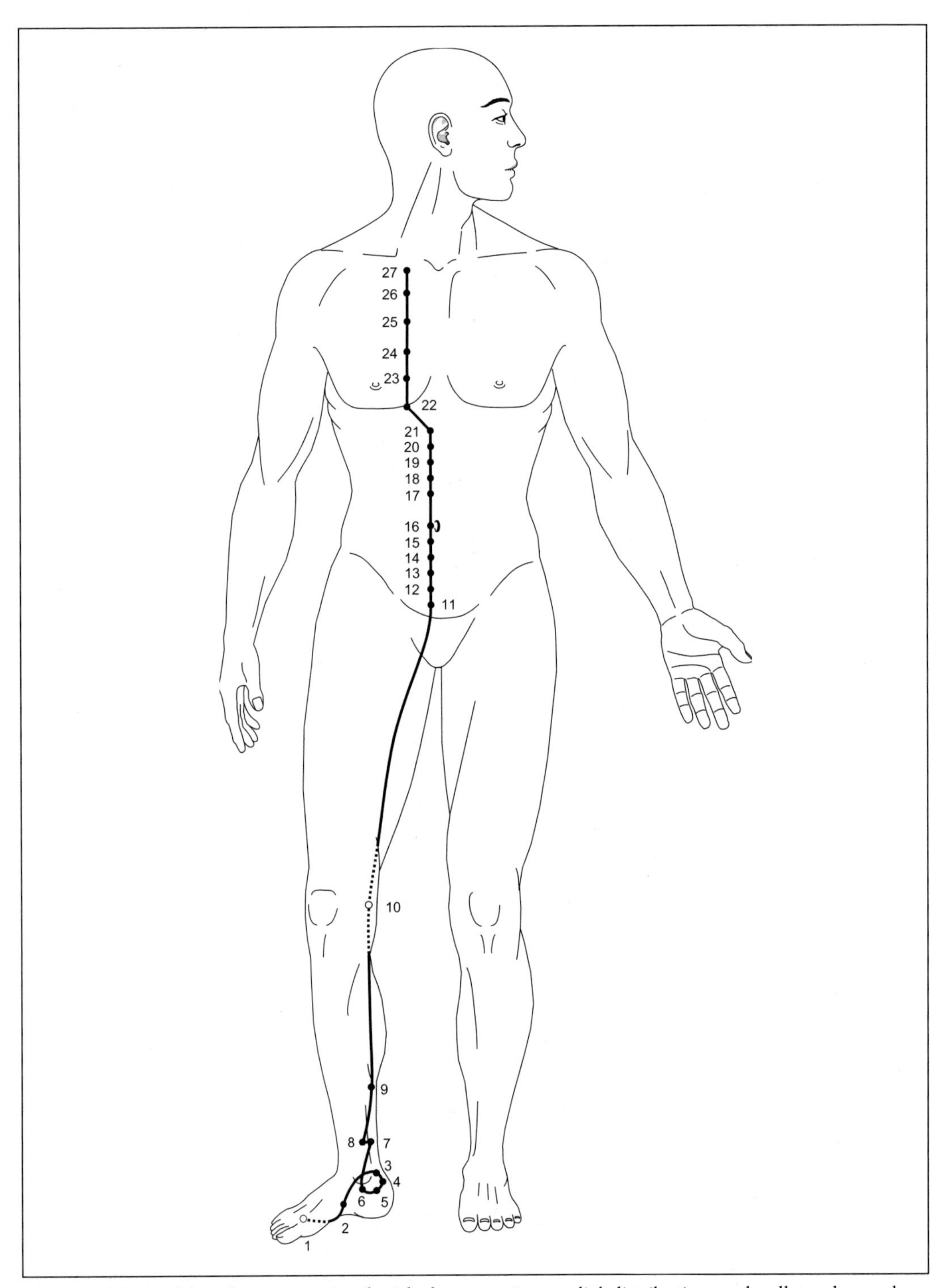

Figure 11.8 Nodal pathway associated with the posterior medial distribution and collateral vessels of the lower extremity (foot *shaoyin*), related to the kidneys.

palmar artery] following along the radial aspect of the little finger to its extremity [proper palmar digital artery].

Disorders due to circulation in the heart distribution vessel and the heart itself are noted in Table 11.3.

When the above diseases are abundant [excess] disorders, the patient's pulse at Taiyuan [LU 9] will be three times as great as at the neck pulse at Renying [ST 9]. If the diseases are hollow [deficient] disorders, the patient's pulse at Taiyuan [LU 9] will conversely be smaller than the neck pulse at Renying [ST 9].

Vessels of Posterior Lateral Hand: Small Intestine

The distribution vessel of the posterior lateral aspect of the upper extremity [small intestine] arises at the extremity of the little finger [dorsal digital veins]. It then follows along the outer side of the hand upward to the wrist, where it reaches the head of the ulnar bone [dorsal venous network and basilic vein]. It follows directly up along the lower border of the ulna, reaching the medial side of the elbow [basilic vein] between the two tendons [space between the medial epicondyle and the olecranon]. It then follows upward along the posterior aspect of the humerus to reach the shoulder joint [axillary vein], where it winds around to the scapula [venous branches to the scapula].

Simultaneously it continues up the shoulder to enter the region of the supraclavicular fossa [subclavian vein], where it makes a collateral connection with the heart [coronary veins]. It follows along the larynx [vena cava] to below the diaphragm to reach the region of the stomach [inferior vena cava], and makes connections with the small intestine [portal vein then superior mesenteric veins].

Table 11.3 Indications for the two main distribution (*jing*) vessels of the upper extremity, supplying the posterior body superficial area (heart and small intestine).

Jing *Vessel*	*Indications*
Heart	Posterior Medial Upper Extremity (Hand *Shaoyin*)
Vessel	Dry throat; cardialgia; thirst with desire to drink, which is due to upstream flow of vital substance in arms.
Heart Organ	Yellowish eyes; pain in chest; pain and cold sensations along medial posterior aspect of upper and lower arms; and fever and pain in palm.
Small Intestine	Posterior Lateral Upper Extremity (Hand *Taiyang*)
Vessel	Sore throat; swelling in region of chin; inability to turn neck; shoulder feels seized; and upper arm feels broken.
Body Fluids	Deafness; yellowish eyes; swollen cheeks; and pain along lateral posterior aspects of neck, chin, shoulder, upper arm, elbow, and forearm.

A branch of this vessel travels up the neck from the supraclavicular region [external jugular vein] to the cheek [retromandibular vein] until it reaches the outer canthus of the eye [middle temporal vein], where it turns back to enter the ear. Another branch of this vessel goes up from the cheek to the cheekbones, reaching the nose and continuing to the inner canthus of the eye, and then obliquely branching to the cheekbones.

Disorders due to circulation in the small intestine distribution vessel and in body fluids controlled by the small intestine are noted in Table 11.3.

When the above diseases are abundant [excess] disorders, the patient's neck pulse at Renying [ST 9] will be three times as great as at Taiyuan [LU 9]. If the diseases are hollow (deficient) disorders, the patient's neck pulse at Renying [ST 9] will conversely be smaller than the pulse at Taiyuan [LU 9].

Vessels of Posterior Lateral Foot: Bladder

The distribution vessel of the posterior lateral aspect of the lower extremity [bladder] arises at the inner canthus of the eye, and travels upward [supratrochlear artery] over the forehead to reach the vertex. A branch of this vessel travels from the vertex until it reaches the top of the ear [parietal branch, superficial temporal artery]. A direct branch [branches of occipital artery] travels from the vertex, down the back of the head, and joins the collateral vessels [vertebral arteries] distributed to the brain [basilar artery], where these vessels turn around to exit as a branch that travels down the neck [vertebral arteries]. From here it follows out to the underside of the scapula and distributes on each side of the spine equally [intercostal arteries] until it reaches the lumbar region.

Deeper [internally] it follows the spine [abdominal aorta] to form collateral branches with the kidneys [renal arteries], and joins with the bladder [superior vesical arteries].

A branch from the lumbar region travels downward on each side of the spine to penetrate the buttocks [superior and inferior gluteal arteries], and continues down [first, second, and third perforating arteries of the deep femoral artery] to the popliteal fossa [popliteal artery].

Another branch from the medial border of the right and left scapulae follows downward in a continuous line from the scapular region, traveling on each side of the spine [perforating branches of the costal arteries] to the region of the greater trochanter [hip joint], then following along the medial posterior aspect of the thigh [deep femoral artery perforating branches] below to the popliteal fossa, where it joins the former branch.

From here it continues downward passing through the deep regions of the gastrocnemius muscle [peroneal artery] to reach the posterior aspect of the lateral malleolus. It then follows along the tuberosity of the fifth metatarsal bone [dorsal and plantar metatarsal arteries] to the lateral side of the small toe [dorsal and plantar digital arteries].

Disorders due to circulation in the bladder distribution vessel and muscles controlled by the bladder are noted in Table 11.4.

When the above diseases are abundant [excess] disorders, the patient's neck pulse at Renying [ST 9] will be three times as great as at Taiyuan [LU 9]. If the diseases are hollow [deficient] disorders, the patient's neck pulse at Renying [ST 9] will conversely be smaller than the pulse at Taiyuan [LU 9].

Table 11.4 Indications for the two main distribution (*jing*) vessels of the lower extremity, supplying the posterior body superficial area (bladder and kidneys).

Jing *Vessel*	*Indications*
Bladder	Posterior Lateral Lower Extremity (Foot *Taiyang*)
Vessel	Throbbing headache; sensation like eyeball is being pushed out; seized neck; back pain; low back feels like it is broken; inability to bend (extend) thigh; sensation like popliteal fossa is bound up; sensation like gastrocnemius is split, due to an upsurge of vital substance from region of lateral malleolus.
Influence on Muscles	Hemorrhoids; malaria; madness; mental derangement; headache; pain in top of head and pain in nape of neck; yellowish eyes; lacrimation; rhinitis and nosebleed; pain in all areas including the nape of neck, back, lumbar region, buttocks, popliteal fossa, gastrocnemius, and feet; and stiffness and dysfunction of small toe.
Kidneys	Posterior Medial Lower Extremity (Foot *Shaoyin*)
Vessel	Hunger with no desire to eat (anorexia); face black as a burnt offering; coughing and spitting up blood; uproarious heavy breathing (asthma); sitting with desire to stand up; inability to focus the eyes (blurred vision); and mind feels anxious, like in the case of a starving condition.
Functional Deficiency	Great fright, with mind exhibiting extreme cautiousness like a military general in combat, all of which is due to an upsurge of activities in the bones.
Kidney Organs	Hot mouth with dry tongue; swollen throat; belching; pain reaching throat; mental vexations (depression); cardialgia; jaundice; bloody stools; pain in back and inner posterior aspect of thigh; paralysis (flaccidity) with cold limbs and addiction to sleeping; and burning pain on the bottom of foot (causalgia).

Vessels of Posterior Medial Foot: Kidneys

The distribution vessel of the posterior medial aspect of the lower extremity [kidneys] arises at the plantar aspect of the small toe [plantar digital veins], where it deflects through the sole of the foot [lateral plantar vein] to reach below the tuberosity of the navicular bone [Rangu, KD 2]. It then follows up behind the medial malleolus, where a branch reaches the calcaneous. The main vessel continues upward into the gastrocnemius muscle [posterior tibial vein] and continues up to the medial aspect of the popliteal fossa [sural vessels and popliteal vein].

Following upward to the medial posterior aspect of the thigh, it passes through to the backbone to join collateral vessels [superior vesical veins] to the bladder. A straight or direct vessel continues upward from the kidneys [renal vein] to pass through the liver [vena cava] and diaphragm, and enters the central region of the lungs [pulmonary arteries]. It then follows along the larynx to reach both sides of the root of the tongue [jugular vein, superior thyroid vein, sublingual vein]. A branch of this vessel travels from the lungs to exit in the collateral branches [pulmonary veins] to the heart, which are concentrated in the center of the thorax.

> The application of moxibustion can strengthen the appetite and rebuild the flesh. The patient should loosen their belts and unroll their hair for the treatment. Also, they should use a big cane or staff, and wear heavy shoes to aid walking.

Disorders due to circulation in the kidney distribution vessel, the kidneys themselves, and kidney vital substance deficiency are noted in Table 11.4.

> When the above diseases are abundant [excess] disorders, the patient's pulse at Taiyuan [LU 9] will be three times as great as at the neck pulse at Renying [ST 9]. If the diseases are hollow [deficient] disorders, the patient's pulse at Taiyuan [LU 9] will conversely be smaller than the neck pulse at Renying [ST 9].

Medial and Lateral Vessel and Nodal Pathways

The medial and lateral aspect in the Chinese anatomical orientation of the arms, legs, side of the head, and side of the trunk are supplied by four major distribution vessels that serve the pericardium, internal membrane system, gallbladder, and liver, and give rise to nodal pathways that traverse this region of the body. The distribution pathways are discussed below individually for these vessels, along with pathology affecting the vessels themselves or along the vessel pathway, in addition to problems of the organs or their related tissues or functions. Table 11.5 summarizes this information for the vessels of the pericardium and internal membrane; Table 11.6 for the gallbladder and liver.

The pericardium vessel is an outflowing artery that supplies the medial aspects of the arms. Internally it consists of the pericardiacophrenic arteries and the gastroepiploic and other membrane arteries. The internal membrane (*sanjiao*, 三焦) vessel is a return-flowing vein supplying the lateral aspects of the arms, and it drains the regions supplied by the pericardium vessel, except for regions of the shoulder, neck, and face. Internally it consists of the pericardiacophrenic veins and the gastroepiploic and other membrane veins.

The pericardium distribution pathway has nine nodes starting with Tianchi (PC 1), which is located in the fourth intercostal space, 1 cun lateral to the nipple. From here the pathway swings slightly up in order to course down the anterior portion of the arm, crossing the palm and ending at the extremity of the middle finger at Zhongchong (PC 9) (Figure 11.9).

The internal membrane vessel distribution pathway has twenty-three nodes starting at the medial extremity of the fourth finger at Guanchong (SJ 1). From here the pathway continues up the dorsum and posterior arm, continuing up to the posterior shoulder and then the lateral neck. Here it courses around the auricle to terminate in the depression at the lateral end of the eyebrow at Sizhukong (SJ 23) (Figure 11.10).

The gallbladder is an outflowing artery that supplies the head, shoulders, lateral trunk, and lateral legs. Internally it consists of the hepatic and cystic arteries. The liver vessel is a return-flowing vein supplying the medial aspects of the lower extremity, and it drains the regions supplied by the gallbladder vessel in the leg and feet areas. Internally it consists of the proper hepatic and cystic veins. The gallbladder vessel distribution pathway contains forty-four nodes, and begins 0.5 cun lateral to the outer canthus of the eye at Tongziliao (GB 1). From here it courses over and around the auricle and then back to the forehead, where it then travels over to the back of the head in the lateral aspect. It then distributes down to the shoulder, passing in front of the arm to continue down the entire lateral aspect of the body. It moves on to the foot, ending at the lateral extremity of the fourth toe at Zuqiaoyin (GB 44) (Figure 11.11).

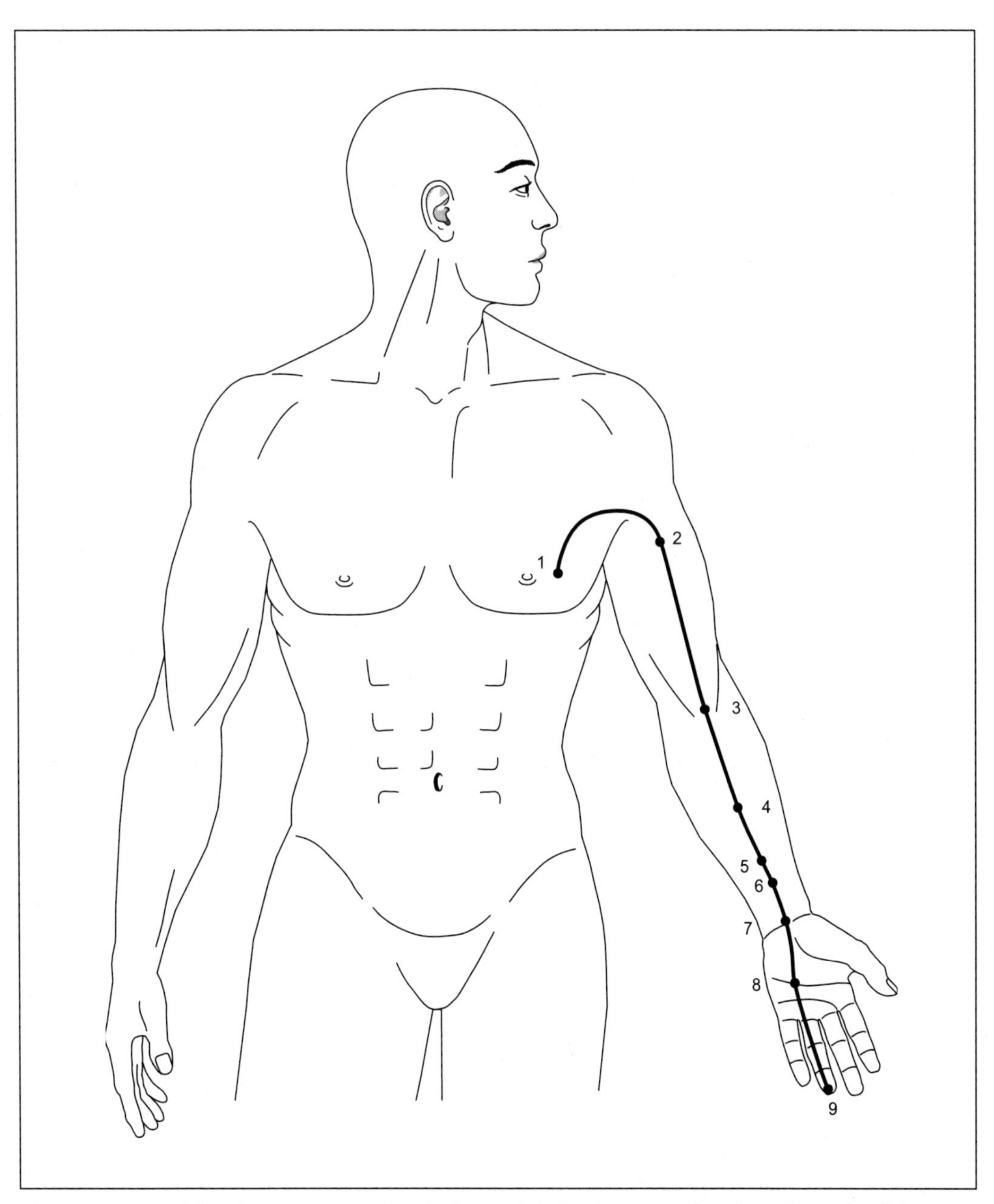

Figure 11.9 Nodal pathway associated with the medial distribution and collateral vessels of the upper extremity (hand *jueyin*), related to the pericardium.

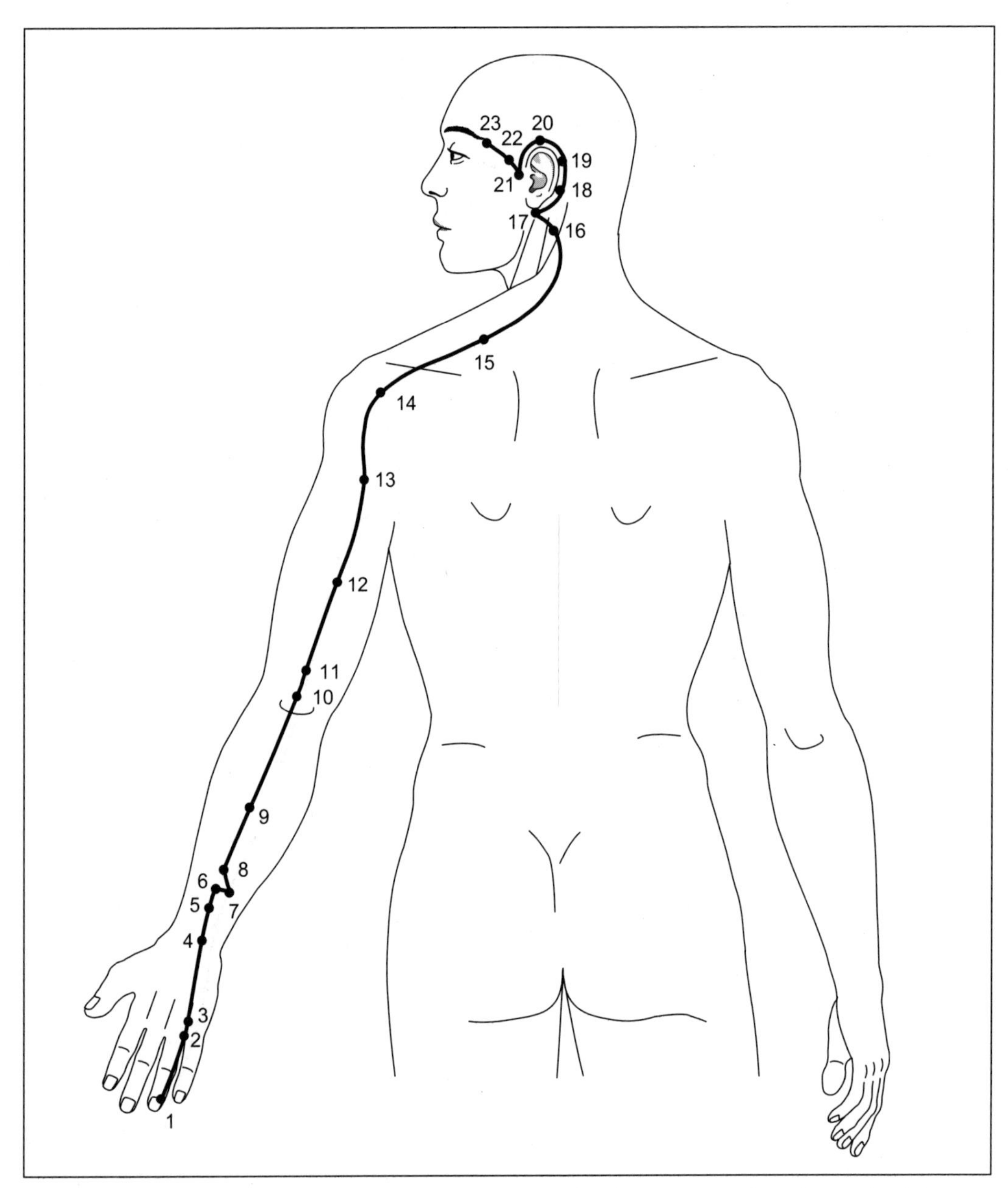

Figure 11.10 Nodal pathway associated with the lateral distribution and collateral vessels of the upper extremity (hand *shaoyang*), related to the internal membrane (*sanjiao*).

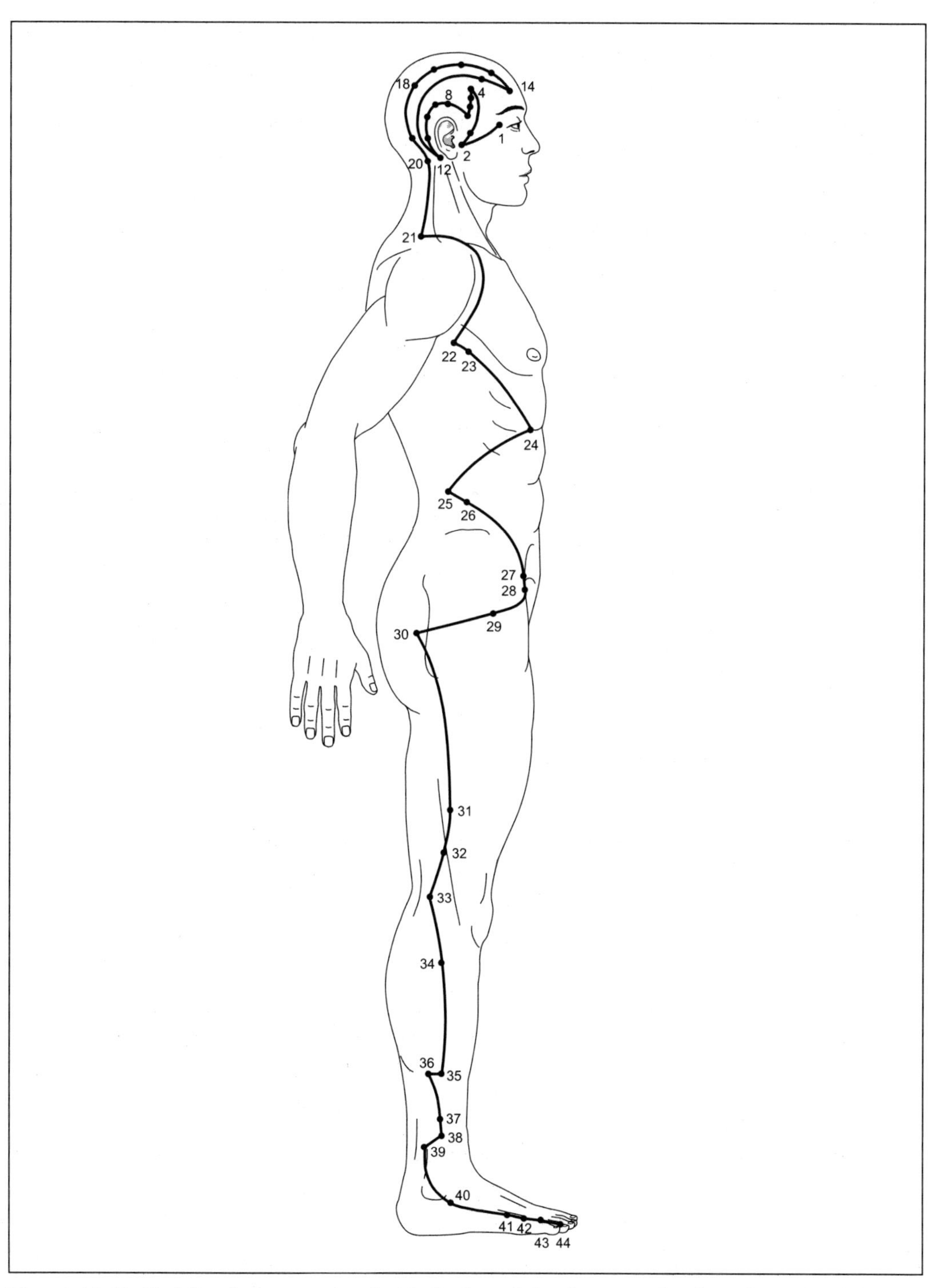

Figure 11.11 Nodal pathway associated with the lateral distribution and collateral vessels of the lower extremity (foot *shaoyang*), related to the gallbladder.

The liver vessel distribution pathway contains fourteen nodes starting with Dadun (LV 1), located at the lateral extremity of the big toe. From here it travels up the dorsum anterior to the medial malleolus, traveling up the anterior medial aspect of the leg. It passes on to the abdominal regions and terminates in the sixth intercostal space directly in line with the nipple at Qimen (LV 14) (Figure 11.12).

Vessels of Medial Hand: Pericardium

> The distribution vessel of the medial aspect of the upper extremity [pericardium] of the external membrane of the heart arises in the center of the thorax cavity, where it reaches and joins the pericardium [pericardiacophrenic arteries]. It travels down through the diaphragm to form collateral branches [gastroepiploic arteries and other membrane arteries] to all three segments of the visceral peritoneum [sanjiao] system.
>
> A branch of this vessel [lateral thoracic artery] follows along the thorax to reach the ribs 3 cun below the armpit to distribute from the axilla above [axillary artery]. It then follows down along the medial aspect of the humerus [brachial artery], traveling between the anterior medial hand [lung] and posterior medial hand [heart] distribution vessels, where it reaches the cubital fossa. It travels down the forearm [common interosseous artery] between the two tendons [flexor carpi radialis tendon and palmaris longus tendon] to enter the palm, and then follows along the middle finger to reach its extremity [common proper palmar artery, proper palmar digital arteries]. A branch of this vessel distributes to the little finger [radial side] and the fourth finger to reach their extremities [proper palmar digital arteries].

Disorders due to circulation in the pericardium distribution vessel and general blood circulation controlled by the pericardium are noted in Table 11.5.

Table 11.5 Indications for the two main distribution (*jing*) vessels of the upper extremity, supplying the medial and lateral body superficial area (pericardium and internal membrane system).

Jing *Vessel*	*Indications*
Pericardium	Medial Upper Extremity (Hand *Jueyin*)
Vessel	Infection of palm; acute contractions of elbow and upper arm; swelling of axilla; and in very serious conditions, congested chest, violent throbbing of heart, red face, yellowish eyes, and joy of laughing without ceasing.
Blood Circulation	Mental vexations, cardialgia, and a hot sensation in the palms.
Internal Membrane	Lateral Upper Extremity (Hand *Shaoyang*) (*Sanjiao*)
Vessel	Deafness; diminished hearing due to ringing in ears and humming in ears; and swollen throat with sore larynx.
Vital Substance	Sweating; pain in eye and outer canthus; pain in lateral aspect of region behind ear, shoulder, upper arm, elbow, and forearm; dysfunction and stiffness in little finger and fourth finger.

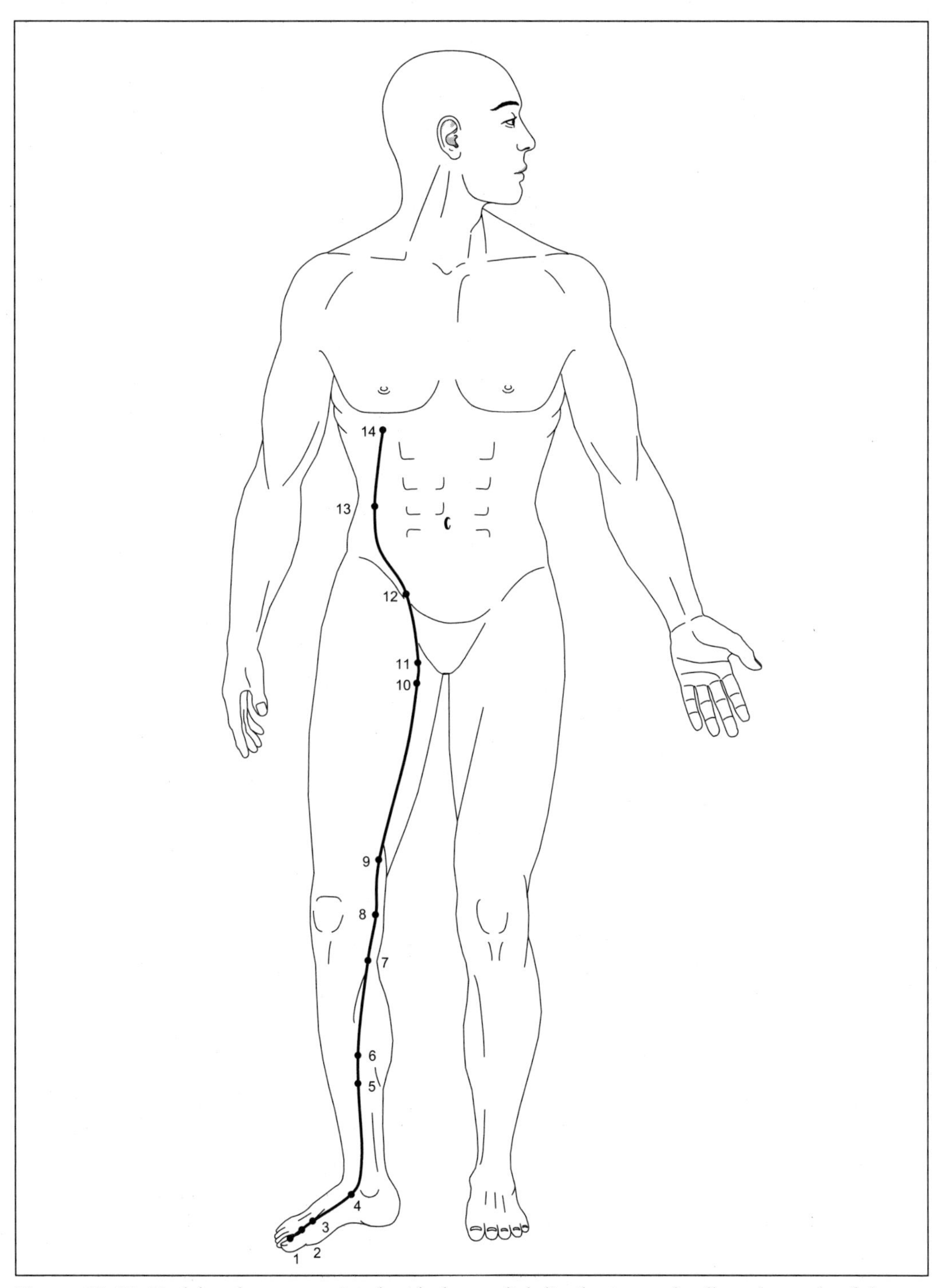

Figure 11.12 Nodal pathway associated with the medial distribution and collateral vessels of the lower extremity (foot *jueyin*), related to the liver.

When the above diseases are abundant [excess] disorders, the patient's pulse at Taiyuan [LU 9] will be twice as great as at the neck pulse at Renying [ST 9]. If the diseases are hollow [deficient] disorders, the patient's pulse at Taiyuan [LU 9] will conversely be smaller than the neck pulse at Renying [ST 9].

Vessels of Lateral Hand: Internal Membrane

The distribution vessel of the lateral upper extremity [internal membrane] arises at the extremities of the little finger [radial side] and fourth finger [dorsal digital veins]. Above, it reaches between the fourth and fifth fingers to follow along the dorsum of the hand to the wrist [dorsal venous network]. It then continues along the lateral aspect of the forearm, traveling between the ulnar and radial bones to enter the elbow. It then travels along the posterior aspect of the humerus to reach the shoulder above. Here it crosses behind the lateral foot [gallbladder] vessel and enters the supraclavicular fossa [junction of jugular vein and subclavian vein].

From here it spreads through the center of the thorax to disperse into the visceral pericardium [pericardiacophrenic veins]. Below this it passes through the diaphragm to join the three segments of the visceral peritoneum [sanjiao] [gastroepiploic veins and other membrane veins].

A branch of this vessel travels from the center of the thorax, up to the supraclavicular fossa, continuing up the nape of the neck [external jugular vein], and going up behind the ear [posterior auricular vein] to reach the area above the tip of the ear. From here it bends down around [superficial temporal vein] in front of the ear to the cheek, and then continues to the cheekbone [transverse facial vein]. Another branch from behind the ear travels to the internal ear region and exits to travel in front of the ear, traveling over in front of the node Kezhuren [Shangguan, GB 3], crossing the cheek to reach the outer corner of the eye [zygomaticoorbital vein].

Disorders due to circulation in the internal membrane distribution vessel or disturbances along the vessel, or in vital substances controlled by the internal membrane, are noted in Table 11.5.

When the above diseases are abundant [excess] disorders, the patient's neck pulse at Renying [ST 9] will be twice as great as at Taiyuan [LU 9]. If the diseases are hollow [deficient] disorders, the patient's pulse at Taiyuan [LU 9] will conversely be smaller than the neck pulse at Renying [ST 9].

Vessels of Lateral Foot: Gallbladder

The distribution vessel of the lateral lower extremity [gallbladder] arises at the outer angle of the eye [zygomaticoorbital artery]. Above, it reaches the temporal region [superficial temporal artery], where it travels behind the ear [branches of the superficial temporal and posterior auricular arteries] to follow along the neck [ascending cervical artery], then traveling in front of the internal membrane [sanjiao] lateral hand vessel at the top of the shoulder [superficial branch, traverse cervical artery]. From here it drives back to cross behind the internal membrane [sanjiao] lateral hand vessel, entering the supraclavicular fossa [subclavian artery].

Another branch of this vessel travels from behind the ear to enter the internal ear, and then exits to travel in front of the ear, continuing to the posterior aspect of the outer angle of the eye [maxillary and deep temporal arteries].

Another branch travels from the outer angle of the eye [transverse facial and external carotid arteries] downward to Daying [ST 5] [facial artery]. It also joins with the visceral peritoneum [sanjiao] lateral hand vessel to reach the cheekbone. Continuing below, it reaches the masseter [Jiache, ST 6] and then continues down the neck to join its main vessel at the supraclavicular fossa [common carotid artery].

It then continues down through the center of the thorax [aorta] to pass through the diaphragm, where it distributes a collateral branch to the liver [hepatic artery] and joins the gallbladder [cystic artery]. It continues downward internally, following below the ribs to reach the vital substance street [Qichong, ST 30] [external iliac artery], where it winds around the pubic hair region [external pudendal arteries]. A transverse branch enters the region of the greater trochanter [medial femoral circumflex artery and trochanteric network].

A separate branch travels from the supraclavicular fossa [axillary artery] to below the axilla [thoracodorsal artery], following along the rib cage to reach the lower ribs [perforating branches of costal and subcostal arteries]. Below [superficial circumflex iliac artery], it joins its former branch at the greater trochanter.

It then follows below along the outer thigh [descending branch, lateral femoral circumflex artery] to reach the lateral aspect of the knee [inferior lateral genicular and anterior tibial recurrent arteries], continuing down along the lateral anterior aspect of the fibula [branches of anterior tibial artery]. It travels straight down to reach the extremity of the fibula [perforating branch of peroneal artery]. Below, it reaches the ankle to travel in front of the lateral malleolus [anterior lateral malleolar artery], following along the dorsum of the foot [lateral tarsal artery] to enter between the small toe and the fourth toe [dorsal metatarsal artery]. Another branch goes across the dorsal aspect of the foot [arcuate artery] to reach the joint of the big toe, following along the lateral side of the bone juncture to reach its extremity [lateral dorsal digital artery of the big toe]. Here it distributes to the big toenail and reaches the hair on the proximal phalanx of the big toe.

Disorders due to circulation in the gallbladder distribution vessel or disturbances along the vessel, or the bones controlled by the gallbladder, are noted in Table 11.6.

When the above diseases are abundant [excess] disorders, the patient's neck pulse at Renying [ST 9] will be twice as great as at Taiyuan [LU 9]. If the diseases are hollow [deficient] disorders, the patient's neck pulse at Renying [ST 9] will conversely be smaller than the pulse at Taiyuan [LU 9].

Vessels of Medial Foot: Liver

The distribution vessel of the medial lower extremity [liver] arises at the big toe in the margins of the hair on the dorsum of the toe [lateral digital veins of the big toe]. From

Table 11.6 Indications for the two main distribution (*jing*) vessels of the lower extremity, supplying the lateral and medial body superficial area (gallbladder and liver).

Jing *Vessel*	*Indications*
Gallbladder	Lateral Lower Extremity (Foot *Shaoyang*)
Vessel	Bitter taste in mouth; frequent sighing; pain in ribs and heart with inability to turn upper body; a serious condition where complexion appears as if patient has fine dust on their face; skin of body not oily or moist (dry and dull skin).
Bones	Headache; pain in chin; pain in eye and outer angle of eyes; pain and swelling in supraclavicular region; swelling below axilla; axillary and cervical lymphadenitis resembling a saber or string of beads; perspiration with shivering; malaria; pain in all sites along thorax, lateral side of ribs, hypochrondrum, thigh, knee, lateral aspect of the tibia, distal end of fibula, and anterior region of lateral malleolus; and dysfunction and stiffness in small toe and fourth toe.
Liver	Medial Foot Lower Extremity (Foot *Jueyin*)
Vessel	Low back pain with inability to bend or lift head; conditions in males that could include incarcerated hernia, ulcerative lesion of external genitalia, swelling and pain or nodulation and numbness of scrotum; in females, lower abdominal swelling; and a very serious condition characterized by dry throat, dusty-appearing face, and faded complexion.
Liver Organ	Fullness of chest with vomiting and lienteric diarrhea; inguinal hernia; enuresis and dysuria.

there it follows up the dorsal aspect of the foot to pass within 1 cun of the medial malleolus and continues upward [anterior tibial vein] to cross behind the spleen–anterior medial foot vessel 8 cun above the malleolus.

It continues up through the medial aspect of the popliteal fossa following along the inner aspect of the thigh to enter the region of the pubic hair [external pudendal veins]. It travels over to the genitalia [dorsal vein of penis and scrotal veins in males, dorsal vein of clitoris and labial veins in females].

It enters the lower abdomen [external iliac vein], travels up to the stomach [inferior vena cava] and joins with the liver [proper hepatic vein], with a collateral vessel traveling to the gallbladder [cystic vein]. Above this, it passes through the diaphragm and spreads in the costal region [superficial perforating veins on abdomen and lower ribs].

It follows behind the larynx to enter the jugular foramen [internal jugular vein] to link with the eye connections [superior ophthalmic and ophthalmic veins], above which it exits [nasofrontal vein] at the forehead [supratrochlear vein] to distribute to the governing [du] vessel, meeting at the vertex. A branch from the eye connections descends to the inside of the cheek, circling around the inside of the lips. Another branch travels from the liver, passes through the diaphragm, and pours into the lungs [vena cava].

Disorders due to circulation in the liver distribution vessel or disturbances along those vessels, or due to the liver itself, are noted in Table 11.6.

When the above diseases are abundant [excess] disorders, the patient's pulse at Taiyuan [LU 9] will be twice as great as at the neck pulse at Renying [ST 9]. If the diseases are hollow [deficient] disorders, the patient's pulse at Taiyuan [LU 9] will conversely be smaller than the neck pulse at Renying [ST 9].

Deep Singular Vessel Nodal Pathways

The deep singular vessels consist of the thoroughfare (chong aorta), allowance (ren), and governing (du)—these vessels are discussed in Chapter 9. Internally the thoroughfare is the chong aorta. The allowance (ren) vessel consists of the vena cava, and all the major veins supplying the head are considered secondary branches of this vessel. The governing (du) vessel consists of the azygos, hemiazygos, and ascending lumbar veins, which drain the posterior portion of the body, including the intercostal veins. The role of these major vascular structures in the circulatory system is to support the main distribution vessels (Figures 9.1 and 10.1). Both the allowance (ren) and governing (du) vessels have important nodal pathways that respectively traverse the anterior and posterior central body line. The thoroughfare vessel (chong aorta) has superficial arterial pathways on the lower abdomen that are coincident with the kidney distribution vessel superficial venous route. Hence nodes of the thoroughfare vessel are coincident with kidney node locations on the lower abdomen. Nodal locations and pathways for these three singular vessels were originally discussed in *NJSW 59* (*On the Storehouses of Vital Substances*).

Thoroughfare Vessel

The thoroughfare vessel (chong aorta) has eleven nodes 0.5 cun lateral to each side of the abdominal midline, starting 1 cun below Jiuwei (RN 15), with six sites down to the umbilicus, coincident with Youmen, KD 21; Futonggu, KD 20; Yindu, KD 19; Shiguan, KD 18; Shangqu, KD 17; and Huangshu, KD 16. Continuing on the same line from 1 cun below the umbilicus, for each cun down to the pubic bone there are five locations coincident with Zhongzhu, KD 15; Simen, KD 14; Qixue, KD 13; Dahe, KD 12; and Henggu, KD 11 (Figure 11.8). Counting each side there are twenty-two nodes in all.

Allowance Vessel

The allowance (ren) vessel distribution pathway contains twenty-four nodes that course up the anterior centerline of the body. The pathway starts at Huiyin (RN 1) located between the anus and the scrotum in males, or between the anus and the posterior labial commissure in females. From here it travels up the body to end below the lower lip in the mentolabial groove at Chengjiang (RN 24) (Figure 11.13).

Governing Vessel

The superficial course of the governing (du) vessel traverses along the midline of the back, starting below the tip of the coccyx and traveling over the head to end in the upper mouth. The importance of the governing (du) vessel is that all the nodes exist at locations where nerve branches meet from both sides of the body. Stimulation of these sites activates both right and

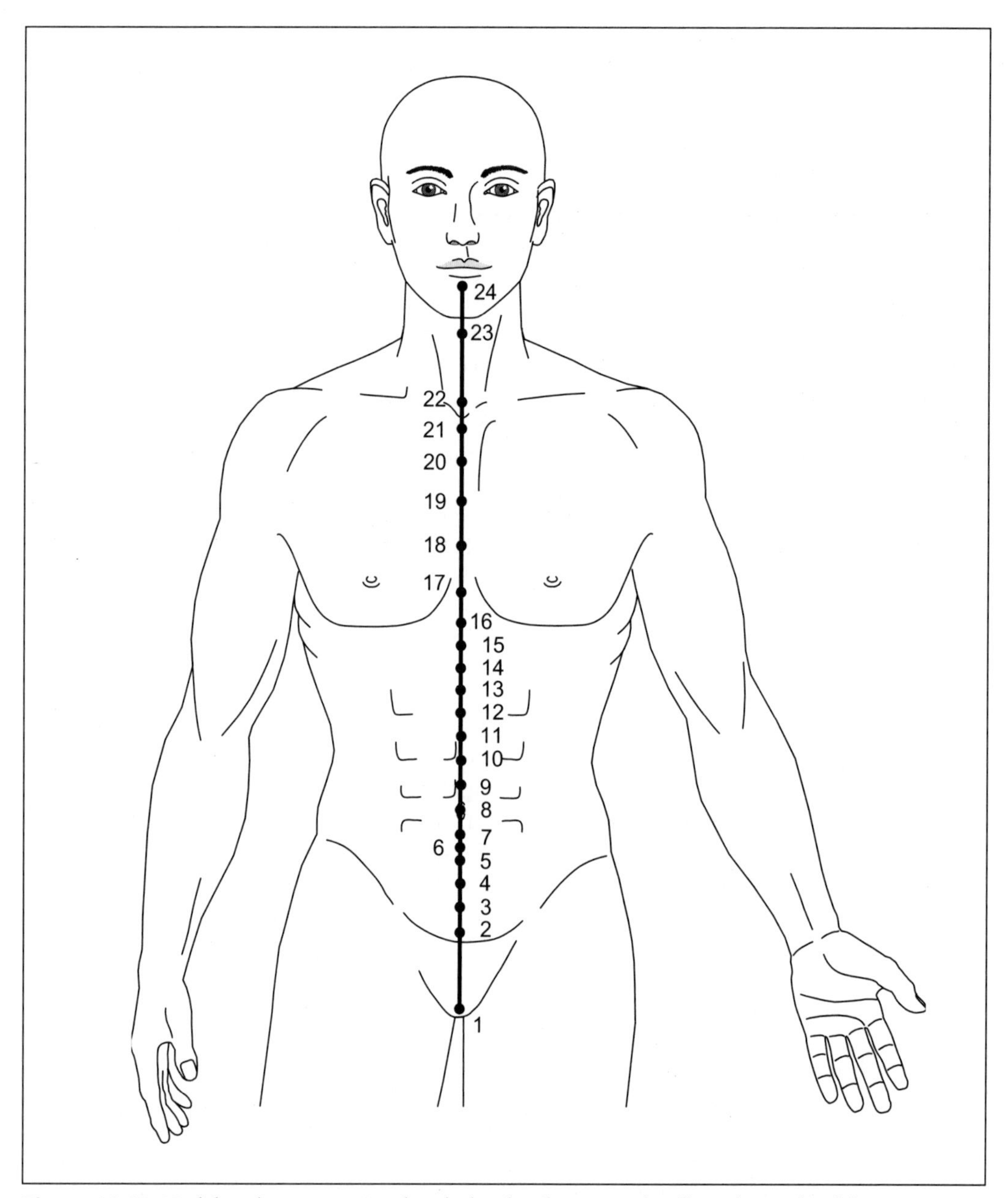

Figure 11.13 Nodal pathway associated with the distribution and collateral vessels of the anterior centerline, related to the allowance (*ren*) singular vessel.

left afferent pathways. Nodes along the spinal column are primarily innervated by posterior rami nerve branches, while sites on the allowance (ren) vessel are represented by anterior rami. For these reasons the location of both the governing (du) and allowance (ren) vessels has a significant influence on the internal organs. Also, several of these nodes are important integration or crossing sites for the other vessels, such as Dazhui (DU 14) and Zhongji (RN 3).

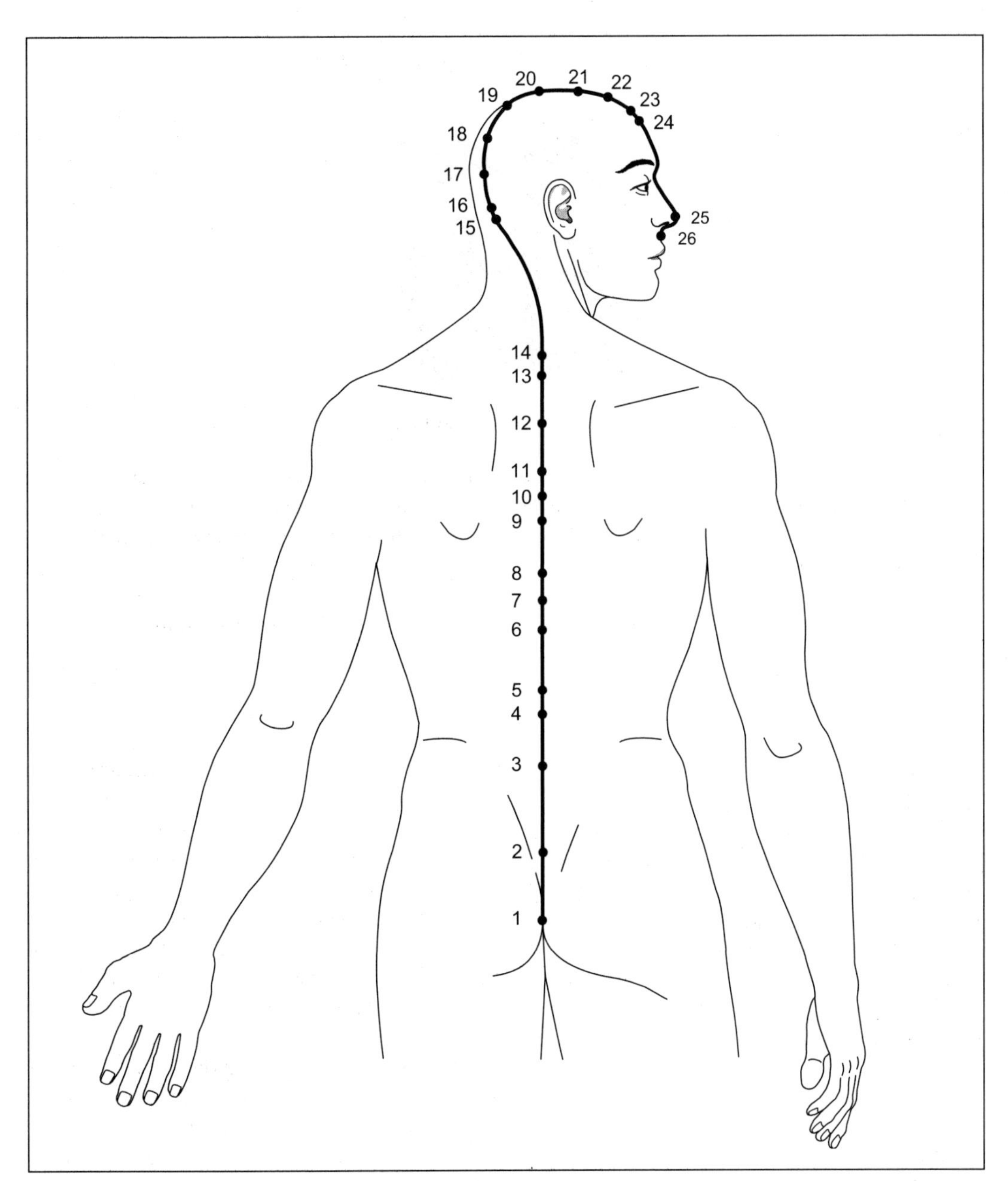

Figure 11.14 Nodal pathway associated with the distribution and collateral vessels of the posterior centerline, related to the governing (*du*) singular vessels.

The governing (du) vessel distribution pathway contains twenty-eight nodes, starting midway between the coccyx and the anus at Changqiang (DU 1). From here it travels up the centerline of the back, over the top of the head, and down the center of the face to end inside the upper lip at the junction of the gum and frenulum at Yinjiao (DU 28) (Figure 11.14).

12

Muscle Distributions

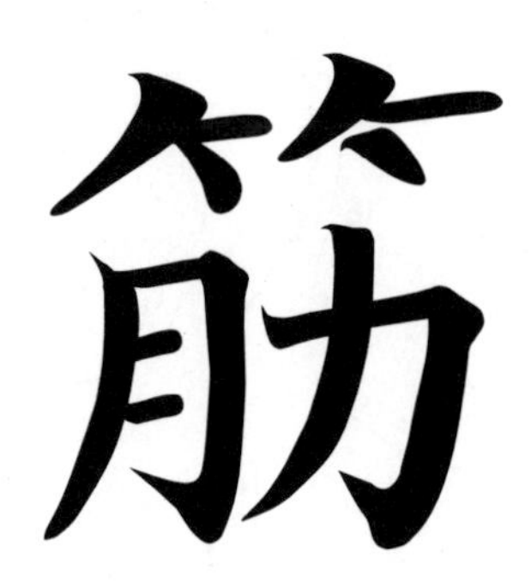

Jin: Muscle

> I have heard that the sages of ancient times understood the logic of the human body, … discovered and named the sites for needling, determined the distribution of muscles and their attachments to the bones, and all of the origins of these muscles, and also identified the skin zones.
>
> Yellow Emperor,
> *NJSW 5 (Great Treatise on the Proper Representation of Yin and Yang)*

Muscles act on specific joints of the body to provide movement and are organized in longitudinal distribution patterns in the same twelve yin-yang anatomical regions as their related distribution vessels (Chapter 11). Unlike the vessels, muscles relate only indirectly to specific internal organs—except for the diaphragm and the lungs—through their pairing with specific distribution vessels. Muscles can, however, develop spasm, cramps, and pain as a result of organ problems. Muscles are classified as being part of the external body, and most musculoskeletal problems are external disorders, unless an internal organ is the primary source of the problem. The description of the twelve muscle distributions in *NJLS 13* (*Muscle Distributions*) demonstrates a thorough understanding of the muscular system. Even before the Zhou Dynasty, the ancients had already identified all the muscles and their attachments to specific bones. Muscles are supplied by specific longitudinal distribution vessels and nerves associated with certain regions of the body. Needling-induced propagated sensations (PS) travel along the superficial muscle and vessel pathways, while the development of sensitive locations due to musculoskeletal pathology usually distribute along these same muscle pathways. Sensitive sites can reflect organ pathology as well.

The Chinese for muscle distribution is *jingjin* (经筋), where the word *jing* (经), meaning longitudinal distribution, is applied to all distribution vessels. The character *jin* (筋)[1] is a complex ideograph for skeletal muscle, including muscle tissue, fascia, and tendons (Figure 12.1). The primary element of the character has two components: the first being *rou* (肉), which is a pictographic representation of flesh or muscle tissue; the second element, *li* (力), depicts a tendon or sinew, and is often used to denote strength. When combined, these two components indicate muscle tissue with its fascia and tendons. The components rou and li together make the character *lei* (肋), which denotes the costal region and intercostal muscles.

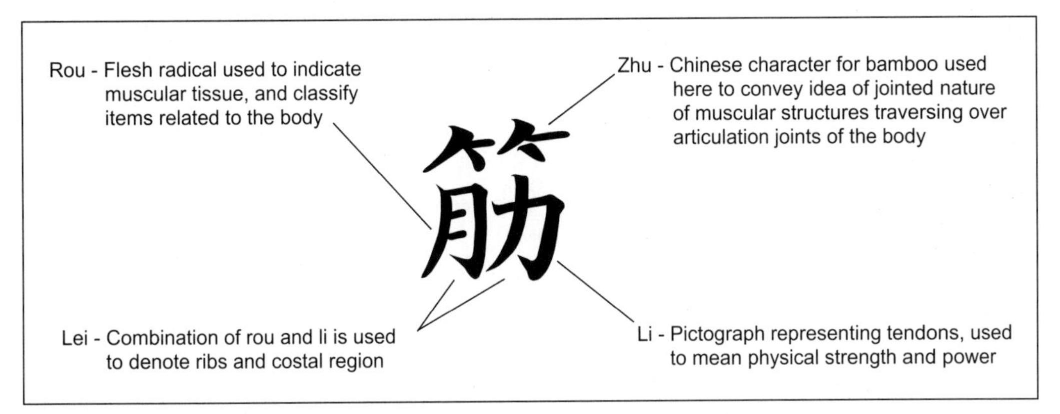

Figure 12.1 Derivation of the Chinese character *jin* for skeletal muscles.

To convey the idea of skeletal muscles connecting over articulation joints, the radical for bamboo, *zhu* (竹), is added to form jin. Bamboo has segmented joints: by analogy this indicates the longitudinal muscle fibers and tendons traversing from joint to joint. Jin therefore represents the muscles and fascia, along with their connecting tissue fibers, the tendons. This view of muscles is totally consistent with Western terminology. Muscles of motion can only function by directing a contractile force from the bone where the muscle originates over a joint to the bone where its tendon inserts. Thus, the Chinese ideograph jin is as fully descriptive as the Western concept of muscle. Sometimes this character is interpreted to represent musculotendinous or tendinomuscular structures.

Features of the Muscular System

The muscular system, comprised mostly of muscle tissue, has several unique features aside from the function of moving the body. First, many muscles have different capabilities to perform their specific function, related to the speed of the muscle and its inherent strength. It is now know that muscles are composed of different types of tissue fibers to mediate their respective functions (Table 12.1). The ancient Chinese may have appreciated the subtle differences between the muscles, borne out by the fact that nodal sites in muscles are usually found in the slower muscles and are not found in fast muscles. Muscles are arranged in longitudinal pathways, and sensitive sites within these routes are useful for diagnosis and assessment of treatment. Temperature and color variations in the cutaneous regions that overlie the muscle and vessel distribution pathways are also useful for diagnosis.

Longitudinal Organization

Metaphorically, the longitudinal organization of the muscular system is thought of in terms of streams and valleys, as noted in *NJSW 58* (*Vital Nodes*), where large gatherings of muscles are the valleys and small gatherings are the streams. Spaces between the striated muscles are the meetings of streams and valleys. The importance of muscle and vessel associations along longitudinal pathways is that pathology and muscle dysfunction can be reflected along these routes. Hence diagnosis, assessment, and formulation of treatment approaches are facilitated

Table 12.1 Characteristics of fast-, intermediate-, and slow-twitch muscle fibers.

Phasic (Fast-Twitch)	*Intermediate*	*Tonic (Slow-Twitch)*
Pale in color	Red in color	Red in color
Few mitochondria	Many mitochondria	Many mitochondria
Poorly vascularized	Richly vascularized	Richly vascularized
Anaerobic metabolism (uses glycolysis)	Both oxidative (myoglobin) and anaerobic (glycolysis) metabolism	Oxidative metabolism (myoglobin)
Quick contraction and relaxation	Intermediate range of contraction and relaxation	Slow contraction and relaxation
Fatigue easily	Medium range of fatigability	Resistant to fatigue
Develop wide range of tensions	Average tension range	Develop tension over narrow range of displacement
Suited for high-intensity, short-duration muscle activity	Suited for muscles of motion where wide range of performance activity is crucial	Suited for long-term contraction, such as needed in maintaining posture

by the longitudinal relationships. Knowing the particular muscle pathway involved in a musculoskeletal problem provides an immediate indication of the related vessel. Since nodes are distributed along specific vessel pathways, selection of candidate sites for treating a problem is a logical process.

Motor Points versus Nodal Sites

In comparing the location of nodes to known neuromuscular attachment sites, or motor points as they are often called, it is obvious that there is not a perfect one-to-one correlation. Motor points are areas of enhanced concentration of sensory and motor nerves; however, not all of these locations are good needling sites, indicated by the fact that these are not assigned nodal sites. As an example of good candidates for needling, Feiyang (BL 58) and Zhubin (KD 9) are respectively located at the lateral and medial motor points of the soleus muscle, which is a strong, tonic muscle in the lower leg that is important to posture and must therefore be able to withstand long-term contractions without being fatigued. The lateral and medial portions of the soleus are assigned to the bladder (Figure 12.2) and kidney (Figure 12.6) muscle distributions, respectively. The lateral and medial heads of the gastrocnemius are also respectively assigned to the bladder and kidney muscle distributions; however, this muscle, which has to respond quickly, is classed as an intermediate-twitch muscle and will fatigue more easily than the soleus. Even though the gastrocnemius has a motor point on each head, neither of these are treatment nodes.

The same situation applies to the biceps brachii, which is also an intermediate muscle. Here the lateral part of the biceps (long head) and the medial portion (short head) are respectively assigned to the large intestine (Figure 12.10) and lung (Figure 12.11) muscle distributions. Both heads of the biceps have motor points that are not nodes. Needling the motor points and sensitive points of fast or intermediate muscles can produce local fatigue and soreness.

Sensitive Locations in Muscles

Sensitive or painful *ahshi* (阿是) sites can develop spontaneously in the muscle tissue, or known nodes can become painful. These ahshi sites often form along the course of the muscle distribution that has a problem; many are motor points, others develop where there may not be any obvious reason for their existence. When located, these sensitive areas can be used to diagnose and treat musculoskeletal problems. The patient may report a sensation of pain at specific locations, or a sensitive location may be detected by gentle palpation of the body surface. Palpation of sensitive sites is normally a part of the examination process. This routine is repeated each time the patient returns for further treatment, and the disappearance of sensitive locations indicates how well the treatment is proceeding. Sensitive sites were first investigated in the West by the Huneke brothers in 1928, when they developed a technique of injecting these areas with local anesthetics. They called this practice neural therapy; a variation of the technique is referred to as trigger point therapy (Dosch: 1985; Travell and Simons: 1983).

Cutaneous Regions

Regions of the skin that overlie the longitudinal route of the distribution vessels and muscle pathways are associated with those particular structures, as named by the yin-yang anatomical divisions. Abnormalities reflected on the skin are used in diagnosis. Temperature variations in the skin regions, either hotter or colder than normal, or other differences in the surrounding areas, provide useful information; the coloration and texture of the skin also provides important clues to possible pathology. Areas of pain, sensitivity, and numbness can indicate a problem associated with the vessel, muscles, and possibly their related viscera.

Muscle Distribution Disorders

Most musculoskeletal problems are due to environmental and other influences on the superficial and deep vessels, since these structures supply all the vital air containing oxygen and nutrients to the muscles and joints. Muscle distributions are also affected by physical stress, wear and tear, and injury, including injury to nerves. Musculoskeletal disorders are often viewed in terms of obstructive (*bi*, 痹) syndromes and flaccid (*wei*, 痿) syndromes. Problems associated with obstructive conditions are the result of impairment in the distribution of nutrients, other essential substances, and vital air to the muscles, and are generally classified as rheumatism. Injury, trauma, and physical strain are other major sources of pain and dysfunction, often leading to wei disorders. Wei syndromes involve flaccid conditions, atrophy of muscle tissue, injuries to muscles, and pain, including neurogenic pain. Both wei and bi syndromes are influenced by environmental factors that affect particular body tissues and by internal organ conditions. Certain organs also have a specific influence on the muscles and tendons.

Visceral Influence on Muscular System

In Chinese physiology the kidney organ is considered to have a profound influence on the bones, and on the tendons and ligament attachments to the bone (Chapter 3). The bladder distribution vessel is thought to have an influence on muscles and tendons (Chapter 10). The liver has a principal role in processing and dispersing nutrients and other vital substances. For this reason the liver has a dominant influence on the muscles, tendons, and joint ligaments. The gallbladder distribution vessel is thought to have a special influence on the bones. The spleen-pancreas helps supply nutrients to the muscle tissue, notably the uptake of glucose in muscle cells as controlled by insulin. The stomach distribution vessel is considered to have a special influence on the formation of blood and therefore assists the spleen to distribute nutrients to muscle tissue.

Longitudinal Distribution of Muscles

Muscles are assigned in *NJLS 13* to longitudinal distributions for each of the twelve yin-yang anatomical regions of the body. Each specific group of muscles is served, both in terms of blood circulation and neural innervation, by one of the twelve distribution vessels (Chapter 11). Muscle distributions are associated with the same internal organs that are related to the distribution vessels. The muscle pathways discussed in the treatise are a clear depiction of all of the body's skeletal muscles—some are specifically identified by name, such as the gastrocnemius, quadriceps, sternocleidomastoid muscles, and the diaphragm. Other muscles throughout the body are accurately described but not specifically named, such as the temporalis, occipitalis, frontalis, pectoralis, deltoids, and trapezius. The location of particular muscles and their areas of insertion and origin are anatomically correct. However, some muscles are mentioned only vaguely, and several are not specifically noted. The ancients did not make the subtle distinction between insertion and origin related to place of attachment and area of action, instead they simply classified all major sites of tendon and muscle attachment as insertion, knotting, or tying locations. The remaining muscles are described by their distribution pathways, origins, and area of insertion. This method of describing muscles is a logical one—in the West the practice of naming each specific muscle in the body did not come into being until the nineteenth century.

Viewing the organization of the muscles in terms of longitudinal pathways is key to understanding both muscle pathology and treatment approaches, as is understanding the function of muscles in relation to specific joints or articulations. When pathology can be attributed to a specific muscle distribution and vessel, the selection of nodes for treatment is easily determined. Most important, however, may be the fact that the muscle distributions, especially in the arms and legs, are easily correlated with currently known spinal nerves at specific segments of the spinal cord. This helps trace the source of the problem and determine whether it is locally influenced or involves upper motoneurons distributing from the motor cortex.

The *NJLS 13* presents the twelve muscle distributions starting with the lower extremity posterior lateral, lateral, and anterior lateral muscle distributions, which comprise the bladder, gallbladder, and stomach. This is then followed by the three lower extremity medial distributions, then the three upper extremity lateral and three hand medial distributions. Muscles are most usefully viewed in terms of their medial-lateral (yin-yang) pairs to best understand their functional roles and disorders in particular joints or body regions. Western names for the muscles described in this chapter are included in brackets in the translations. Pain and dysfunction along the muscle pathways, as well as other manifestations related to each muscle distribution, are summarized in Tables 12.2 and 12.3, listed according to their medial-lateral (yin-yang) pairs by foot and hand distributions.

A recommended treatment method given in *NJLS 13* (apart from nodal selection) is common to all the muscle distributions, with a recommendation to palpate sensitive locations to determine the success of the treatment, as follows:

> To treat these disorders [of the specific distribution], quick insertion with a heated needle of indefinite duration should be employed. Working out the duration and frequency of treatment involves assessing treatment effectiveness by palpation of painful and sensitive locations along these muscle pathways.

Table 12.2 Indications for the six lower extremity muscle distributions (*jingjin*) of the yin-yang body regions (Chinese anatomical orientation).

Muscle Distributions	*Indications*
Posterior Lateral Foot (*Taiyang*): Bladder	Pain and swelling in small toe and heel region; contractions in back of knee; abnormal curvature in back; muscle spasms in nape of neck; inability to raise shoulders due to pain; cramp-like pain in axilla extending to supraclavicular fossa; inability to turn upper body left or right.
Posterior Medial Foot (*Shaoyin*): Kidneys	Acute cramps in bottom of feet; pain and cramps at major insertion sites (ankle, heel, knee, pubic region, back, and nape of neck) for these muscles; epilepsy; alternating contraction and relaxation of limbs leading to tetanus or convulsions.
Anterior Lateral Foot (*Yangming*): Stomach	Acute cramps and spasms in middle toe and along tibia; foot tremors; acute cramps and spasms in rectus femoris muscle; swelling and edema in anterior aspect of thigh; incarcerated hernia; contractions of abdomen (spasms); stretching sensation from supraclavicular fossa to jaw; unexpected or sudden deviation of mouth, with acute condition where the eye cannot close (Bell's palsy).
Anterior Medial Foot (*Taiyin*): Spleen	Pain in big toe and medial ankle; acute cramps and pain in medial knee with pain in upper medial fibula; stretching pain sensation along inner thigh; cramping pain around genitalia; stretching pain from below umbilicus extending up through ribs on each side; stretching pain extending from breast around to spine.
Lateral Foot (*Shaoyang*): Gallbladder	Acute cramps and spasms in fourth and fifth toes; stretched muscles and acute cramps in lateral aspect of knee; knee unable to bend or extend; contractions in back of knee, with tightly stretched muscles in anterior aspect of thigh, and posteriorly in sacral region, and extending above to cause pain in lateral abdomen and hypochondrium, extending further upward causing spasms in breast, supraclavicular region, and neck muscles and tendons.
Medial Foot (*Jueyin*): Liver	Pain in big toe and anterior region of medial malleolus; pain in medial aspect of fibula; pain and acute cramps of inner thigh; dysfunction of sexual organs, including impotence in case of internal injury.

Table 12.3 Indications for the six upper extremity muscle distributions (*jingjin*) of the yin-yang body regions (Chinese anatomical orientation).

Muscle Distributions	*Indications*
Anterior Posterior Hand (*Yangming*): Large Intestine	Pain, spasms, and acute cramps along hand *yangming* traveling route; inability to raise shoulders due to pain; inability to turn neck left or right to look either direction.
Anterior Medial Hand (*Taiyin*): Lungs	Acute cramps and spasms along hand *taiyin* traveling route; severe pain causing dyspnea affecting region of the cardia; spasms in sides of ribs; spitting or vomiting blood.
Lateral Hand (*Shaoyang*): Internal Membrane	Acute cramps and spasms along hand *shaoyang* traveling route; acute cramps and spasms causing tongue to curl up.
Medial Hand (*Jueyin*): Pericardium	Acute cramps and spasms along hand *jueyin* traveling route; pain in anterior region of chest with dyspnea related to region of cardia.
Posterior Lateral Hand (*Taiyang*): Small Intestine	Pain in little finger, posterior aspect of medial epicondyle of elbow following along inner aspect of arm to enter below the axilla, causing pain below axilla; pain in posterior aspect of axilla; pain wrapping around scapula leading to neck; pain and ringing in ears leading to pain in chin; heavy sensation in eye after having been closed for some time; spasms in neck muscles causing fistula of these muscles; swelling in neck.
Posterior Medial Hand (*Shaoyin*): Heart	Acute cramps and muscle pain in muscles along hand *shaoyin* traveling route; condition called *fu liang*,[1] causing pressure on heart and a sensation in arms like a net wrapped around the elbow.

1. *Fu liang* is a name from ancient times that describes a condition involving epigastric fullness due to a fixed abdominal mass, possibly indicating cancer or tumor, that puts pressure on the cardiac region.

A reduction or elimination of sensitive sites (ahshi locations) indicates that the selected treatment protocol is on track. It should be noted that the quote above about using sensitive locations for assessment is often incorrectly referred to as a justification for needling any sensitive area.

Other general comments from *NJLS 13* on treating muscle problems include:

> With regard to disorders in any of the longitudinal muscle distributions, when it involves a cold condition, there will be abnormal muscle curvature and contractions. In the case of heat conditions, there will be abnormal muscle relaxation with the inability to contract [atony], and dysfunction of the sexual organs [impotence]. When cramps occur in the more superficial muscles of the back it will cause abnormal backward curvature of the back. If the contractions occur in the deeper muscles of the back, then the back will be bent forward with an inability to straighten the body. A fire-hot needle can be used to treat acute cold disorders; however, in hot diseases where the muscles are flaccid and unable to contract, use of the heated needle is not indicated.

Muscles of Posterior Lateral Foot: Bladder

The longitudinal distribution of the muscles and related tendons belonging to the posterior lateral lower extremity [bladder] arises at the small toe [flexor digiti minimi brevis], above which it ties into the lateral malleolus [peroneus brevis]. From here it bends around the anklebone to deflect upward [peroneus longus and brevis] to tie into the knee. A branch [abductor digiti minimi] follows along the lateral aspect of the foot and inserts into the heel. From the calcaneus [tendo calcaneus] it continues upward [along the course of the peroneus longus and brevis] to insert into the posterior aspect of the knee [lateral soleus, plantaris, and popliteus]. Another branch [from the calcaneus bone to the popliteal fossa] forms the lateral gastrocnemius muscle. From the medial corner [semitendinosus] and lateral aspect [biceps femoris, long head] of the popliteal fossa these muscle pathways travel upward side-by-side to tie into the region of the buttocks [quadratus femoris, gemellus inferior, obturator internus, gemellus superior, and piriformis]. Above this [gluteus maximus] it travels up each side of the spine [erector spinae muscles, including the iliocostalis lumborum, thoracis, and cervicis; longissimus thoracis, cervicis, and capitis; and spinalis thoracis, cervicis, and capitis; and also the serratus posterior superior and inferior muscles] to the nape of the neck. Here a branch enters into the root of the tongue [styloglossus]. The muscles [semispinalis capitis, splenius capitis, splenius cervicis, longissimus capitis, and trapezius] distribute straight up the neck to insert into the occipital bone. Above [occipitalis], it travels over the head [galea aponeurotica] to descend to the face, tying into the nose [procerus]. From here a branch forms a network around the upper part of the eye [orbicularis oculi, upper palpebral, and orbital parts], and below it ties into the zygoma. A branch at the level of the axilla from the lateral posterior aspect of the back ties into the shoulder [trapezius]. Another branch from the back enters below the axilla [latissimus dorsi]. Above this region a branch travels up from the supraclavicular fossa to tie into the mastoid process [sternocleidomastoid]. Another branch travels out from the supraclavicular fossa, slanting upward to reach the lower border of the zygoma [platysma].

Symptoms associated with this [bladder] muscle distribution are called midspring rheumatism [corresponds to March].

See Figure 12.2 for the bladder muscle distribution; Table 12.2 for muscle problems associated with this distribution.

Muscles of Lateral Foot: Gallbladder

The longitudinal distribution of the muscles and related tendons belonging to the lateral lower extremity [gallbladder] arises at the small toe and at the fourth toe [4th dorsal interosseous], and above it ties into the lateral malleolus [extensor digitorum brevis]. It then follows up along the tibia to insert into the lateral aspect of the knee [peroneus tertius]. Another branch arises along the upper medial aspect of the fibula [biceps femoris, short head] and travels above the thigh. An anterior branch of this muscle pathway [iliotibial tract, tensor fascia latae, and gluteus minimus] ties into the rectus femoris [at the anterior superior iliac spine], while the posterior branch ties into the sacral region [gluteus medius]. Another branch travels straight up between the iliac crest and

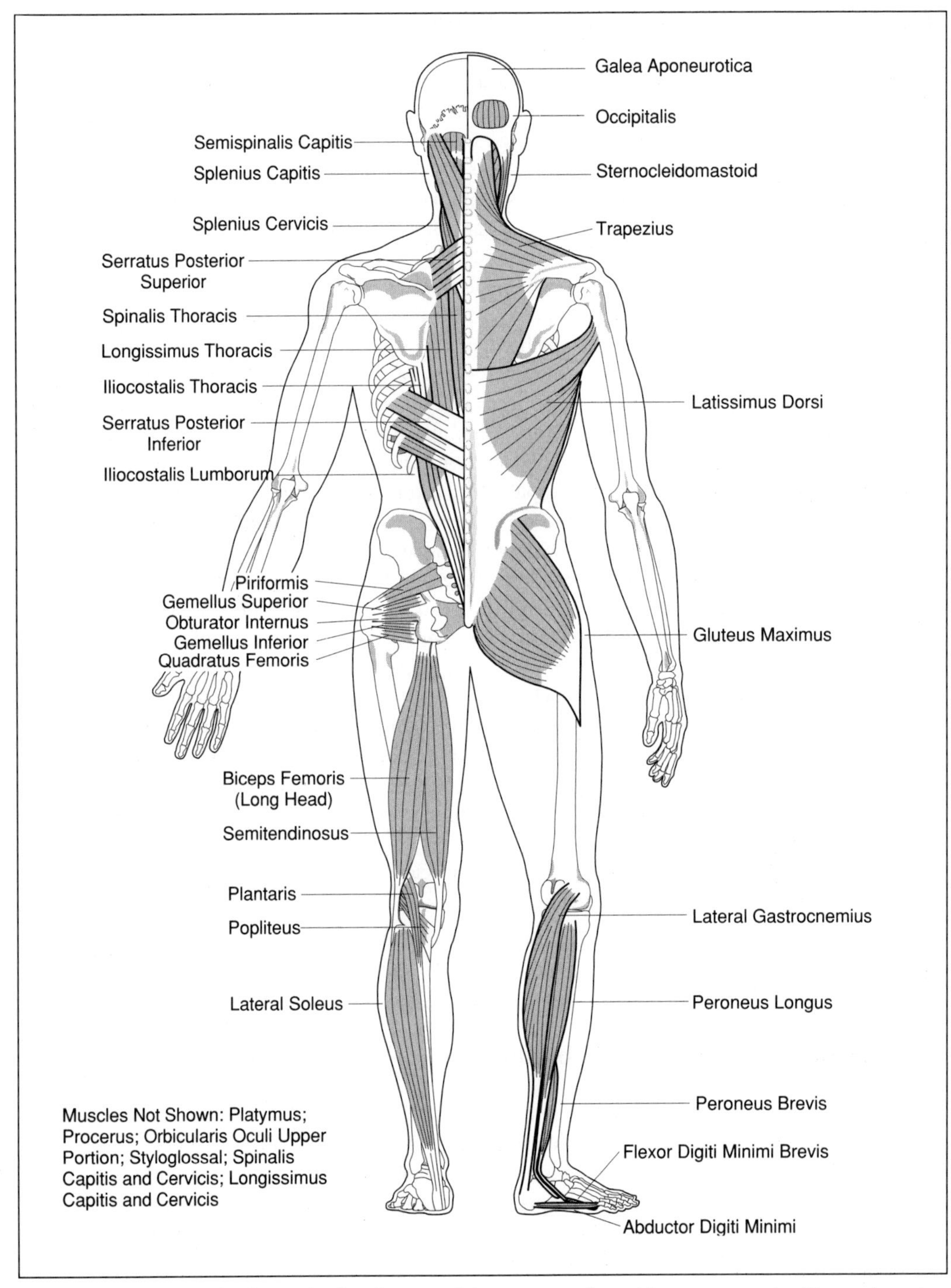

Figure 12.2 Longitudinal muscle distribution of the posterior lateral lower extremity (foot *taiyang*), related to the bladder (upper portion of the orbicularis oculi muscle and the platysma muscle not shown).

hypochondrium [external oblique, internal oblique, and transverse abdominis], continuing up to the anterior aspect of the axilla to tie into the region of the breast [external oblique], and above this pathway inserts into the supraclavicular fossa [superior serratus anterior]. Another branch moves up and out from the axilla region to pierce the supraclavicular fossa [scalenus anterior], moving out anterior to the bladder-taiyang muscle distribution [splenius capitis and trapezius], following up behind the ear and up to the frontal eminence [temporalis]. This muscle [temporalis] crosses the zygoma up to the vertex and below to the chin, above which it ties into the zygoma. Another branch ties into the lateral corner of the eye, forming a connective tendon of the outer canthus.

If the spasms extend from left to right, the right eye will not be able to open because the [right side] of this muscle pathway extends up along the right side of the forehead where it combines with the lifting [*qiao*, 蹺] vessel distribution. Since the muscle and tendons on the left side connect with those on the right [frontalis muscle], when the left aspect of the head is injured it can result in paralysis of the right foot.[2] This is called the mutual relationship of the muscle connections.

Symptoms associated with this [gallbladder] muscle distribution are called early-spring rheumatism [corresponds to February].

See Figure 12.3 for the gallbladder muscle distribution; Table 12.2 for muscle problems associated with this distribution.

Muscles of Anterior Lateral Foot: Stomach

The longitudinal distribution of the muscles and related tendons belonging to the anterior lateral lower extremity [stomach] arises in the region surrounding the third toe [2nd and 3rd dorsal interosseous] and inserts into the dorsum of the foot [extensor hallucis brevis], then deflects laterally upward [extensor digitorum longus] to attach to the fibula, and inserts above in the lateral aspect of the knee. It then extends straight upward [vastus intermedius and rectus femoris] to insert into the greater trochanter, and continues above this to follow along to the ribs and join the backbone [psoas major and minor, and iliacus]. Another branch [tibialis anterior] follows up along the tibia to insert at the knee. A segment of this muscle inserts at the lateral aspect of the fibula where it meets the muscle distribution of the *shaoyang* [少阳, gallbladder: biceps femoris, short head]. A branch above this [vastus lateralis] follows up along the rectus femoris muscle to insert into the thigh above, and then distributes around the sexual organs [obturator externus]. It then travels above where it spreads along the abdomen [rectus abdominis], and continues up to tie into the supraclavicular fossa [sternohyoid, sternothyroid, and thyrohyoid], and then further upward [mylohyoid, mentalis, and depressor labii inferior] to clasp around the mouth [orbicularis oris]. From here it joins the lower border of the zygoma [zygomaticus major], and below it ties into the nose [zygomaticus minor]. Above this [levator labii and levator labii superioris alaeque nasi] it joins the posterior lateral foot [bladder] muscles. The posterior lateral foot [bladder] muscles form a network around the upper part of the eye [orbicularis oculi, upper palpebral, and orbital parts], and the anterior lateral foot [stomach] distribution forms the muscles around the lower part of the eye [orbicularis oculi, lower palpebral, and orbital parts]. Another branch from the cheek [masseter] inserts above, anterior to the ear.

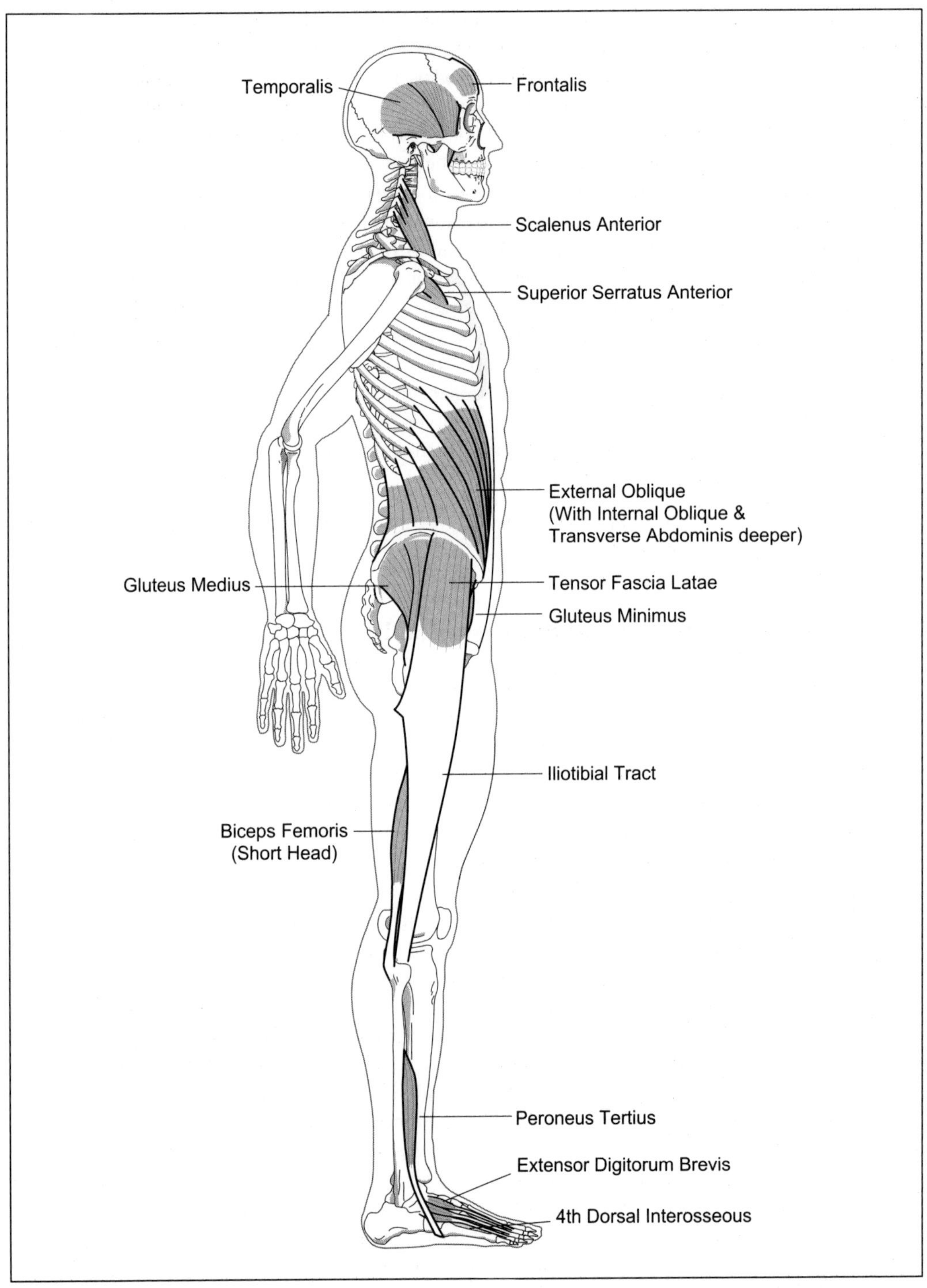

Figure 12.3 Longitudinal muscle distribution of the lateral lower extremity (foot *shaoyang*), related to the gallbladder.

With respect to this last disorder [facial paralysis], if the condition is caused by heat, the muscles will be relaxed and the eye will not be able to open [ptosis of the eyelid]. If the muscles of the cheek have a cold sensation, it will cause acute drawing of the cheeks and alterations or movements in the mouth. If heat conditions are present it will result in relaxation and release of the muscles, with an inability to contract and a consequent deviation of the mouth.

To treat these conditions an ointment made from horse fat can be applied in the case of contractions [spasms and cramps], while white wine mixed with cinnamon can be applied to the areas in the case where the muscles are flaccid. A hook made of mulberry wood can be used to support the drooping of the mouth. Mulberry wood coals can also be placed in a pit, whose depth and size is dictated by how long it takes to warm the patient when they are seated over or next to the coals.

Apply the ointment like ironing the spastic muscles of the cheeks, and the patient can meanwhile drink good wine and eat roasted meat. Even if they do not normally drink, they can make an effort to do so and thereby enhance the effect of massage that is applied to bring about a cure.

Symptoms associated with this [stomach] muscle distribution are called late-spring rheumatism [corresponds to April].

See Figure 12.4 for the stomach muscle distribution; Table 12.2 for muscle problems associated with this distribution.

Muscles of Anterior Medial Foot: Spleen

The longitudinal distribution of the muscles and related tendons belonging to the anterior medial lower extremity [spleen] arises at the medial aspect of the extremity of the big toe [abductor hallucis] and above this ties into the medial malleolus. From here a branch connects with the knee [tibialis posterior and flexor digitorum longus] and medial aspect of the fibula [flexor hallucis longus]. It travels upward, following along the inner aspect of the thigh, and ties into the femur [vastus medius and sartorius] and then distributes around the sexual organs [pectineus]. Above this [linea alba] it ties into the umbilicus, following an interior path along the abdomen to tie into the lower ribs [hypochondrium], where it spreads out into the chest [internal intercostals]. Internally these travel around to connect to the spine [external intercostals].

Symptoms associated with this [spleen] muscle distribution are called early-autumn rheumatism [corresponds to August].

See Figure 12.5 for the spleen muscle distribution; Table 12.2 for muscle problems associated with this distribution.

Muscles of Posterior Medial Foot: Kidneys

The longitudinal distribution of the muscles and related tendons belonging to the posterior medial lower extremity [kidneys] arises below the small toe [flexor digiti minimi brevis, plantar interosseous, and lumbricals] and travels at a slant [quadratus plantae, flexor digitorum brevis, adductor hallucis, and flexor hallucis brevis] to combine with the muscles

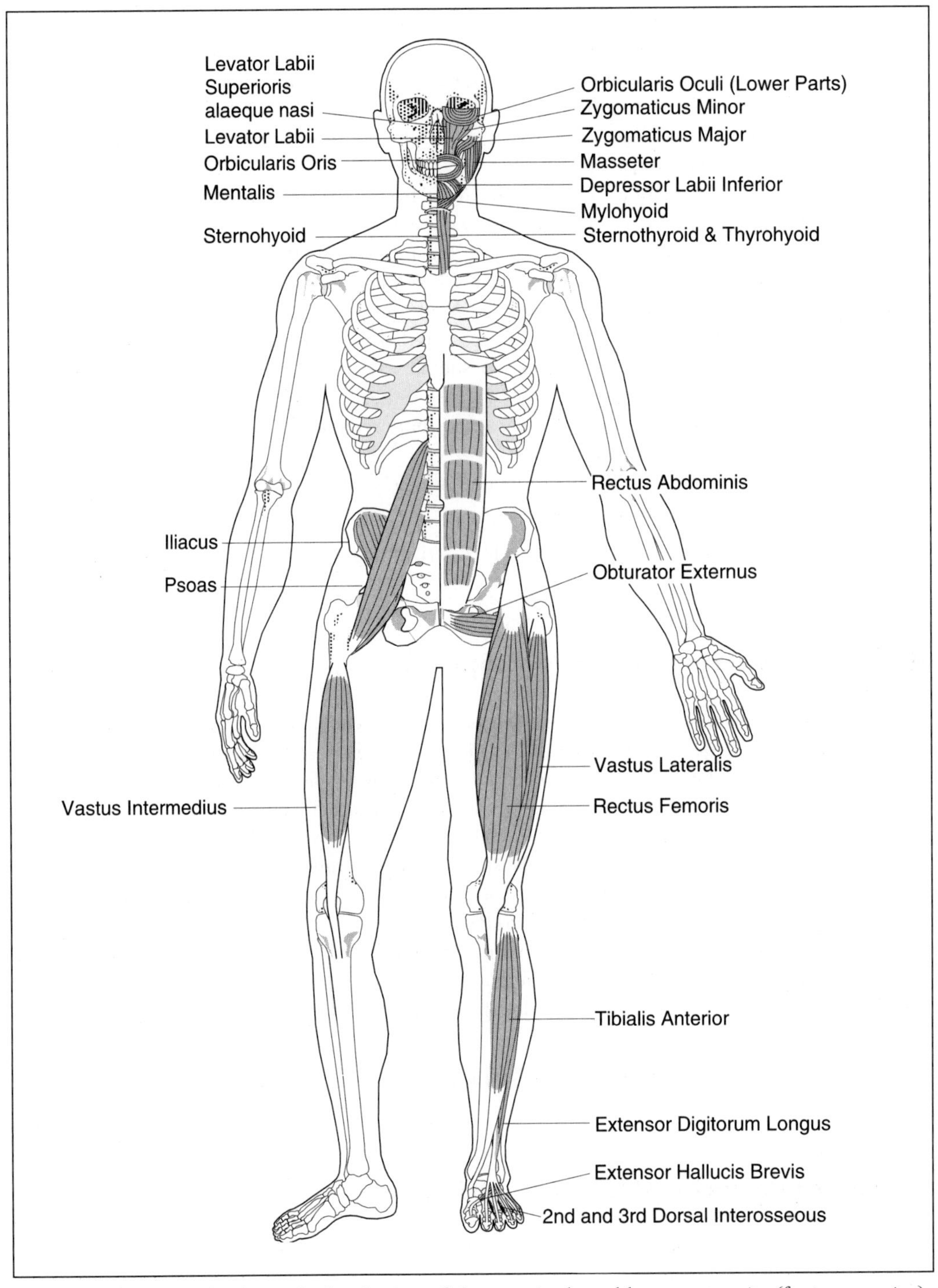

Figure 12.4 Longitudinal muscle distribution of the anterior lateral lower extremity (foot *yangming*), related to the stomach.

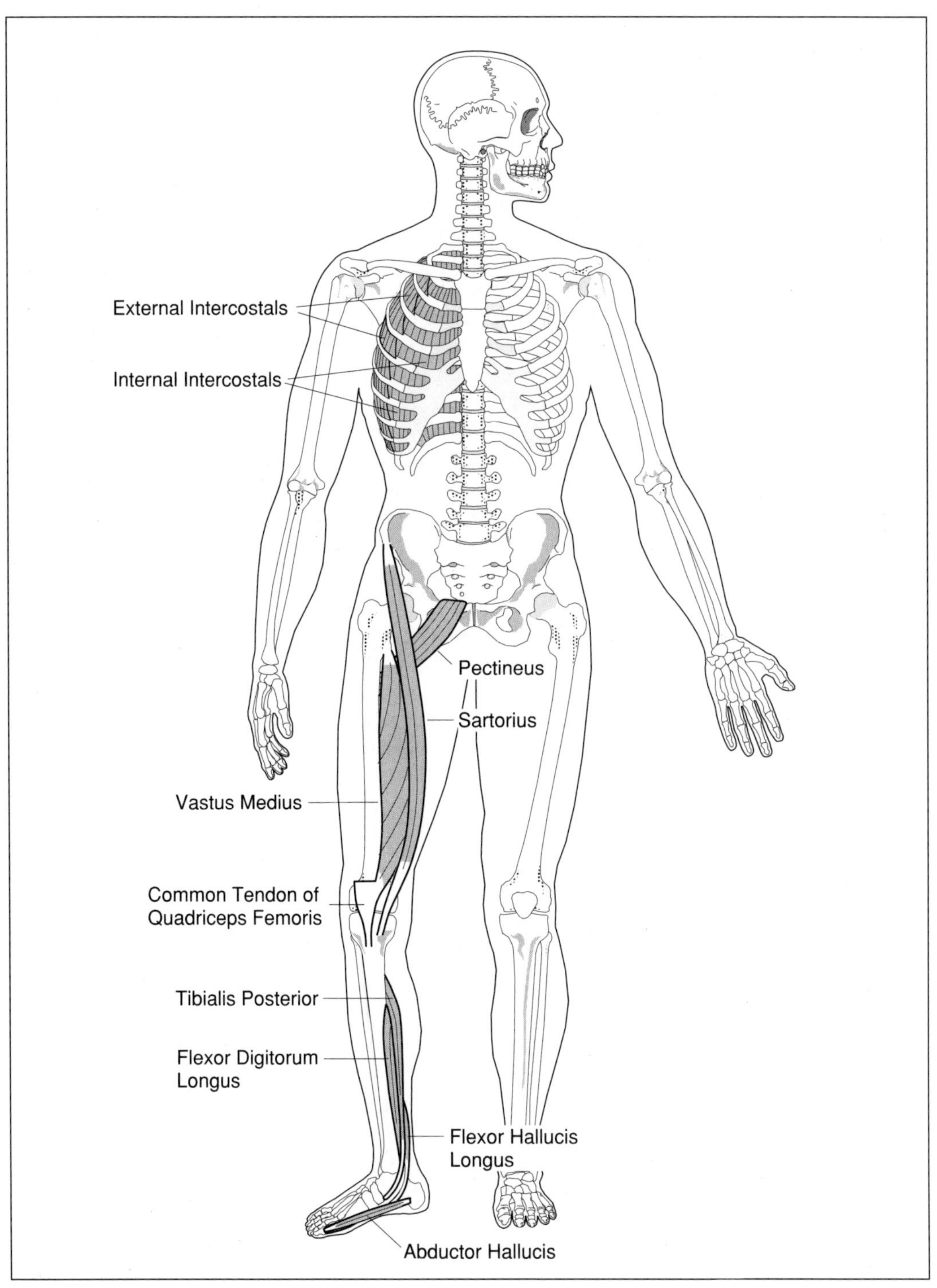

Figure 12.5 Longitudinal muscle distribution of the anterior medial lower extremity (foot *taiyin*), related to the spleen.

of the anterior medial foot [spleen] below the medial malleolus, and then to tie into the heel. From here, it [medial soleus and medial gastrocnemius] joins to insert above at the medial aspect of the fibula, below the head of the fibula. It then combines with the anterior medial foot [spleen] muscles to follow up along the thigh [semimembranosus, adductor magnus, adductor longus, and adductor brevis] to insert at the region of the sexual organs [deep transverse perineal and iliococcygeus]. It then follows along the inner aspect of the spine [coccygeus and quadratus lumborum], clasping each side of the backbone [transversospinal group of muscles, including semispinalis cervicis and thoracis, rotatores thoracis, levatores costarum brevis and longi, intertransversarii, and multifidi muscles], and traveling up until it reaches the nape of the neck [obliquus capitis inferior] to insert into the occipital bone [obliquus capitis superior, rectus capitis posterior major and minor, longus colli, longus capitis, rectus capitis anterior, and rectus capitis lateralis]. These muscles join to participate with and support the muscles of the posterior lateral lower extremity [bladder].

If this latter disorder [tetanus or convulsions] involves the more superficial muscles of the back, the patient will be unable to bend forward. If it involves the deeper muscles of the back, the patient will be unable to bend their head backwards. Therefore, if it is a yang disorder, it will cause abnormal curvature in the lumbar region [because of contraction of the superficial muscles], resulting in the inability to bend forward. If it is a yin disorder, it will result in the inability to bend backwards [because of contraction of the deeper muscles].

If these disorders occur internally [deeper muscles of the back], they can be relieved by stretching exercises and drinking herbal remedies. When the kidney-assigned muscles are in contraction and seized, and if this seized condition is a very dominant feature of the disorder, the disease is incurable [possible discussion of tetanus].

Symptoms associated with this [kidney] muscle distribution are called midautumn rheumatism [corresponds to September].

See Figure 12.6 for the kidney muscle distribution; Table 12.2 for muscle problems associated with this distribution.

Muscles of Medial Foot: Liver

The longitudinal distribution of the muscles and related tendons belonging to the medial lower extremity [liver] arises on the upper region of the big toe [tendon of extensor hallucis longus] and then [1st dorsal interosseous] ties into the anterior region of the medial malleolus. Above this it follows the tibia to insert medially below the head of the fibula [extensor hallucis longus]. It continues upward, following along the inner thigh [gracilis] to tie into the region of the sex organs [pubococcygeus]. Here it makes connections with all the other muscles in this local region.

These disorders are treated by promoting the circulation of water and clearing the sexual organ vital substance.

Symptoms associated with this [liver] muscle distribution are called late-autumn rheumatism [corresponds to October].

See Figure 12.7 for the liver muscle distribution; Table 12.2 for muscle problems associated with this distribution.

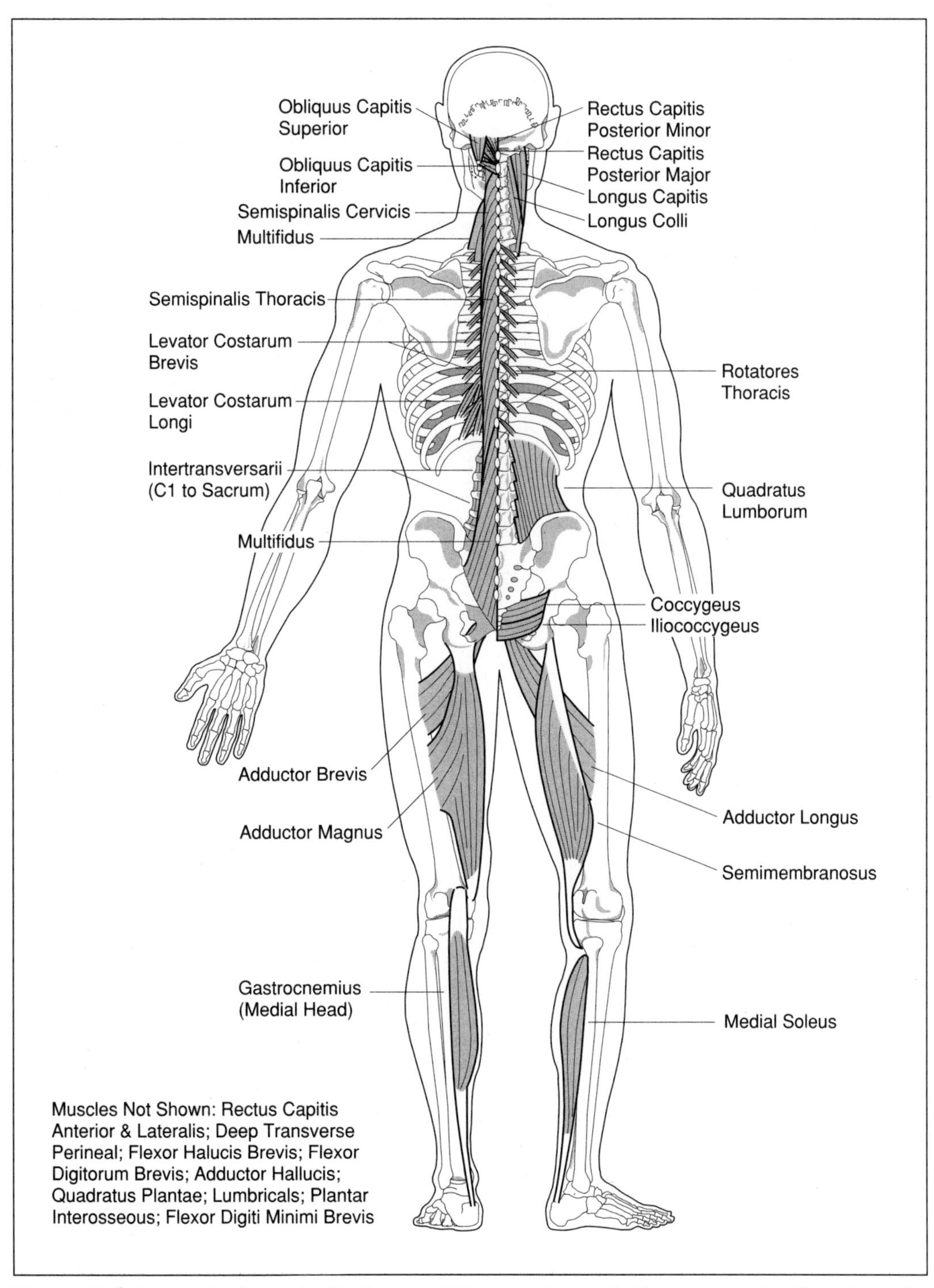

Figure 12.6 Longitudinal muscle distribution of the posterior medial lower extremity (foot *shaoyin*), related to the kidneys (related muscles in the feet not shown).

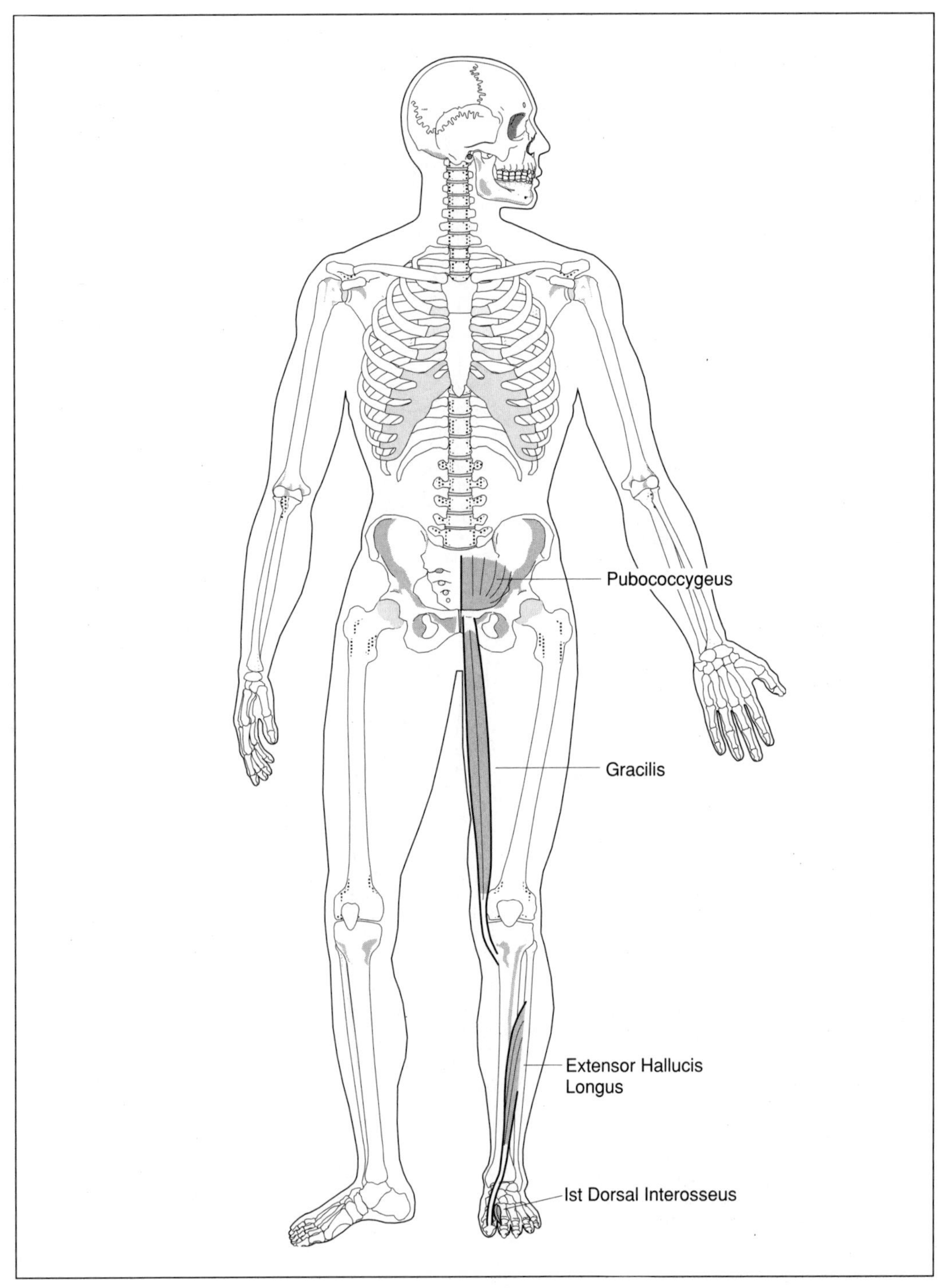

Figure 12.7 Longitudinal muscle distribution of the medial lower extremity (foot *jueyin*), related to the liver.

Muscles of Posterior Lateral Hand: Small Intestine

> The longitudinal distribution of the muscles and related tendons belonging to the posterior lateral upper extremity [small intestine] arises at the superior border of the little finger and then ties into the wrist [abductor digiti minimi]. It then follows up along the medial aspect of the forearm [flexor carpi ulnaris] to tie into the elbow at the posterior aspect of the medial epicondyle of the humerus. Snapping the tendon at this location will cause a response that will radiate down to the little finger. From here it continues upward and ties in just below the axilla [triceps brachii, long head]. A posterior branch travels behind the axilla [teres major and minor] to wind upward around the scapula [infraspinatus], to then follow along the neck [levator scapulae] where it travels outward and anterior to the muscles of the posterior lateral foot [bladder: splenius capitis and trapezius]. It ties into the mastoid process behind the ear. Another branch ties into the ear itself [auricularis posterior], with a straight path outward [auricularis anterior] and upward [auricularis superior] from the ear. Below it ties into the chin [digastric, posterior belly] and above it connects with the lateral canthus of the eye.
>
> When there are cold or hot sensations in the neck, they should be treated by quick insertion with a heated needle for an indefinite duration. Working out the duration and frequency of treatment involves assessing treatment effectiveness by palpation of painful and sensitive locations. If there is swelling, this should be treated by use of very sharp needles. In addition, since this muscle pathway passes through the angle of the jaw, follows anterior to the ear, connects with the outer canthus of the eye and upper jaw, and ties into the temporal region, there can be pain along these traveling areas, as well as acute cramps.
>
> Symptoms associated with this [small intestine] muscle distribution are called midsummer rheumatism [corresponds to June].

See Figure 12.8 for the small intestine muscle distribution; Table 12.3 for muscle problems associated with this distribution.

Muscles of Lateral Hand: Internal Membrane

> The longitudinal distribution of the muscles and related tendons belonging to the lateral upper extremity [internal membrane, *sanjiao*, 三焦] arises at the extremities of the little finger and the fourth finger. From here [4th dorsal interosseous] it ties into the wrist and follows along the center of the forearm [extensor indicis, extensor digiti minimi, and extensor carpi ulnaris] to tie into the elbow [anconeus]. Above it wraps around the lateral aspect of the upper arm [triceps brachii, lateral head] up to the shoulder [posterior deltoid], and then [supraspinatus] travels to the neck [scalenus posterior] where it joins the muscles of the posterior lateral upper extremity [small intestine: levator scapulae]. A branch at the angle of the jaw [stylohyoid] travels down the cheek to enter and fasten to the root of the tongue [hyoglossus and genioglossus]. Another branch travels up over the angle of the jaw to follow anterior to the ear [temporoparietalis], and then connects [galea aponeurotica] with the outer canthus of the eye and the muscle above [gallbladder: temporalis], which travels from the chin to tie into the lateral forehead.

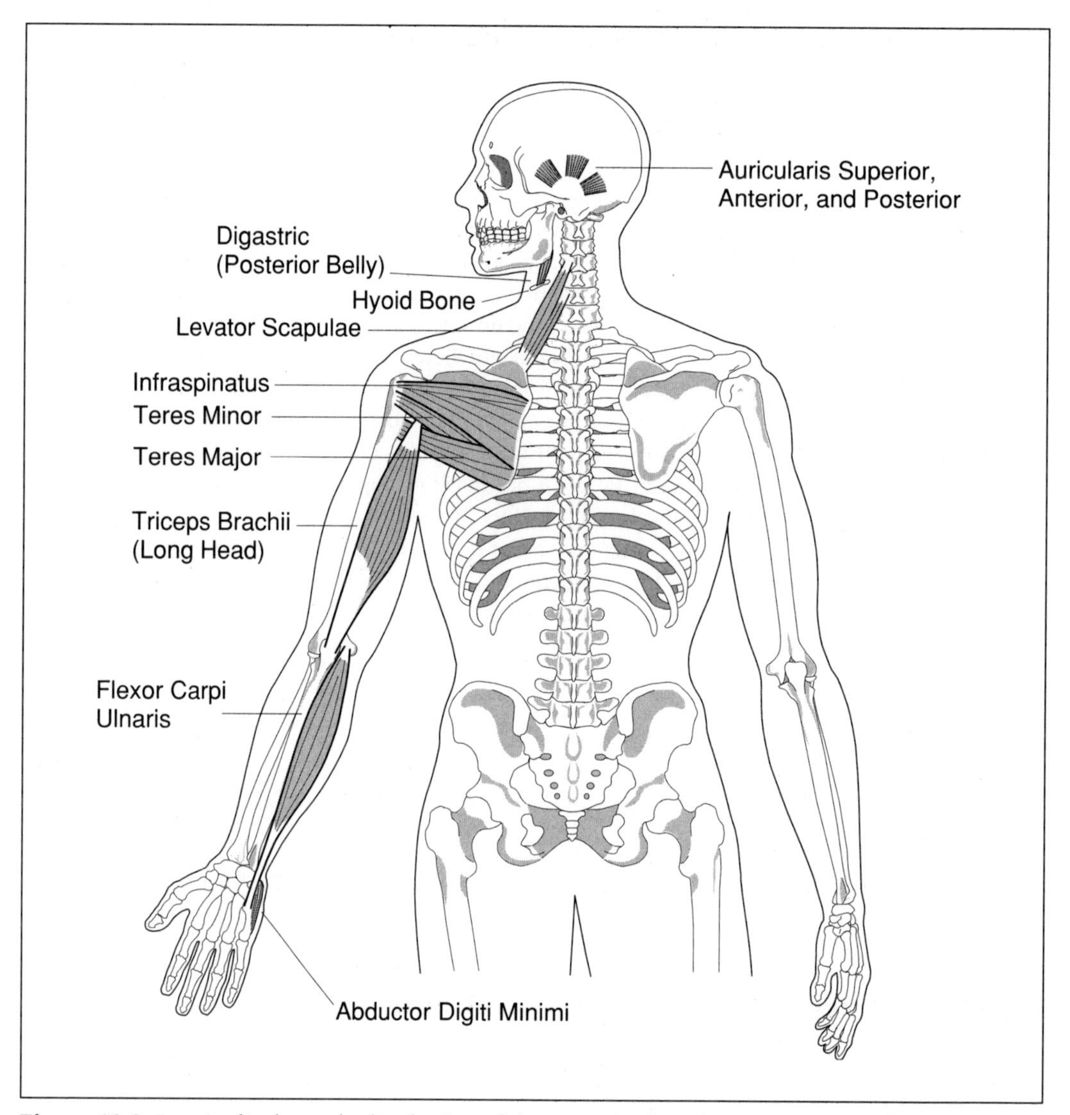

Figure 12.8 Longitudinal muscle distribution of the posterior lateral upper extremity (hand *taiyang*), related to the small intestine.

> Symptoms associated with this [internal membrane] muscle distribution are called late-summer rheumatism [corresponds to July].

See Figure 12.9 for the internal membrane (sanjiao) muscle distribution; Table 12.3 for muscle problems associated with this distribution.

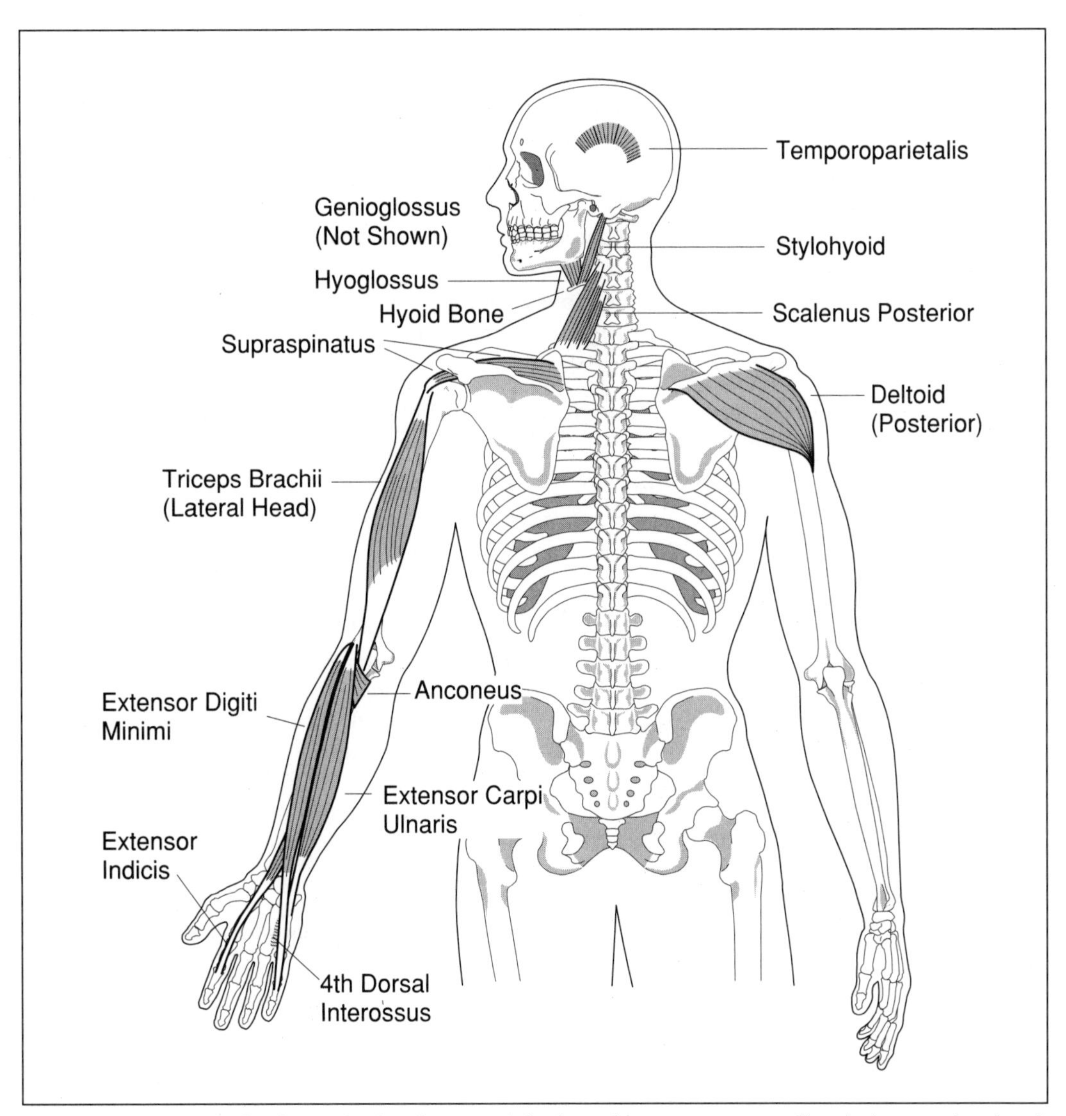

Figure 12.9 Longitudinal muscle distribution of the lateral upper extremity (hand *shaoyang*), related to the internal membrane (*sanjiao*).

Muscles of Anterior Lateral Hand: Large Intestine

The longitudinal distribution of the muscles and related tendons belonging to the anterior lateral upper extremity [large intestine] arises at the extremities of the thumb and forefinger and ties into the wrist [1st dorsal interosseous, adductor pollicis, abductor pollicis longus, and extensor pollicis longus and brevis]. Above it follows the forearm to tie into the lateral aspect of the elbow [extensor digitorum communis, extensor carpi radialis longus, extensor carpi radialis brevis, and the supinator], and above this to the humerus [biceps brachii, long head] to tie into the acromion [middle deltoid]. A branch winds around to the scapula [subscapularis] to insert into the spine [rhomboid major and minor]. A branch from the shoulder [middle deltoid] travels up to the neck [omohyoid], and this branch continues up [digastric, anterior belly] to the cheek [depressor anguli oris and risorius] and then ties into the lower border of the zygoma [buccinator]. Another branch traveling straight upward [scalenus medius] moves out anterior to the posterior lateral hand [small intestine: levator scapulae] muscles and travels upward to the protuberance to the left [sphenoid bone] [or the right if viewing the left aspect of the face], attaching to the head [lateral pterygoid] and traveling down to the right [or left, on the opposite side of the body] to the chin [medial pterygoid].

Symptoms associated with this [large intestine] muscle distribution are called early-summer rheumatism [corresponds to May].

See Figure 12.10 for the large intestine muscle distribution; Table 12.3 for muscle problems associated with this distribution.

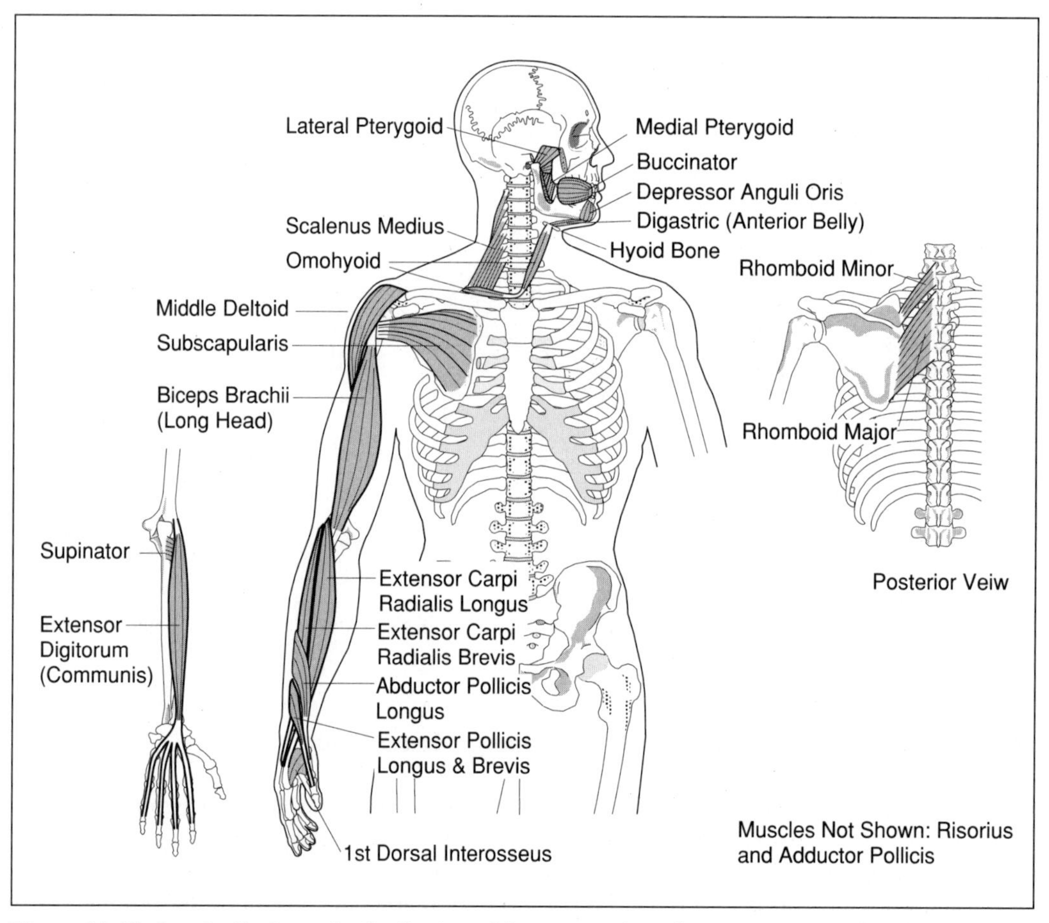

Figure 12.10 Longitudinal muscle distribution of the anterior lateral upper extremity (hand *yangming*), related to the large intestine (cutaway view of zygomatic arch and mandible to show pterygoid muscles; cutaway of rib cage to show the subscapularis muscle).

Muscles of Anterior Medial Hand: Lungs

> The longitudinal distribution of the muscles and related tendons belonging to the anterior medial upper extremity [lungs] arises at the superior aspect of the thumb to distribute above and tie in behind the thenar region [opponens pollicis, abductor pollicis brevis, and flexor pollicis brevis, superficial and deep head], and then distributes to the lateral side of where the radial pulse is detected. It then follows up along the forearm to tie into the center region of the elbow [flexor pollicis longus and brachioradialis]. It continues up the medial aspect of the upper arm [biceps brachii, short head] to enter the region below the axilla, and moves out to the supraclavicular fossa and ties into the shoulder anterior to the acromion extremity [anterior deltoid]. Above it ties into the supraclavicular fossa [coracoid process of scapula]. Below it ties into the interior region of the chest [pectoralis minor], where it spreads [transversus thoracis] to pass through the cardia [diaphragm], joining the cardia below [crura of the diaphragm] and then supporting the hypochondrium.
>
> Symptoms associated with this [lung] muscle distribution are called midwinter rheumatism [corresponds to December].

See Figure 12.11 for the lung muscle distribution; Table 12.3 for muscle problems associated with this distribution.

Muscles of Medial Hand: Pericardium

> The longitudinal distribution of the muscles and related tendons belonging to the medial upper extremity [pericardium] arises at the middle finger [1st and 2nd palmar interosseous and associated lumbricals] and, along with the muscles of the anterior medial upper extremity [lungs], combines to travel up to tie into the medial aspect of the elbow [flexor carpi radialis, flexor digitorum profundus, and includes the pronator quadratus lower on the forearm]. Above it follows the inner aspect of the upper arm [coracobrachialis] to tie in below the axilla. Below this it spreads anteriorly and posteriorly to clasp to the upper ribs on the sides [serratus anterior]. Another branch enters the region of the axilla to spread to the center of the chest [pectoralis major, clavicular and upper sternal portions] and inserts into the humerus.
>
> Symptoms associated with this [pericardium] muscle distribution are called early-winter rheumatism [corresponds to November].

See Figure 12.12 for the pericardium muscle distribution; Table 12.3 for muscle problems associated with this distribution.

Muscles of Posterior Medial Hand: Heart

> The longitudinal distribution of the muscles and related tendons belonging to the posterior medial upper extremity [heart] arises at the inside surface [radial side] of the little finger [3rd palmar interosseous and associated lumbrical]. From here it ties into the pisiform bone [flexor digiti minimi brevis, opponens digiti minimi, and palmaris brevis] and travels above to tie into the medial aspect of the elbow [flexor digitorum superficialis, palmaris

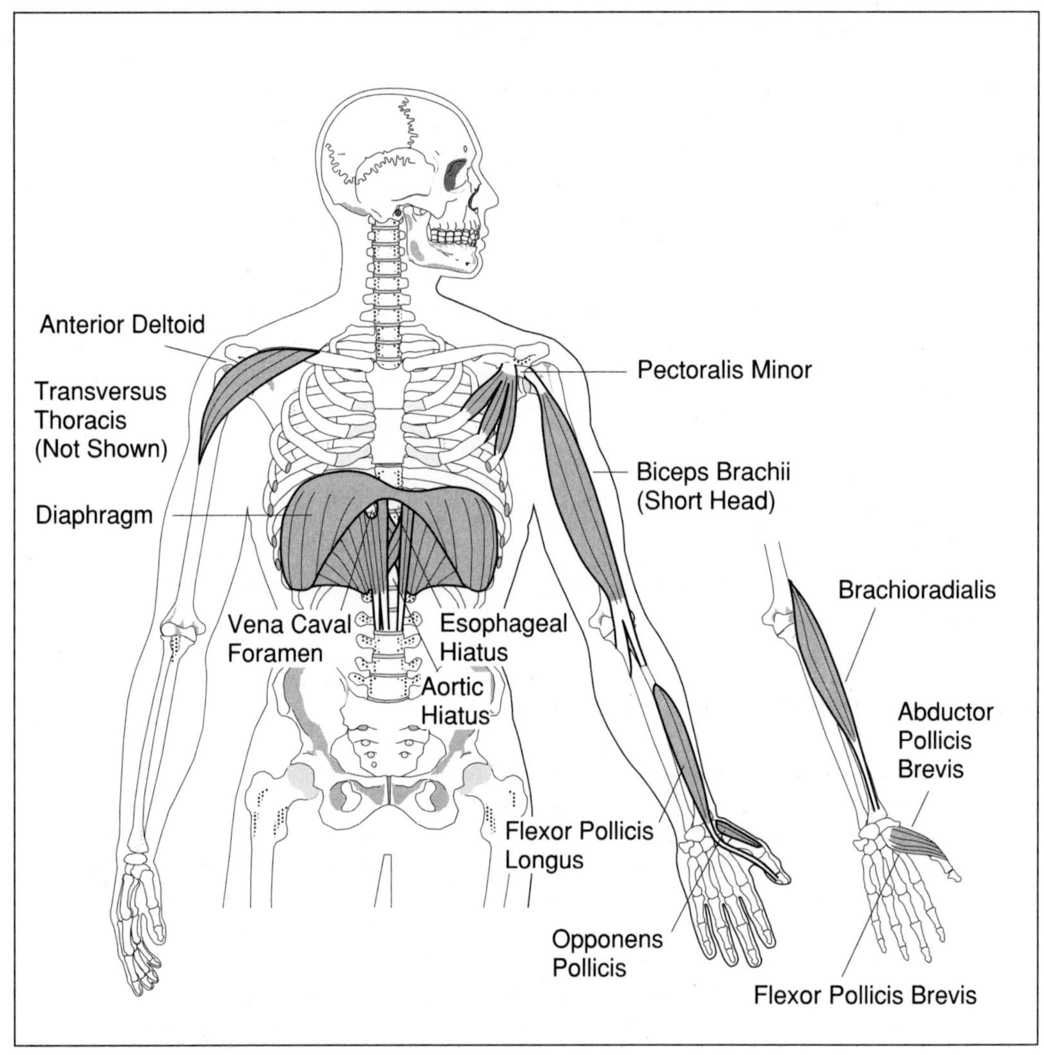

Figure 12.11 Longitudinal muscle distribution of the anterior medial upper extremity (hand *taiyin*), related to the lungs (cutaway view of rib cage and sternum to show the diaphragm).

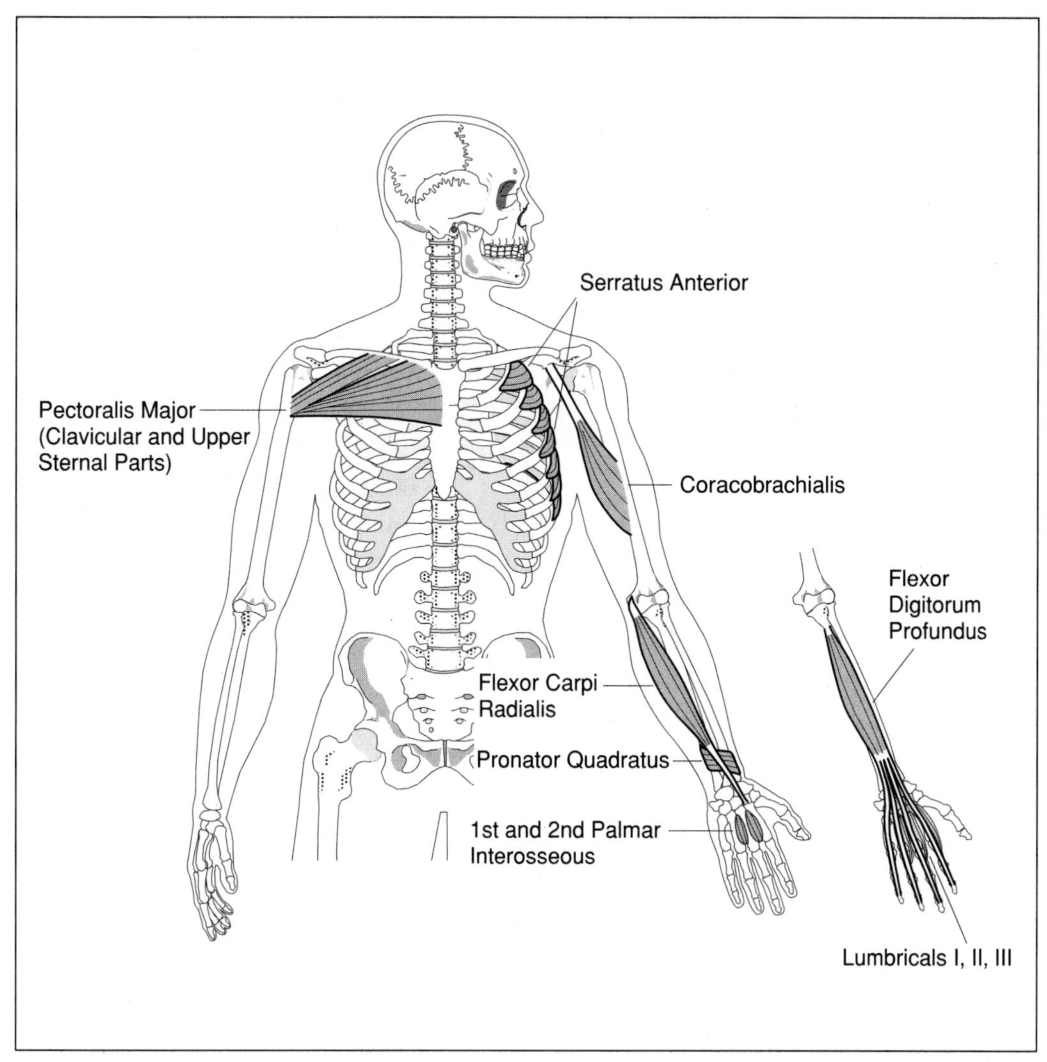

Figure 12.12 Longitudinal muscle distribution of the medial upper extremity (hand *jueyin*), related to the pericardium.

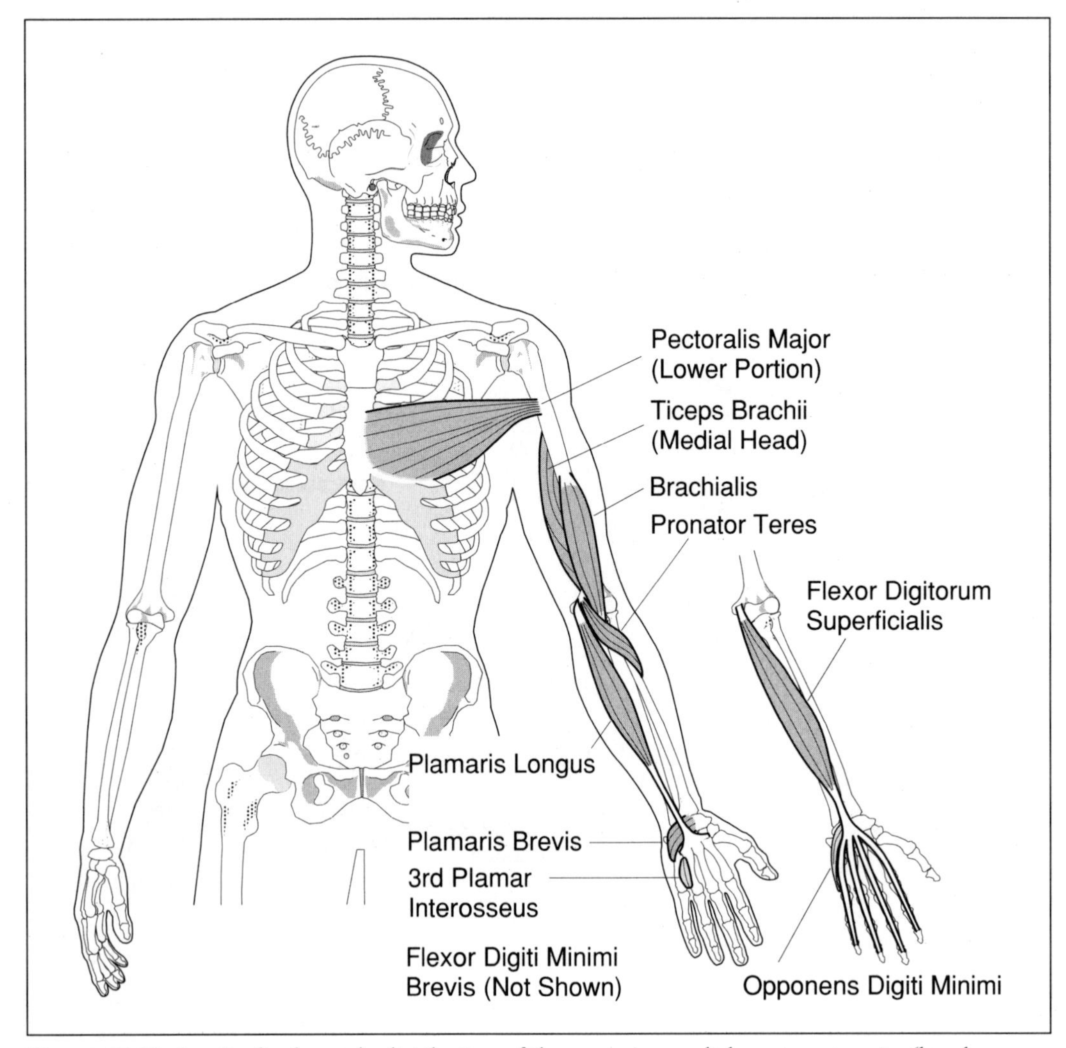

Figure 12.13 Longitudinal muscle distribution of the posterior medial upper extremity (hand *shaoyin*), related to the heart.

longus, and pronator teres]. From here it ascends to enter the region of the axilla [brachialis and triceps brachii, medial head] where it crosses with the muscles of the anterior medial upper extremity [lungs: point where the pectoralis major crosses the biceps brachii]. It travels across the bosom under the breast and ties into the center of the chest [pectoralis major: lower sternal, costal, and abdominal portions], and has its insertion in the upper arm [brachii]. From here it is fastened to the ligaments that descends to the umbilicus [costoxiphoid and linea alba ligaments].

Symptoms associated with this [heart] muscle distribution are called late-winter rheumatism [corresponds to January].

See Figure 12.13 for the heart muscle distribution; Table 12.3 for muscle problems associated with this distribution.

13
View of Health and Disease

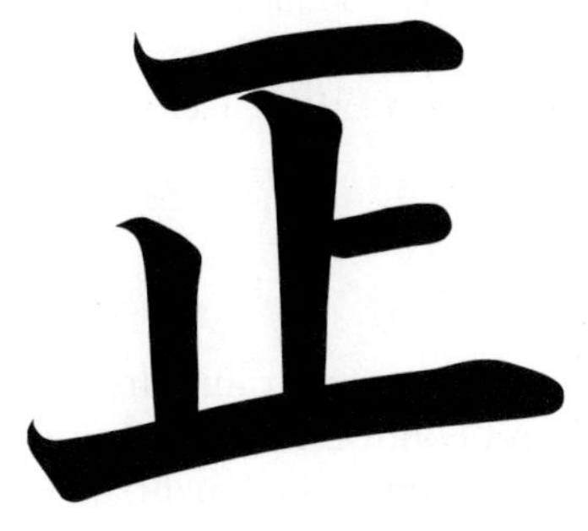

Zheng: Normal

All diseases originate from the environmental conditions of wind, rain, cold, and heat; from seasonal changes; excess joy and anger; from what one drinks and eats; the condition of one's residence; and by incessant worry and sudden fear.

Qibo*, NJLS 28 (Verbal Inquiry)*

The key to health is for each person to maintain a balance with their environment, including such factors as weather conditions, seasonal changes, emotional stress, and physical stress. Health requires a constancy in daily activity patterns, moderation in eating and drinking habits, not being reckless, not worrying to the point of fatigue, not being consumed by grief, remaining calm and unperturbed, and not overachieving. This view of health is truly holistic in the sense that the human condition is thought to be the result of how individuals function in their total environment. All external and internal stressors are considered, even the condition of one's residence—both the location of the residence and the state of tranquillity among family members are regarded as significant. The ancient Chinese understood that the strain of living in civilized communities is a major cause of much disease (Chapter 2); factors held responsible include the environment (periontogenic disease), emotions, and diet.

Physiological Balance and Homeostasis

Maintaining a state of health is viewed in terms of a continuing physiological balance or homeostasis (*zheng*, 正) (Figure 2.3). Normally, homeostasis is maintained over a relatively wide range of internal and external conditions. Only when adverse factors become overpowering, or when the body is weak, do problems result. Life was frequently harsh in ancient times and the Chinese observed that disease is related to environmental, emotional, dietary, and physical factors, as summarized in *NJLS 28* (*Verbal Inquiry*):

All diseases originate from the environmental conditions of wind, rain, cold, and heat; from seasonal changes; excess joy and anger; from what one drinks and eats; the condition of one's residence; and by incessant worry and sudden fear. These factors cause disease by separating blood and vital substances, damaging and counteracting bodily function, exhausting the distribution vessels and collaterals, impeding circulation along the vessel pathways, going against the mutual relationships of vital substances and function, restricting defensive function, emptying the distribution vessels, or by obstructing the circulation of blood and vital substances. All of these factors cause a deviation from normal physiological function.

Disrupting Bodily Function

A deviation in normal physiological function impairs the body's homeostatic process of maintaining biological balance and control. If this impairment is more than transitory, then pain, dysfunction, and disease can result. Functional balance must be maintained constantly under all extremes of external factors, as discussed in Chapter 2 (Figure 2.3). Under normal conditions of health and function, the body responds to external demands without impairing homeostasis. However, disease will occur both in an excess condition, where exposure can be excess in terms of time, magnitude, or both, and when the body is in a state of deficiency, often as result of long-term or chronic exposure.

External factors are thought to damage the body directly, whereas emotions, diet, or internal factors damage vital processes, which then leads to disease conditions. Blood and vital substances are circulated in both the deep and superficial regions of the body, like an endless ring. Hence the entire body can be adversely affected by external and internal forces. Externally, environmental factors directly influence or attack the superficial regions of the body; internally, both emotions and dietary intake affect the functional activity of the viscera and bowels. Physical stress and trauma can directly damage the body and impair the circulation of blood and vital substances, and thereby have a profound effect on the state of health or disease.

Modern Correlation

From the Chinese view of physiology it is apparent that the ancient concept of homeostasis is consistent with twenty-first century thought. The main difference from Western ideas lies in the Chinese emphasis on the circulation of blood, nutrients, defensive substances, and oxygen from vital air, and on the importance of maintaining overall physiological or functional balance. Homeostasis involves most physiological aspects of the body, as mediated by the internal organs, metabolism, blood circulation, nerves, and lymphatics. The relationship between metabolic components serving physiological function and overall homeostatic balance is illustrated in Figure 13.1.

Metabolic processes rely on the normal functioning of the internal organs. Conversely, the internal organs rely on metabolic substrates. This is part of the dual nature of biological systems where function (classed as yang) depends on substance (classed as yin), and substance itself depends on function. Consequently, the dynamic interplay of homeostatic processes can also be viewed in terms of yin and yang properties.

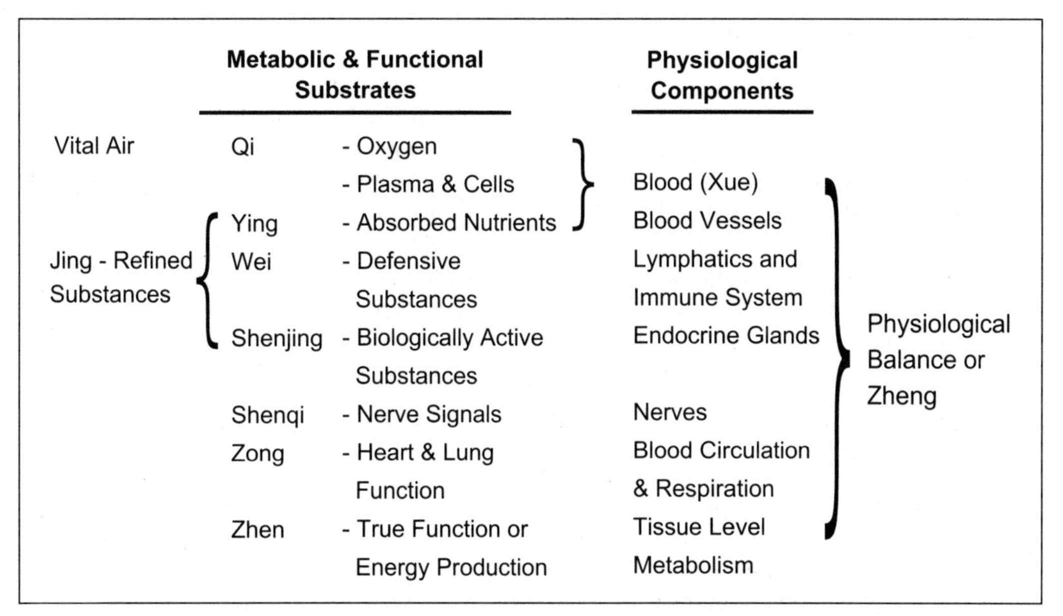

Figure 13.1 Physiological processes and components that comprise the Chinese concept of physiological or homeostatic balance (*zheng*), or antipathogenic function.

External and Internal Assault

Environmental conditions and dietary habits (Chapter 6), as well as emotional strain (Chapter 7), are considered detrimental to health under certain circumstances, as are several other miscellaneous factors. External and internal disease-causing factors have a profound effect on the body's physiological processes. Either excessive factors or internal weakness in conjunction with normal factors lead to pathogenesis. There is a constant struggle between external forces and the internal balance of the body. The body's homeostatic or internal balance is also described as the antipathogenic function.

External Factors in Disease

Environmental forces of wind, damp, heat, summer heat, dryness, and cold are the primary external factors in disease (Tables 6.1 and 6.2). Each of the six sky-airs predominates at a different season, and may become pathogenic if it is abnormal, excessive, or occurs outside its expected predominating time period. If a body is weak, even environmental conditions that are not excessive can cause disease.

Other external disease-causing elements include overconsumption of certain flavors (Table 6.5), pestilential agents, and miscellaneous factors, such as physical stress and lack of exercise. Collectively, these are classified as secondary external factors. Traumatic injuries, including contusions, sprains, scalds, burns, surgical incisions, wounds, animal and reptile bites, and insect stings or bites, are in this category as well. Classifying these factors as miscellaneous does not imply they are insignificant—some, such as physical stress and overstrain, are recognized as critical.

Internal Factors in Disease

Emotions are generally a normal response to external stimuli and do not represent a problem. However, when emotional strain and other influences, including environmental and dietary factors, become excessive, emotions become the primary internal factor in disease. Pathogenic emotions disrupt normal physiological processes and functional activity, resulting in disease and dysfunction (Tables 7.1, 7.2, and 7.3). Emotions harm the body indirectly, while environmental conditions cause injury to the body directly.

Other conditions such as the formation of phlegm fluids or blood stagnation, which may become pathological, are considered secondary internal factors. Often they occur as a result of another pathogenic source. Additionally, internal disorders that mimic environmental conditions such as cold, heat, and damp can develop in the body.

Excess and Deficiency

Another fundamental concept of Chinese medicine is to view disease as being either solid (excess) or hollow (deficient). An excess or solid disorder is when disease, pain, or dysfunction is a result of excessive environmental factors, poor diet, pestilence, or miscellaneous factors overwhelming the antipathogenic function. Here, homeostasis is optimal, but is in a state of struggle with the excessive external factors (Figure 2.3). If the pathogenic assault continues to the point where it causes a disruption in homeostasis, it is then classified as a deficiency or hollow condition. A hollow disorder also occurs when the internal balance is deficient for any reason, including emotional factors or poor diet, but the external factors are normal.

Excess is generally associated with an abundance or surplus of external atmospheric or pathogenic factors, while deficiency is more concerned with the internal balance of the body involving the internal organs. This is discussed in *NJSW 28* (*Comments on Hollowness and Solidness*):

> When the environmental pathogenic factors [*xie*, 邪] are overabundant they cause solidness. Deprivation of refined substances [*ying*, 营; *wei*, 卫; and *shenjing*, 神精] and vital air [*qi*, 气] causes hollowness.

Environmental Pathogenic Routes

Western medicine recognizes that extreme environmental conditions can potentially be fatal. However, the Chinese further understood that even subtle influences of external forces can cause ailments and dysfunction. The means by which environmental or periontogenic factors influence the internal body is through their effect on the distribution vessels and related nerves in the superficial regions (Chapter 11). These structures mediate changes in the skin and provoke responses to external stimuli that are normal protective processes common to most species. The same protective mechanisms provide the anatomical means for superficial influences to penetrate the internal regions. Superficial vessels and nerves form connections to the internal organs, and this ultimately provides a pathway through which environmental forces can affect the body internally.

Effect on Superficial Regions

Anatomical features and characteristics of the superficial skin have evolved so that appropriate adjustments occur in response to environmental changes, injury, and damage such as through animal and insect bites. Many of these responses involve simply contracting or dilating the superficial blood vessels in the skin to conserve or release excess heat. Severe environmental exposure producing conditions such as hypothermia or heat prostration obviously have detrimental or even fatal consequences. On the other hand, subtle environmental changes or exposure can lead to disorders that might not obviously be correlated with the environment.

Development of facial paralysis (Bell's palsy) after riding in an automobile with the window rolled down, or the development of chronic sinusitis because an air-conditioning vent is blowing on the back of a person's neck, are two common examples of environmentally induced problems where the patient may not be aware of the cause. While most cultures have realized that people who live in cold, damp dwellings typically suffer joint and muscle disorders, sometimes complicated by pneumonia, many individuals may never have understood that their environment was the direct cause of their suffering.

Another example of the subtle way that seasonal changes can induce disease is the reduced sunlight in the Northern Hemisphere during the winter months—seasonal light deprivation has a profound effect on the pineal gland, affecting the mood, emotional state, and behavior of some individuals. This can manifest as manic depression and obesity due to carbohydrate craving.

The transmission of environmental pathogenesis to the internal organs is possible because of the continuous communication between the internal and external body through the superficial blood and lymphatic vessels and related nerves. When disease attacks, it first assaults the fine vessels (arterioles, capillaries, and venules) and collaterals in the skin. The body may simply respond without developing a significant disorder. However, if the pathogenic factors are hyperactive (excess condition) or the antipathogenic function is weak (deficiency condition) then disease develops that can eventually be transmitted to the interior of the body (Figure 13.2). Reference to environmental factors initially affecting the vessels in the skin is provided in *NJSW 56* (*Skin Zones*):

> The twelve distribution vessels and their collateral branches serve the skin zones. Therefore, the beginning of all diseases first starts in the skin and body hair. When environmental forces attack the pores open up, which allows the pathogenic factor to enter the body as a guest of the collateral vessels. If it does not leave, the pathogenic factor then moves on to the distribution vessels. If it remains in the body further without leaving, then the pathogenic factor moves on to enter the bowels and stays in the intestines and stomach.

The fine vessels (arterioles, capillaries, and venules) that are affected by external environmental factors are the principal means of distributing nutrients and defensive substances to the tissues (see quote from *NJSW 58: Vital Nodes*, cited in Chapter 8). Excess pathogenic forces can delay or obstruct these vital substances, causing accumulation of blood, fever, and impaired internal function. When pathogenic forces obstruct vital substances in the muscles, this causes heat in the blood vessels, withering of muscles, formation of pus, bone and marrow depletion, and damage to knee joints. Retention of cold restricting the availability of nutrients and defensive substances causes curling of the flesh, muscle contraction, restricted movement of the ribs and elbows, bone rheumatism, and numbness.

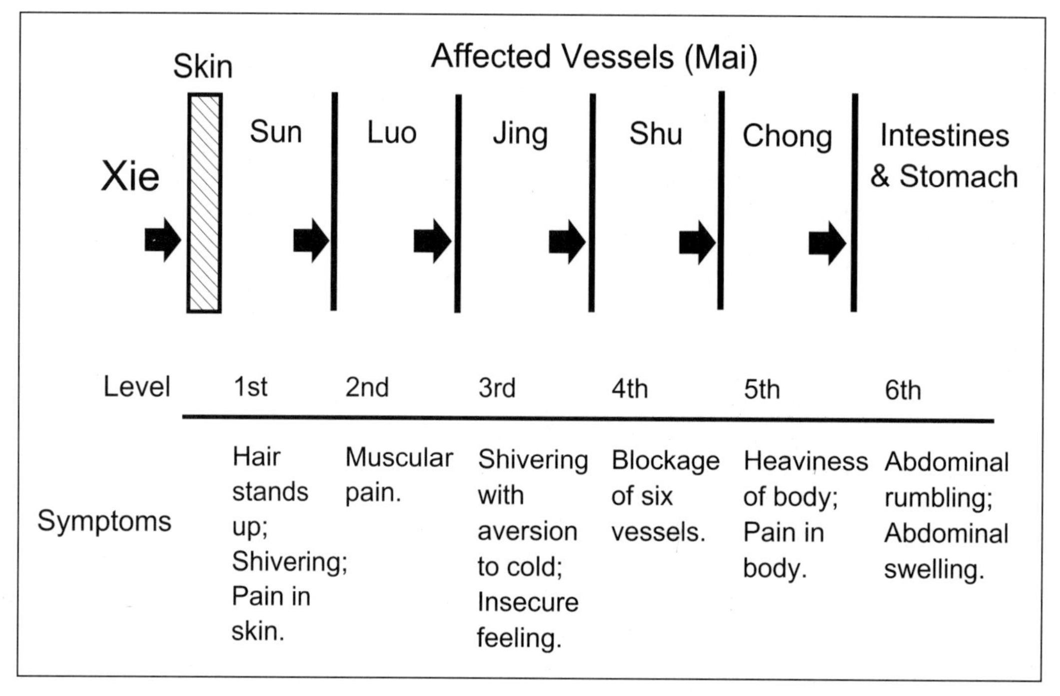

Figure 13.2 Schematic diagram of the progressive penetration of external pathogenic factors into the internal body along vessel pathways.

Internal Transmission

A detailed account of the disease conditions resulting from a progressive penetration of external pathogenic forces into the body (Figure 13.2) is provided in *NJLS 66* (*Origins of All Disease*):

> Environmental agents initially attack the skin and the fine vascular structures [*sunmai*, 孙脉: venules, capillaries, and arterioles] producing symptoms of body hair standing up, shivering, and pain in the skin. When one takes no protective action, these environmental effects continue to impact deeper structures. The collateral vessels [*luomai*, 络脉] are then affected, resulting in the development of muscle pain. If the attack continues to penetrate further into the body, the pathogenic factor then affects the main longitudinal distribution vessels [*jingmai*, 经脉], resulting in shivering with aversion to cold and the development of a sense of insecurity. If no action is taken to rid the body of the pathogenic factor, it then affects deeper regions. The communication vessels [*shumai*, 输脉: carotid, brachial, and femoral arteries] are then involved, which block the six vessels [bladder, stomach, gallbladder, lungs, heart, and pericardium distribution vessels]. When impaired, these distribution vessels fail to supply the four extremities, causing pain in the joints and stiffness of the lower back. As the attack moves deeper, the pathogenic factor then affects the aorta [*chongmai*, 冲脉] itself, producing a sense of heaviness and pain in the body. In the deeper stages, the environmental factor then affects the stomach and intestines, producing rumbling and swelling in the abdomen. If cold predominates,

> abdominal rumbling and diarrhea containing undigested food results. If heat predominates, a sticky, muddy, and thin diarrhea, similar to rice pulp, results. After this point the rest of the body, including the muscles, internal organs, internal membrane system, and blood circulation becomes involved, producing a variety of diseases.

The sensory nerve processes in the superficial regions are also directly affected by environmental factors, and indirectly affected through the influence of environmental factors on the superficial vessels. The proprioceptive muscle sensory fibers are sensitive to both local temperature and pressure—environmentally induced temperature changes, or increases and decreases in atmospheric pressure, influence proprioceptive fibers, and hence propagated signals along the vessel and muscle pathways. Therefore the free transmission of normal signals along these neurovascular pathways can be impaired or blocked by cold or increased atmospheric pressure, and overexcited by heat or low atmospheric conditions.

Locally induced environmental changes can cause significant harm upstream or downstream of the affected area, and account for the development of both pain and dysfunction in muscles that occur when cold attacks local collateral vessels. Afferent nerve signals from an organ to the brain require an input from a corresponding somatic nerve related to some specific area of the body. Impairment of the afferent signals from the body area affected by environmental factors directly influences the related internal organ as well.

Progression of Assault

External syndromes refer to pathological conditions resulting from the invasion of the superficial portion of the body by exogenous pathogenic factors. Here the principal environmental factors, at least initially, are cold and wind. These attack the six main vessel distribution regions because of the physical location of their pathways on the body.

The bladder-*taiyang* (太阳) vessel, which distributes over the head and down the neck, the posterior region of the arms and back, and the posterior medial regions of the legs, is the initial target. The stomach-*yangming* (阳明) vessel, which distributes to the area of the face, is the second region to be affected. As the attack continues and affects the body more deeply, it moves on to the remaining four vessel distributions: gallbladder-*shaoyang* (少阳), spleen-*taiyin* (太阴), kidney-*shaoyin* (少阴), and liver-*jueyin* (厥阴).

Pathological indications for these six vessel distribution regions are analyzed at various developmental stages of the disease. The stages of disease are classified as taiyang, yangming, shaoyang, taiyin, shaoyin, or jueyin syndromes, according to their unique characteristics. The first three are referred to as the three yang syndromes, while the latter three are the three yin syndromes (Table 13.1).

The progression of attack by wind and cold on the six vessels is described in *NJSW 31* (*Hot Diseases*), giving the stages of febrile diseases. Here the Yellow Emperor asks:

> Nowadays hot diseases all belong to the category of injury by cold. People may either recover from it or die. If they die, death always occurs between six or seven days. If they recover, it takes more than ten days, what about this?
>
> Qibo replies: All the yang regions and vessels are subordinate to the great yang [taiyang], and their vessels [bladder, stomach, and gallbladder] join at Fengfu [DU 16]. Thus they serve all the primary yang vital functions. When a person is attacked by cold, it results in a hot disease. The heat may be very intense, but the person may not die. However,

Table 13.1 Indications of six-day developmental stages of exogenous pathogenic factors reflected in the vessels of the six regions.

Day	*Region*	*Indications*
1.	*Taiyang*	Fever, aversion to cold, headache, pain in nape of neck, stiffness in lower back and spine.
2.	*Yangming*	High fever, profuse sweating, extreme thirst, flushed face, soreness of eyes, dryness of nose, inability to lie down.
3.	*Shaoyang*	Alternate chills and fever, fullness and pain in the costal and hypochondriac regions, deafness.
4.	*Taiyin*	Abdominal fullness and dryness of the mouth.
5.	*Shaoyin*	Aversion to cold, dry and parched mouth, dryness of tongue, thirst.
6.	*Jueyin*	Irritability, abdominal fullness, contraction of the scrotum.

if they develop cold sensations associated with the disease deep in the body, they will certainly die.

The injurious cold is received on the first day in the great yang superficial region and vessels. This results in symptoms of headache with pain in the nape of the neck, as well as intractable stiffness in the lower back and spine.

On day two the injurious cold is received in the sunrise yang [yangming] region and vessels. The sunrise yang dominates flesh and its vessels are intimately associated with the nose, as well as collateral branches traveling up to the eyes. Therefore, symptoms of heat in the body, soreness of the eyes, and dryness in the nose result, along with the inability to lie down.

On day three the injurious cold is received by the lesser yang [shaoyang] region and vessels. The lesser yang dominates the gallbladder and its vessels follow along the ribs with collateral branches traveling to the ears. Therefore, symptoms of pain in the thorax and ribs can result, along with deafness. When the three yang vessels and collateral branches are all affected by the disease, but it has not yet entered the viscera, it can be treated at this stage by inducing perspiration.

On the fourth day the injurious cold is received in the great yin [taiyin] region and vessels. The great yin vessels [spleen] spread out over the stomach with collateral branches ascending to the throat. Thus, symptoms of abdominal fullness and dryness in the mouth are observed.

On day five the injurious cold is received in the lesser yin [shaoyin] region and vessels. The lesser yin vessels [kidney] pass through the kidneys, with collateral branches to the lungs and with attachments to the root of the tongue. Thus, symptoms of a dry and parched mouth with dryness of the tongue result, along with thirst.

On day six the injurious cold is received by the transitional or decreasing yin [jueyin] region and vessels. The decreasing yin vessels [liver] travel to the genitalia, with collateral branches to the liver. Therefore, symptoms of irritability, abdominal fullness, and contraction of the scrotum are observed.

> When the three yin and the three yang vessels, and the five viscera and the six bowels all suffer from the disease, nutrients and defensive substances cannot circulate freely. Hence the five viscera cannot perform their proper function, and death results.

Transformation of Disease

Morbid diseases of the viscera can transform into problems affecting the other organs. Outward symptoms are observed to determine if a condition is showing signs of moving on to another organ. The order of transformation generally follows the five-phase victorious modes. If the disease proceeds to a final phase before receiving treatment, the patient is likely to die. However, if treatment is provided before the terminal stage the patient can recover, even if several organs are already involved in the disorder. The *NJSW 65* (*Symptoms, Root Cause, and Transformation of Disease*) describes transformation patterns for each of the five viscera, the stomach, and the bladder. One example is the transformation pattern for serious heart disease as explained by Qibo:

> When the heart is diseased, first there is pain in the heart, and in one day it results in coughing [lungs], within three days there is pain in the ribs [liver], and in five days there is blockage causing pain and heaviness in the body [spleen]. If the patient does not recover in three days, death will ensue. In winter the patient will die at midnight, and in summer at noon.

Manifestations of Disease

The Chinese pathogenic model is broad based and complex, emphasizing physiological or functional balance as mediated by vascular circulation of vital substances, mainly involving nutrient-based materials. Understanding the Chinese model requires a detailed knowledge of physiology, including the internal organs, circulatory system, muscle distributions, and factors of disease and their manifestations. In addition, it is essential to grasp innumerable details in order to truly understand how to diagnose and treat disorders. As with other medical systems, it is necessary to reduce this data into guiding principles. These generalized concepts then provide a starting point in the diagnostic process. When properly applied, the guiding principles consistently lead to a correct diagnosis and treatment of a presenting problem.

A logical diagnostic process allows the practitioner to focus quickly on the likely cause of a patient's problem. Rarely, if ever, would a patient report that their homeostasis is out of balance, or their antipathogenic function is weak, or that they have a spleen deficiency. Presenting complaints in ancient times were basically the same as they are in the twenty-first century: patients may complain of pain, fever, insomnia, upset stomach, stress, fatigue, depression, and other symptoms. The practitioner may initially recognize some overall general conditions of a true heat problem; an attack of the superficial regions; disharmony of emotions, lifestyle, or seasons; stagnation of blood and vital substances; or an imbalance in yin and yang attributes. Initially, the ailment can be viewed in terms of three general aspects of the pathogenic model: ongoing attack by pathogenic forces; disharmony of yin and yang attributes; and impairment in physiological function affecting the distribution of vital nutrients.

Struggle Between Antipathogenic and Pathogenic Forces

Environmental conditions are considered the primary causative factors in disease. Hence it is critical to determine whether these are involved in the presenting complaint. If so, then it is important to determine how deeply these influences have penetrated into the body and the severity of the ongoing active struggle of the body's natural defenses. If fever is present then a pathogenic or pestilential organism may be involved. In ancient times, just as it is in twenty-first century clinics, infectious disease was given immediate attention. Certain precautions may be required and the treatment approach may vary.

The struggle between the body's antipathogenic function (zheng) and the external environment (xie) is a continuing and constant process. The degree of conflict is a measure of the resistance to pathogenic factors. The response magnitude to external factors must be discerned at the onset of disease as it is indicative of the progression and transformation of the disorder.

An invasion or attack by pathogenic forces activates an antipathogenic response, which has the overall effect of disrupting the harmony between yin and yang aspects of the body. Consequently there is a functional disturbance of the internal organs and vessels, disorder of blood and vital substances, and derangement of ascending and descending function. The net effect is pathological changes and the development of disease. These changes manifest as either excess or deficiency syndromes.

Excess syndromes occur if antipathogenic forces are strong and the pathogenic forces are hyperactive. Deficiency syndromes, or syndromes of deficiency mixed with excess, occur when the antipathogenic function is weak and pathogenic forces are either excessive or at the normal background level (Figure 2.3). As stated in *NJSW 28* (quoted in Physiological Balance and Homeostasis, see page 239), overabundant environmental or pathogenic factors cause excess, but it is deprivation of refined substances (ying, wei, and shenjing) and vital air (qi) that causes deficiency. Insufficient refined substances and vital air causes impairment in homeostasis or antipathogenic function (Figure 13.1).

Therefore excess refers to pathological conditions due to hyperactivity of pathogenic factors. Excess exists in the early or middle phases of diseases that result from the invasion of external pathogenic factors. Excess is also the case in diseases caused by retention of either food or phlegm fluid, or by stagnant blood and retained water, or dampness. Deficiency on the other hand refers to pathological conditions resulting from the impairment of homeostasis or antipathogenic function (zheng). Deficiencies are seen in diseases resulting from prolonged weakness of body constitution, long-term emotional strain, or poor dietary habits. Such lingering diseases result in inadequate function of the internal organs and deficiency of blood, vital substances, and body fluid.

An active struggle between zheng and xie represents the relative state of the body's immune response. A review of symptoms related to the six regions and their vessels provides a clue on how deeply the pathogenic factors have penetrated into the body (see Progression of Assault, page 245). Conditions that produce a true fever are heat syndromes, which usually involve pathogenic or pestilential organisms. If the disorder is contained within one of the three body cavities and has symptoms of damp heat, it can be differentiated by internal membrane (*sanjiao*, 三焦). Specific organs, including the lungs, large intestine, stomach, spleen, liver, gallbladder, and bladder, can also be the focus of heat or damp heat disorders.

Disharmony of Yin and Yang

Fundamental to the physiological model is that health depends on maintaining homeostasis. Presenting complaints are therefore viewed with respect to impaired functional balance, often expressed in terms of yin and yang attributes. Viewing disease and dysfunction in this manner is helpful in characterizing a wide range of problems affecting individual internal organs, and disease is thus often diagnosed and treated in terms of an imbalance or disharmony in yin and yang qualities.

All aspects of physiology can be viewed in terms of yin and yang characteristics (Chapter 4). The interdependent opposition of yin and yang is mutually balanced in a state of health, hence either an impairment of vital substances (yin) or disturbances in functional activities (yang) can be viewed in terms of disharmony of yin and yang. Understanding this crucial yin-yang opposition, which underlies the basic processes of disease, is rudimentary to identifying the source of disease. All pathological conditions, including those of the internal organs, can be characterized in terms of yin and yang attributes. The overall functional activity of an organ (visceral qi) is viewed in terms of yin substance, including refined substances, and yang function, which can include vital air and metabolism as well.

Ailments do not occur unless the body is invaded by external pathogenic forces or functionally impaired by internal factors that cause derangement of the yin-yang balance. Disharmony of yin and yang suggests that one quality is excess or deficient, manifesting as cold or heat syndromes: excess yang properties generally produce heat syndromes of the excess type; excess yin qualities usually produce cold syndromes of the excess type. Deficiency of yang properties produces deficiency cold syndromes; deficiency of yin qualities produces deficiency heat syndromes.

Excess heat syndromes result from the inflammatory (yang) aspect of defensive function (*weiqi*, 卫气) mounting a reaction against an invading organism. In contrast, deficiency heat syndromes include reduced output of anti-inflammatory substances (yin substance) from the adrenal cortex failing to control the inflammatory processes.

Excess cold syndromes indicate that pathogenic cold (yin factor) has invaded the body, restricting the flow of blood and vital substances. This impairs the warming function of vital substances, involving nutrients (ying), defensive substances (wei), vitality substances (shenjing), and oxygen from vital air (qi). Deficiency cold syndromes can result from metabolic dysfunction, such as hypofunction of the thyroid gland (yang deficiency), resulting in reduced vigor.

Abnormal Distribution and Function

Homeostasis also depends on the overall function of the body, with metabolism and blood circulation being of major significance. When disease conditions involve impairment in the distribution of blood and vital substances, or are the result of impaired functional activity, the problem is viewed in terms of abnormal distribution and function. Abnormal function can be classified as a failure of either ascending or descending function. Many conditions associated with the internal organs, distribution vessels, circulation, and muscle distributions are considered within the broad framework of abnormal distribution and function.

Internal organ function and the processes of distributing blood, nutrients, defensive substances, vitality substances, and vital air (qi) are discussed in terms of ascending and descending (for organ functional direction), and outward and inward movement (for arterial and venous flow). For example, the stomach and intestines pass food through the body: their function descends. The lungs oxygenate the blood, which is dispersed throughout the body: lung function is said to descend and disperse. The spleen is responsible for sending the absorbed nutrients on to the heart via the liver: its function ascends. The liver, which processes nutrients received via the portal vein and subsequently passed on to the vena cava and heart, has an ascending and dispersing function.

Abnormal ascending and descending function refers to pathological conditions of the internal organs when their normal state or direction of function is impaired. Abnormal ascending or descending function and impaired or altered distribution of blood and vital substances affects all the internal organs, as well as the internal and the external regions of the body, causing numerous pathological changes. Failure of the lung function to descend and disperse vital air results in coughing, asthmatic breathing, and a suffocating sensation in the chest. An abnormal ascending function of the stomach causes belching, nausea, vomiting, and acid reflux. Failure of the spleen's ascending function, and dysfunction of the transportation and transformation function of the spleen, results in loose stools and diarrhea.

Even though all the internal organs are involved in ascending and descending functions and the distribution of blood and vital substances, the functional activities of the spleen and stomach play a key role. In the Chinese view, the spleen (including the pancreatic function) and stomach have the task of processing food and distributing the acquired materials for maintenance and bodily function. The spleen and stomach are contained in the abdominal cavity (middle *jiao*), which connects with the other internal organs in the thoracic, abdominal, and lower abdominal cavities (upper, middle, and lower jiao)—for this reason the spleen and stomach are considered pivotal to the ascending and descending of blood and vital substances. The spleen and stomach are also important in the production of blood.

Organ functional activity, characterized as visceral qi, has both yin-substance and yang-function components, and is greatly affected by supplied nutrients—hence the spleen and stomach help to sustain functional activity. Diet also makes a crucial contribution to supporting functional activity or causing dysfunction by overconsumption of certain flavors. One feature unique to the Chinese medical system is the conception of functional activity in terms of direction: any disturbance in direction of normal flow, often called perverse or inverse function (*niqi*, 逆气), causes pathological conditions.

Because vessels distribute blood and vital substances to the extremities and internal organs, the normal outflow of arterial blood and return flow in the veins is critical. Superficial body regions are directly susceptible to environmental influences that can impede the outward and inward flow. Impairment in this distribution function can manifest in pathology related to specific distribution vessels. The superficial body regions supplied by the vessels are mainly the musculoskeletal structures. Hence impaired distribution of blood, nutrients, oxygen, and other vital substances results in pain and pathology in the muscle distributions.

Clinical Presentation

Determining the cause of a disease requires a systematic diagnosis and differentiation of presenting symptoms. As to be expected, both the diagnostic process and the treatment strategies are consistent with the pathogenic model. Without the benefit of modern laboratory tests or diagnostic imaging capability, the ancient Chinese physicians were able to discern and treat the acute superficial symptoms (*biao*, 表) and chronic root cause (*ben*, 本) of all diseases afflicting their patients. Some present-day practitioners do use modern diagnostic tests as an adjunct to the Chinese diagnostic method. However, the challenge remains to sort through presenting complaints and outward symptoms to determine the most likely cause of a problem. To this end sophisticated diagnostic routines are applied, consisting of inquiry; observing the patient; auscultation (listening) and olfaction (smelling); and palpating body regions and pulses. Information gathered via the latter three methods is used to confirm the suspected disease profile determined by the inquiry phase of the diagnosis. Full details of the diagnostic process are beyond the scope of this present text; a summary of the four diagnostic categories is provided below.

Inquiry

Most important in the diagnostic process is questioning the patient about their chief complaint and associated conditions, including the onset of the problem and its history. The patient's status, profession, residence, lifestyle, habits, emotions, and environmental exposures are also taken into account. A family member or companion of the patient may also supply additional facts, especially if the patient is not able to respond. Medical history forms are often used to obtain additional information to assist the practitioner during the inquiry process. These forms may be organized along the same lines as the Chinese system of diagnosis, or may be similar to a Western medical history questionnaire. The inquiry follows a systematic plan involving a standard group of questions to focus on the chief complaint of the patient. A wide range of topics is used and the practitioner is not restricted in what questions are asked. These may include inquiries about the presence of chills and fever; presence or absence of sweating; eating, drinking, and substance-use habits; frequency and quality of defecation and urination; nature and location of pain or possible impairment; sleeping patterns, including times of waking and going to bed; menses, leukorrhea, and obstetric history for women; state of stress and emotional strain; physical activities; and medical history, surgical events, present medication use, and previous injuries.

Inspection and Observation

This aspect of diagnosis involves detecting abnormal changes by visually observing the patient's vitality, color, appearance, body size and structure, movement and posture, and secretions and excretions. With respect to vitality, if the patient is alert and in good spirits, is responsive with a sparkle in the eyes, and is energetic, the prognosis is good and the disease is considered mild. If the patient has dull eyes, is spiritless and sluggish, shows possible mental disturbance, and lacks vigor, the prognosis is poorer and the disease is considered severe. Observation of color involves coloration and luster of the face; color of the body regions, secretions, and excretions; and color of the tongue body and coating. Observation of the tongue involves examination of the tongue body, size, shape, and color, and the presence or absence of coatings and their coloration. The tongue is supplied by collaterals of the heart, spleen, and kidney distribution vessels, and therefore reflects conditions of the internal organs. Each of the sense organs is carefully examined to determine the possible involvement of each of the related viscera (Table 3.2). The condition of the body is observed to determine if the patient is strong or weak, firm or flaccid, or overweight or skinny. Movement and activity are also observed to determine if there is motor impairment or weakness, joint dysfunction, violent movement of the limbs, normal or impaired gait while walking, or slumped or straight posture.

Auscultation and Olfaction

In ancient times auscultation involved detecting and noting certain characteristic sounds that are related to specific organs, and involved attention to speech, to the sound of respiration, and to any cough. Speech is evaluated in terms of loudness or feebleness compared to normal levels, and whether it is incoherent or delirious. Changes in speech, including the inability to speak and whether its onset was sudden or gradual, or related to emotional stress or unconsciousness, are also important to determine. The sound of respiration is evaluated to determine if breathing is feeble, or forced and coarse compared to normal. The sound and characteristics of any cough are also observed and noted. A cough can be weak in a feeble voice or loud in a coarse voice.

Characteristic odors can also be associated with each of the viscera (Table 3.2). Odors of secretions or excretions are evaluated to determine whether they are unusually foul or not, or if they have a sour characteristic, in order to deduce the nature of the disease. The source of any odor is examined to determine the locality of the disease.

Palpation and Articulation

Palpation is a method of physical diagnosis in which pathological conditions are detected by feeling and gently pressing along specific areas of the body. Some conditions of the internal organs or referred pain, and other problems associated with the vessels, muscle distributions, and nodes (acupoints), can be ascertained. The body surface, including along the distribution course of the vessels, muscles, and nodal pathways, is examined to determine sites of sensitivity, temperature variations, lumps and masses, abnormalities in the internal organs, abnormal muscle contractions or knots, and response at painful regions. Palpation proceeds from the localized source of the problem out to the extremity associated with the affected area. Observation of sensitive locations, either distal or proximal to an area involving muscle pain and dysfunction, identifies the muscle distribution affected. Changes in sensitivity of nodes and other regions can be used to assess the effectiveness of treatment.

Articulation involves movement of the joints, whether assisted or not by the practitioner, to assess the functional status of the muscle distributions. Range of motion and ease of articulation are evaluated. The strength of specific muscles, as well as reflex activity, can be determined. Specific diagnosis is performed to differentiate between certain musculoskeletal conditions, and the nature and degree of pain associated with joint movement is also noted.

Feeling the pulses at the wrist location of the radial artery and other specific pulsating locations on the body is an important part of palpation methods. The pulse is measured while observing the breathing, with four heartbeats per respiration cycle assessed as normal. Above this rate the pulse is considered fast; below it, slow. The Chinese formalized the examination of the radial artery (lung distribution vessel) pulse at the wrist and the carotid artery (stomach distribution vessel) pulse on the neck. Comparing the radial artery and carotid pulses provides information for a differential diagnosis to determine whether the presenting condition is internal or external, and which distribution vessel is involved in the disorder (Chapter 11).

Pulses are palpated at nine other regions on the body to confirm which organ may be involved (Table 10.1). Without the aid of instrumentation to measure and record pulse profiles, dedicated practice is needed to develop a high level of proficiency. Modern pulse-measuring devices are very useful, and provide consistent and repeatable information (Wang: 1988; Broffman and McCullock: 1986). These units are helpful in training students and practitioners to become proficient in pulse-taking and diagnosis.

Because it is difficult to perform pulse diagnosis on very young children, a form of pediatric diagnosis involving observation of the veins on the index finger is used with infants in lieu of taking the pulse.

Differentiation of Syndromes

Information gathered after a full diagnosis is systematically evaluated to determine the likely cause of a disorder. Presenting symptoms are compared with disease profiles as they are known to manifest in various body regions or physiological systems. Initially, the presenting complaints are viewed in terms of the three main pathogenic categories: the struggle between antipathogenic and pathogenic factors; disharmony of yin and yang characteristics; and abnormal distribution and function. Any of the three areas of pathogenesis may be involved to some extent. It is important to consider the most likely causative factors. Possible attack by primary external environmental factors suggests some degree of penetration into the body. The presence of true heat indicates an active struggle between pathogenic and antipathogenic forces. Miscellaneous factors, including dietary or internal factors, such as emotions, suggest internal disorders. Some aspects of internal organ involvement manifest as disharmony in yin and yang attributes. Musculoskeletal problems are usually external, and do not necessarily involve the internal organs.

Symptoms can be differentiated within major physiological categories, such as by organ-related distribution vessels (Tables 11.1 through 11.6), their collateral vessels (Table 9.4), and the eight singular vessels (Table 9.2). Specific syndromes of the muscle distributions are analyzed, including through the performance of functional tests, to determine the distribution involved (Tables 12.2 and 12.3). When problems involve a particular articulation joint, the six muscle distribution pathways across the affected joint are examined, including palpating sensitive areas. Problems of the internal organs can be differentiated by syndrome patterns (Table 3.4), and also by examining the wide range of attributes of each organ, including its dominant tissue, sensory organ, sensory function, body orifice, bodily fluids, emotions, endocrine gland, and vitalities (organ spirits). Disparities in functional activities or responsibilities assigned to a particular organ provide additional information for the differentiation of syndromes.

To help the practitioner identify the nature of a disorder, presenting complaints are classified in terms of four sets of opposites: exterior/interior, cold/heat, excess/deficiency, and yin/yang. Most disorders are described using some or all of these classifications. These paired aspects are the eight diagnostic keys noted in the *Neijing* that were popularized by Zhang Zhongjing (150–219). The first step in the process is to determine whether the condition is an internal or an external disorder. If a condition of true heat is present, this problem is examined first. Ultimately, the presenting problem can be categorized as either an excess or a deficiency condition, or determined to be neither. Finally, most conditions can be viewed in terms of yin and yang qualities.

Exterior and Interior

A comparison of external and internal disease manifestations is used to determine the depth of the disorder within the body (Figure 13.2) and its likely direction of development (Table 13.1). The viscera and bowels within the body cavities are interior; the skin, hair, muscles, and their distribution and collateral vessels belong to the exterior portion of the body. Even the deeper vessels reflect exterior conditions. When the five viscera are affected by exterior conditions, it is considered an interior disorder. The demarcation between exterior and interior disorders is not always clear, and syndromes of both conditions can be present at the same time.

Exterior syndromes are often marked by a sudden onset with short duration, as typically seen during the early stages of disease caused by external environmental factors. Clinical presentation may be characteristic of the taiyang syndrome (Table 13.1). Symptoms may vary depending on the strength of the external factor and the fundamental constitution of the individual. Manifestations can include conditions of cold, heat, excess, or deficiency. Distribution vessels reflect significant exterior signs (Tables 11.1 through 11.6). Pain and dysfunction of the muscle distributions manifest mostly as exterior syndromes not involving the internal organs (Tables 12.2 and 12.3).

Interior syndromes are the result of external factors penetrating deep into the body to affect the viscera (after level 6 in Figure 13.2), or from functional disturbance of the internal organs due to other causes. Pathological manifestations may vary to some extent, depending on whether the condition is the result of deep transmission of external factors to attack the internal organs, or is due to dietary factors or emotional strain. Interior syndromes are often differentiated in terms of the internal organs (Table 3.4), or in terms of excess and deficiency.

Cold and Heat

The nature of some disorders can be characterized in terms of cold and heat. Syndromes of cold and heat are often viewed in relation to deficiency and excess in either yin or yang attributes. In general, excess yang produces fever, while excess yin produces cold. Pathological syndromes of true heat are due to an invasion of pathogenic heat factors (usually an infective agent), while false heat is the result of an internal yin substance deficiency in the body. The presence of true heat indicates an active struggle between pathogenic and antipathogenic forces. Of the internal organs, the lungs are particularly affected by heat, and most of the organs, including the internal membrane system, are affected by damp heat. Heat syndromes also manifest in many flaccid syndromes of the muscle distributions. A morbid heat condition can progressively attack the nutrients, defensive substances, and vital air systems, eventually affecting the blood itself, resulting in possible death.

Pathological syndromes due to cold are the result of external cold, or due to a deficiency of internal yang function in the body. Excess cold often results in the development of heat (see Progression of Assault, page 245). The development of internal cold conditions, typified by shaoyin cold, is serious. Many musculoskeletal problems are the result of cold attacking the superficial regions of the body, and most obstructive rheumatism disorders are thought to involve cold.

Excess and Deficiency

Primary to the Chinese homeostatic disease model is the consideration of the relative strength of the pathogenic and antipathogenic forces (Figure 2.3). The resulting balance between these two entities is classified as either an excess or deficiency condition. Pathological syndromes can be differentiated to determine the state of this dynamic interplay. Flourishing environmental factors cause excess, while deprivation of vital substances causes deficiency. Therefore, excess syndromes refer to pathological conditions where external factors are excessive, and the homeostatic balance or the antipathogenic factor is strong. Deficiency syndromes refer to conditions where homeostatic balance or the antipathogenic factor is weak (less than optimum). The deprivation or consumption of vital substances usually results in hypofunction of the internal organs. Deficiency (*xu*, 虛) syndromes can also be expressed in terms of yin and yang attributes. All the viscera can manifest a variety of deficiency disorders, including functional, yin substance, yang function, vital air (qi), and blood deficiencies. Syndromes of blood and vital substance deficiencies can also result. Excess emotions consume vital substances, and overall vitality can be impacted by excess or deficiency conditions.

Yin and Yang

Yin and yang are general terms that can be used to describe most pathological conditions. As such, yin and yang attributes are often applied to summarize each of the preceding three sets of the eight keys. Exterior, excess, and heat are categorized as yang in nature; while interior, deficiency, and cold, are classed as yin. Disharmony of yin and yang qualities often manifests in conditions affecting the five viscera. Yin and yang deficiency syndromes of the internal organs usually predominate over excess disorders. In severe conditions, certain syndromes are characterized as collapse of yin or collapse of yang. However, yin and yang attributes are not sufficient in themselves for an in-depth diagnosis; consequently, the differentiation of syndromes by factors such as internal organs, vessels, vitalities, and muscle distributions is indispensable.

14
Mechanisms of Action

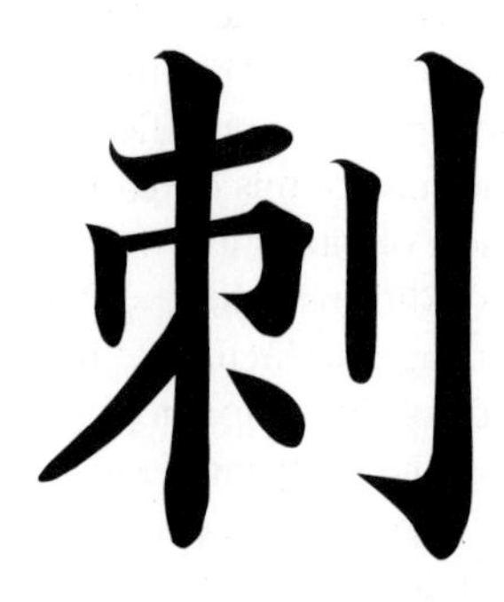

Ci: To Needle

> The scope of needling therapy is principally to regulate vital substances, which are derived from food accumulated in the stomach to form the nutrients [ying] and defensive substances [wei] that are circulated through their respective pathways in the body.
>
> Qibo, *NJLS 75 (Needling Nodes for True Function and Pathogenic Factors)*

Fundamental to the verification of needling (acupuncture) as a viable medical approach is an understanding of the basic mechanisms involved, including a profound appreciation of the Chinese anatomical, physiological, and treatment theories of how inserting fine needles into specific superficial locations produces beneficial results. The most important of these effects are restoring blood, nutrient, and vital air flow; restoring visceral and immune function; promoting physiological and autonomic balance (homeostasis); relieving pain; and promoting tissue healing. Various efforts have proposed possible underlying mechanisms by which needling the superficial body influences the internal organs and brings about pain relief (Pomeranz and Stux: 1988; Kendall: 1989) The first indications of a possible relationship between needle stimulation and internal body pain control was demonstrated when naloxone, a known opiate antagonist, was shown to attenuate the analgesic effect of acupuncture (Chapman and Benedetti: 1977; Chapman et. al.: 1980; Mayer, Price, and Rafii: 1977). Early studies involving morphine and electrical stimulation of the periaqueductal and periventricular gray areas of the midbrain suggested that acupuncture analgesia was mediated by descending inhibitory pathways (Mayer et. al.: 1977). Many biologically active substances, including neurotransmitters, were then identified in acupuncture analgesia (Han et. al.: 1980; Han and Terenius: 1982). A virtual explosion of new research occurred during the 1980s and 1990s, providing additional insight into the complexities of needling stimulation. Even functional magnetic resonance imaging (fMRI) studies have shown that acupuncture stimulates the central nervous system (CNS), including major integration centers in the brain (Cho et. al.: 1998; Fang and Hayes: 1999).

Chinese physicians observed from the earliest times that needle insertion and stimulation often produces an immediate response, called *deqi* (得气) in Chinese. It feels like a small, quick cramping or electrical sensation at the needling site. Pain sensory (nociceptive) neurons in the skin (afferent Aδ and C substance P neurons) are needed to stimulate this initial reaction.

Inhibition of these afferent dorsal root ganglia (DRG) neurons negates the effect of needling therapy. The somatic nociceptive neurons distribute to specific segmental levels of the spinal cord, where they are closely associated with the afferent sympathetic neurons of the viscera and blood vessels that travel to the same cord segment. This close anatomical association potentially gives rise to somatovisceral and viscerosomatic communication (Schott: 1994). Parasympathetic afferents from the viscera are also involved in the mechanisms of needling.

Needling also provokes neural reflexes that cause propagated sensations (PS) along the nodal (acupoint) pathway of the stimulated vessel and muscle distribution. In general, subjects are not aware of these sensations; however, selection of certain needling sites, strength of stimulation, and the patient's condition may result in a conscious awareness of PS. Afferent sensory nerves involved in PS are group II proprioceptive intrafusal neurons of the muscle spindles. These secondary muscle spindles provide static load information for normal function and control of the primary motor nerves; they also participate in complex defensive spinal reflexes, providing the means for quick retraction of a hand, for example, which accidentally encounters a thorn or hot object. Propriospinal reflexes transmit signals to muscles throughout the body to maintain bodily balance and function while instantly pulling the offended limb away from the source of potential injury. Needle insertion provides a controlled means of activating these propriospinal pathways that are essential to promoting restorative processes. The beneficial effects of needling are attenuated or completely eliminated when these propriospinal reflexes are inhibited.

Superficial stimulation affects the internal organs and CNS through three basic anatomical and physiological features. The first involves events at the same segment of the spinal cord that receives sensory input from the needling site. Here, the convergence of somatic and visceral afferent signals initiates somatovisceral responses, activating the ascending spinal cord pathways, and directing supraspinal descending restorative control, including pain relief, from the brain back to the level initially affected by needling stimulation. With this feature in mind, nodes are selected either to treat local and adjacent problems, or because of a specific known nodal property or influence on a particular viscera. The second feature is the stimulation of responses remote from the node location, producing distal and proximal effects. These processes involve the propriospinal system, afferent nociceptive neurons, and participation of autonomic afferents to produce neural reflexes that activate CNS processes and also generate PS. The third feature relates to how a node is stimulated by needling; strength of manipulation and duration of needle retention both influence the response, especially in the treatment of specific disease conditions (Chapter 15). For this reason, it is important to understand the part played by the skin and superficial tissues in mediating CNS responses to needling.

Tissue Response to Needling

Because of the skin's critical role, the body evolved efficient defense and immune functions that provide protection against damage, puncture wounds, pathogenic assault, insect bites, and animal bites. In the Chinese view, the skin controls perspiration and has a primary defensive role, especially against external assault. When impaired by excess environmental or other factors, this defensive function can be activated or restored by needling the neurovascular nodes. Neurological systems are directly involved in cutaneous inflammation and the wound-healing processes that are activated by trauma to the skin, including insertion of a fine needle. It is now recognized that the skin contains a complex neurovasculoimmune regulatory network, involving cutaneous tissues, fine arterial and venous blood vessels (*sunmai*, 孙脉), lymphatic tissue, immune cells, afferent somatic neurons, and sympathetic neurons (Yamada and Hoshino: 1996; Misery: 1996, 1997; Ansel et. al.: 1997; Schulze et. al.: 1997; Panuncio et. al.: 1999; Streilein, Alard, and Niizeki: 1999). The functional integrity of cutaneous immunity is principally mediated by the contribution of mast cells, bradykinin, cutaneous substance P neurons, and sympathetic neurons associated with local blood vessels. A wide range of neuropeptides associated with the skin function as neuromodulators, neurohormones, and hormones (Lotti, Hautmann, and Panconesi: 1995; Berczi et. al.: 1996; Wallengren: 1997; Luger and Lotti: 1998; Misery: 1998; Rossi and Johansson: 1998; Scholzen et. al.: 1998; Streilein, Alard, and Niizeki: 1999). The most important of these with respect to needling responses are the tackykinin substance P, which stimulates neurokinin 1 (NK1) receptors and the kinins, including bradykinin, and related B1 and B2 receptors. Epidermal cytokines are also crucial for the induction and regulation of immune responses of the skin (Luger et. al.: 1996). Cutaneous immune features provide the anatomical and physiological means through which needling stimulates afferent substance P neurons that provoke CNS-mediated effects and antidromic axon reflexes. Central beneficial effects include an influence on the hypothalamus-pituitary-adrenal axis, which is important in maintaining homeostasis and immune system function.

Inserting a needle anywhere in the body will provoke an acute local inflammatory defensive response; however, a greater distribution of skin sensors and cell types are concentrated in critical areas where greater protection is needed. This includes superficial locations of nerves, blood and lymphatic vessels, and neuromuscular attachments, or where vessels and associated nerves penetrate muscle fascia. Likewise, other areas of the skin may be more sensitive to heat or cold for obvious protective reasons. Many of these sensitive locations are coincident with nodes. Anatomical attributes suggest a protective role for these sites, where a pricking or puncture assault could cause more serious damage than a simple superficial wound. Some node locations correspond to motor points or Golgi tendon organs. In comparison with non-node sites, nodes have a higher electrical conductance and a larger concentration of neural and fine vascular components, along with a greater distribution of mast cells[1] (Hwang: 1992; Yu: 1996). Earlier studies confirmed lower electrical impedance at node locations compared to non-nodal sites (Brown, Ulett, and Stern: 1974; Reichmanis, Marino, and Becker: 1975; McCarroll and Rowley: 1979; Zhu: 1981). Electrical conductance has also been found to be higher along the entire pathway compared with non-nodal sites 1 centimeter lateral to the traditional nodal route (Zhu et. al.: 1981; Weng et. al.: 1990). In addition, mechanically tapping along the nodal pathway being stimulated can provoke conscious PS.

The predominant subjective response to needling muscle, tendon, and periosteum is soreness and distension, while needling a nerve branch evokes numbness, or a blood vessel, pain (Lin et. al.: 1985). Progressive blocking of sensations and nerve impulses shows that the sensation of touch and pressure, served by group II neurons, disappears at the same time as the sensation of electroacupuncture stimulation (Dong and Zhang: 1985). A pricking sensation served by Aδ and group III nociceptive neurons disappears at the same time as the sensation of manual needle manipulation. Wang et. al. (1985) found that group II neurons convey numbness, group III distension and heaviness, and group IV soreness. The lightly myelinated cutaneous Aδ neurons (tissue group III) consistently dominate the mediation of needling reactions, followed by unmyelinated cutaneous C neurons (tissue group IV) and then group II fibers. The analgesic effects produced by stimulating these somatic neurons are blocked by the administration of naloxone (Chen et. al.: 1985).

Inserting a fine sterilized needle into a human subject results in a visible reaction on the skin, characterized by a small flare response (reddened area) forming around the needle a short time after its insertion.[2] This response is inhibited by the application of capsaicin, which depletes substance P, indicating that it is mediated by cutaneous nociceptive (substance P) afferents (Jancso, Kiraly, and Jancso-Gabor: 1980; Bernstein et. al.: 1981; Magerl et. al.: 1987; Bjerring and Arendt-Nielsen: 1990; Bunker et. al.: 1991). Capsaicin suppresses substance P–induced joint inflammation in rats (Lam and Ferrell: 1989) and ear edema in mice (Inoue, Nagata, and Koshihara: 1995) due to a reduction in substance P with no loss of NK1 receptor responsiveness. If the nerve function to the site of needling is interrupted, the flare response is absent (Lembeck: 1985) and the therapeutic influence of needling a specific node is negated (He et. al.: 1993). Products from mast cells, including degranulated histamine, platelet activating factor (PAF), and leukotrienes, as well as substance P, are thought to contribute to flare formation. The size and characteristics of the flare and how it spreads or changes over the course of the treatment gives an estimate of the state of hollowness (deficiency) or solidness (excess) of the patient, and whether the treatment has induced a positive effect.

Needling response and local inflammatory reaction involves the participation of superficial substance P nociceptive and sympathetic neurons, and the interaction between the blood coagulation system and the immune complement system[3] (Figure 14.1). In the Chinese system,

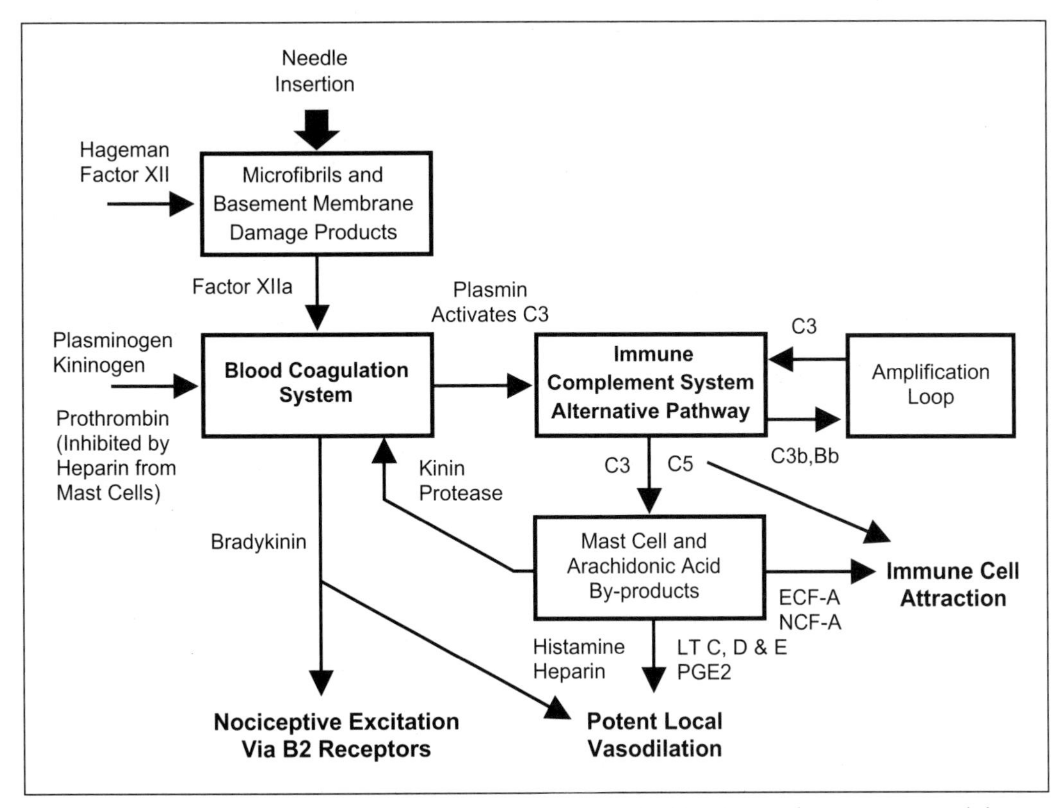

Figure 14.1 Schematic diagram of the interaction between the blood coagulation system and the immune complement system alternative pathway in response to needling.

this response is conceived of as an interaction between nutrients (*ying*, 营) and defensive substances (*wei*, 卫). Two major pathways in the process, involving the activation and production of complement C3 and the release of kinin protease that preferentially produces more bradykinin, allow the reaction to be amplified. However, axon reflex participation of the cutaneous substance P neurons at the needling site is needed to activate and sustain the initial inflammatory process. The reaction covers several discrete time-dependent phases, initially favoring vasodilatation, and later inactivating the inflammatory agents and promoting tissue repair (Table 14.1).

Tissue Reactions: Blood Coagulation System

Tissue reactions are indispensable to needling and other methods that stimulate nodes. Inserting a needle into the skin and superficial regions causes minute local tissue trauma that activates tissue damage and repair mechanisms (Figure 14.1). Electron microscopic analysis of material adhering to needles used to stimulate nodes in the lumbar region was found by Kimura et. al. (1992) to consist of collagen fibers, elastic fibers, fibroblasts, adipocytes, and mast cells. Needling-induced damage products of collagen, microfibrils, and basement membrane activate the blood coagulation Factor XII (Hageman Factor) (Mohammad et. al.: 1984; Packham and Mustard: 1984; Wells and Henney: 1982). Once activated, this factor (XIIa) simultaneously initiates three separate cascading processes that affect the fibrinolytic, kinin, and coagulation features of the blood coagulation system (Rosenburg, R. D.: 1979). One of these processes results in the production of plasmin, which triggers the alternative pathway of the immune complement system by activating complement protein C3 (Cooper: 1982). The immune complement system produces vasodilatation at the needling site and begins clearing needle-damage products.

Table 14.1 Phases of needling-induced tissue reaction.

Reaction[1]	*Activity*
1. Vasodilatory	Degranulation of mast cells, kinin protease, complement, Hageman Factor XII dependent reactants, bradykinin, and substance P released by axon reflex.
2. Nociceptive Excitation	Bradykinin B2 excites substance P Aδ and C fiber, and sustains reaction by axon reflex vasodilatation acting on tissues and sympathetic fibers.
3. Chemotactic	Attracts immune cells, including basophils, neutrophils, monocytes, and eosinophils.
4. Solubility	Activates C3 and C1, lysis of fibrin, inhibits thrombin, disaggregates platelets, and clears needle-damage products.
5. Tissue Repair	Attraction, aggregation, and degranulation of platelets, local vascular constriction, and formation of fibrin and clots.
6. Inactivation	Degradation of Hageman Factor XII, heparin, heparan sulfate, SRS-A (leukotrienes C, D, & E), and histamine to inactivate inflammatory reaction, and cortisol release reduces formation of arachidonic acid.

1. Phases 1, 2, 3, and 4 predominate during the initial stages of the reaction; 5 and 6 predominate during the intermediate and latter stages of the reaction. For more details see Kendall 1989, Table 2.

Blood coagulation is initially reduced by the lysis of fibrin and release of heparin, which inhibits the production of thrombin. Factor XIIa activates kallikrein, which transforms plasma kininogen to bradykinin B1 and B2 (Beck: 1979; Bhoola, Figueroa, and Worthy: 1992; Raidoo and Bhoola: 1998), which serve to activate B2 receptors on substance P nociceptive neurons (Walker, Perkins, and Dray: 1995; Regoli et. al.: 1998). Kallikrein and immune complement protein C5 are both chemotactic and attract immune cells to the site of needle intrusion. The response to needle-damage products is controlled by adenosine triphosphate (ATP), guanosine triphosphate (GTP), and a calcium-dependent cascade modulated in the cytoplasm of the target mast cells and basophils (Benacerraf and Unanue: 1979; Frick: 1982). Reactive products of the blood coagulation system created by the activation of Factor XII are released into the humoral pathway (Beck: 1979; Frick: 1982; Werb and Goldstein: 1982). Many of these are effective only at the needle insertion site, although some exert an influence throughout the body.

Kinins, including bradykinin and kallidin, are peptides produced at the site of needle-induced tissue damage, and produce a variety of effects. These are mediated through B1 and B2 receptors (Walker, Perkins, and Dray: 1995; Regoli et. al.: 1998). The kallikrein-kinin system responds to tissue damage and injury, and is found throughout the body, including in the nervous system (Raidoo and Bhoola: 1998). The action of the kinins in the periphery includes vasodilatation, increased vascular permeability, stimulation of immune cells, and activation of substance P neurons. Bradykinin B2 receptors participate in the classic acute inflammation, while B1 receptors appear to be involved in chronic inflammatory responses (Hall: 1997). Bradykinin B2 receptors are also found on vagal afferent neurons (Krstew, Jarrott, and Lawrence: 1998). The B1 bradykinin receptors are located on cells other than neurons, and may be responsible for releasing mediators that activate or sensitize nociceptive neurons (Davis et. al.: 1996). Bradykinin B2 receptors may play a role in the upregulation of immune cells, including neutrophils and myelocytes (Bhoola: 1996; Kemme et. al.: 1999; Naidoo et. al.: 1999).

Immune Response: Complement Alternative Pathway

Once plasmin provokes the complement alternative pathway a series of complement proteins are activated by C3, resulting in the production of more C3, as well as C5 and C9. Both C3 and C5 are potent vasodilatory agents that degranulate tissue mast cells and their plasma counterpart, the basophils. Mast cells and basophils release the inflammatory agent histamine, along with heparin. Initially, heparin increases blood flow at the needling site by inhibiting the production of thrombin. Mast cells and basophils also release kinin protease, which serves to stimulate the blood coagulation system with the production of more plasmin to activate C3, and bradykinin to continue stimulation of the local substance P neurons. Mast cells and basophils release neutrophilic chemotactic factor of anaphylaxis (NCF-A) and eosinophilic chemotactic factor of anaphylaxis (ECF-A). These chemotactic agents attract neutrophil and eosinophil immune cells to the site of needle insertion, where they play an important role in mediating the controlling and restorative phases of the needling reaction.[4]

Inserting fine needles may not at first appear to produce significant physiological effects, however there are notable potentiating features of this process. The first of these is an amplification loop within the immune complement alternative pathway where C3 produces an intermediate form (C3b, Bb), which in turn activates more C3 (Figure 14.1). The main vasodilatory function of C3 and C5 is to degranulate mast cells and basophils to release histamine and heparin. Kinin protease enzymatically activates more Factor XII, which stimulates the production of plasmin and bradykinin. Plasmin produced in this way activates more C3, which in turn produces even more C3. The additional bradykinin that is produced stimulates the substance P nociceptive neurons, which in turn sustain the needling reaction through the axon reflex affecting the site of needle insertion.

Membrane material from the mast cells and basophils is converted to arachidonic acid by the phospholipase A2 pathway, which in turn leads to the production of prostaglandins and leukotrienes by two different routes. The first of these involves the formation of prostaglandins and thromboxanes from arachidonic acid via the cyclooxygenase-2 pathway (Murakami et. al.: 1999). The other route involves the production of leukotrienes from arachidonic acid via 5-lipoxygenase action. The prostaglandins most important to mediating needling response are PGI2 (prostacyclin), which causes disaggregation of platelets and initially prevents clotting at the needle intrusion site, and the potent bronchodilator and vasodilator PGE2, which regulates tissue microenvironment. Prostaglandin PGE2 also has a possible role in sensitizing and recruiting primary afferent substance P neurons, which have bradykinin B2 receptors, and thereby increasing the proportion of substance P neuron participation (Stucky, Thayer, and Seybold: 1996). Substance P release from the primary afferent neurons by the cytokine interleukin-1 beta (IL-1 beta) is through the cyclooxygenase-2 system (Inoue et. al.: 1999). The prostaglandin-dependent proinflammatory role of IL-1 beta appears to involve sensitization of afferent nociceptive nerve endings (Herbert and Holzer: 1994). Release of PGE2 relies on bradykinin via B2 receptor activity, cyclooxygenase-2, and substrate (arachidonic acid) via activation of phospholipase A2 (Saunders et. al.: 1999).

Thromboxanes (Tx) A2 and B2 are potent regulators of blood coagulation and homeostasis, and participate in the tissue repair phase of the needling reaction. Both bradykinin and substance P have a possible regulatory role in the activation and deactivation of platelets (Gecse et. al.: 1996). Induced ischemia in rabbit kidneys showed an increase in TxA2 and a decrease in PGI2, but electroacupuncture of node Taixi (KD 3) increased PGI2 and decreased TxA2 (Xu: 1993). Relative plasma levels of TxA2, TxB2, and PGI2 correlate with the Chinese concepts of blood stasis and promoting blood circulation (Xu, Liao, and Wang: 1993; Li: 1995; Qin, Jin, and Deng: 1997).

Leukotrienes LTC4, LTD4, and LTE4 are the slow-reacting substances of anaphylaxis (SRS-A) described by Sir Thomas Lewis in 1937 (Lembeck: 1985). These substances are one hundred to one thousand times more potent than histamine in producing bronchospasm and vascular permeability, and are found in the inflammatory fluids from tissues involved in rheumatoid arthritis, gout, and psoriasis (Heavey et. al.: 1986; Higgs: 1986). Leukotriene LTB4 is a potent chemotactic agent comparable to C5, causing delayed onset, long-lasting leukocyte accumulation when topically applied to the skin, and is cyclooxygenase- and prostaglandin-independent (Larkin et. al.: 1995).

Phases of Needling Reaction

Tissue reactions to the microtrauma induced by the needle involve six discrete time-dependent phases (Table 14.1). The first is the activation of the blood coagulation system and stimulation of the immune complement system to mount a defensive reaction to the inserted needle.

Initially, vasodilatation of capillaries at the site of intrusion is greatly enhanced to allow immune cells to egress from blood circulation to fight off the offending object. The net effect of this initial phase is local vasodilatation in the region of the inserted needle. Part of the vasodilatation phase may actually aid in attempting to push out or rid the body of the foreign object. However, the principal result is the initiation of a nonspecific immune defense reaction and simultaneous stimulation of nociceptive (pain sensory) neurons—the second phase. This produces the familiar needle reaction (deqi) that initiates the needling-induced process of stimulating spinal afferent nerves. The third phase attracts immune cells to the needling site, which further augments tissue reaction. In the fourth phase blood solubility products are released, which improves the flow of blood to the needle insertion site. Tissue repair processes are then stimulated in the fifth phase, with thrombin being activated to produce fibrin, while attraction and degranulation of platelets seals up the small tissue intrusion when the needle is removed. Finally, a controlling phase mediated by local tissue processes and supraspinal descending control comes into play, shutting down the inflammatory reactions, normalizing blood flow, inhibiting afferent nerve fibers, and promoting overall homeostasis. Humoral pathways also release substances into the bloodstream and cerebral spinal fluid (CSF). This includes the release of pituitary hormones, including adrenocorticotropic hormone (ACTH) bound with β-lipotropin (LPH).

The strength of needle stimulation and retention time are important parameters to be considered in the treatment of specific problems, as they can potentially enhance certain phases of the tissue response to needling. Strong needle stimulation and short duration of needle retention tends to favor the initial phases of the needling response. This would be considered in the case where a true heat condition may exist, which would necessarily involve pathogenic agents. Hence, strong stimulation enhances the inflammatory component of the immune response. Short retention time prevents overproduction of anti-inflammatory properties. In the case of false heat, needle stimulation is mild, but retention time is longer, thus assuring the production of corticosteroids to increase cell membrane stability and decrease the production of inflammatory substances such as PGE2 and leukotrienes.

Nociceptive Activation

Bradykinin B2 produced in response to needling excites the afferent nociceptive substance P neurons supplying the local site. These dorsal root ganglia (DRG) neurons send high-threshold signals to several laminae of the spinal cord dorsal horn. Here, synaptic junctures stimulate neurons in the dorsal lateral funiculus (DLF), as well as crossing neurons that ascend along the anterior lateral tract (ALT) on the opposite side of the spinal cord. Messages are sent to spinal afferent processing circuits involving various centers of the brain, spinal cord, muscles, blood vessels, and internal organs (Yaksh: 1986). Propriospinal circuits are provoked, which then activates spinal motor reflexes and PS along the body surface. Sympathetic neural reflexes are also provoked. Only a few of the signals produced by the external assault are actually transmitted to the sensory cortex; individuals are therefore generally not conscious of the exact point of needle insertion, nor may they be aware of insertion at all. Most of the information is directed to the brain stem to activate descending control signals that are sent back down the spinal cord. It is these supraspinal signals that bring about restorative descending control processes that play a part in needling therapy.

The initial role of activating the substance P nociceptive neurons is to amplify and sustain the tissue reactions in order to prolong the activation of the spinal afferent processing systems. This is brought about by axon reflex release of substance P from terminal endings of the neuron fibers at the local site of needle insertion and in the paravertebral ganglia. Substance P neurons provide the neurogenic contribution to plasma leakage at the needling site and the activation of sympathetic neurons that cause constriction of slightly deeper veins to enhance plasma leakage from the upstream capillaries and venules. These effects are mediated by the axon reflex, which continues to participate until supraspinal descending control inhibits the nociceptive neurons and restores sympathetic tone.

Enhancing Vasodilatory Response

Mast cells located in the tissue, often found sequestered with fine blood vessels and intimately associated with nerve endings at the needle insertion site, are the primary proinflammatory agents that respond to tissue damage. In addition to the role of complement proteins C3 and C5 in degranulating mast cells, axon reflex release of substance P also plays a major part in degranulating mast cells (Bunker et. al.: 1991; Suzuki et. al.: 1995; Hua, Back, and Tam: 1996). This basic mechanism, along with increased levels of bradykinin through the release of kinin protease from mast cells, sustains the initial needle-induced reaction, and subsides when the CNS provides inhibitory signals to the afferent substance P peripheral neurons and corticosteroids are produced, stabilizing cellular membranes and reducing the formation of arachidonic acid. Basophils, the plasma counterpart to mast cells, are attracted to the site and are also degranulated. The chemotactic action of kallikrein and C5a release ECF-A and NCF-A to attract the granulocytes, eosinophils, and neutrophils, and may be influenced by mast cell degranulation by substance P (Matsuda et. al.: 1989).

Electroacupuncture stimulation of Zusanli (ST 36) in rats increased degranulation of subcutaneous mast cells in nodes Zusanli (ST 36) and Xiajuxu (ST 39), which was attenuated after transection of the sciatic nerve, showing peripheral nerve involvement (Deng et. al.: 1996a). More mast cells were noted in five nodes along the stomach vessel pathway, from the abdomen to the lower leg, compared with non-node sites in rats, and electroacupuncture of nodes Biguan (ST 31) and Zusanli (ST 36) increased the number of mast cells in all five node locations, but had no effect on mast cell numbers in adjacent non-nodal sites (Deng et. al.: 1996b). Some studies have shown more mast cells in rats along the nodal pathways compared to non-nodal locations (Zhu and Xu: 1990), or more mast cells and substance P (Cao and Wang: 1989). Electroacupuncture showed a naloxone-reversible increase in tail-flick reflex thresholds and significant decrease of substance P levels in the skin and plasma.

Sustaining Initial Reaction by Axon Reflex

Superficial substance P dorsal root ganglia (DRG) neurons stimulated by needling-produced bradykinin acting on B2 receptors direct nociceptive signals to the dorsal horn of the spinal cord (Figure 14.2). The signals serve to activate CNS spinal afferent processes. These same substance P neurons send branches that synapse on sympathetic neurons in the paravertebral ganglia that serve deeper blood vessels near the site of activation. Branching fibers are also directed back to the superficial tissues. Both of the branching pathways are activated by antidromic[5] action (reverse direction) when the neuron is stimulated. Substance P released

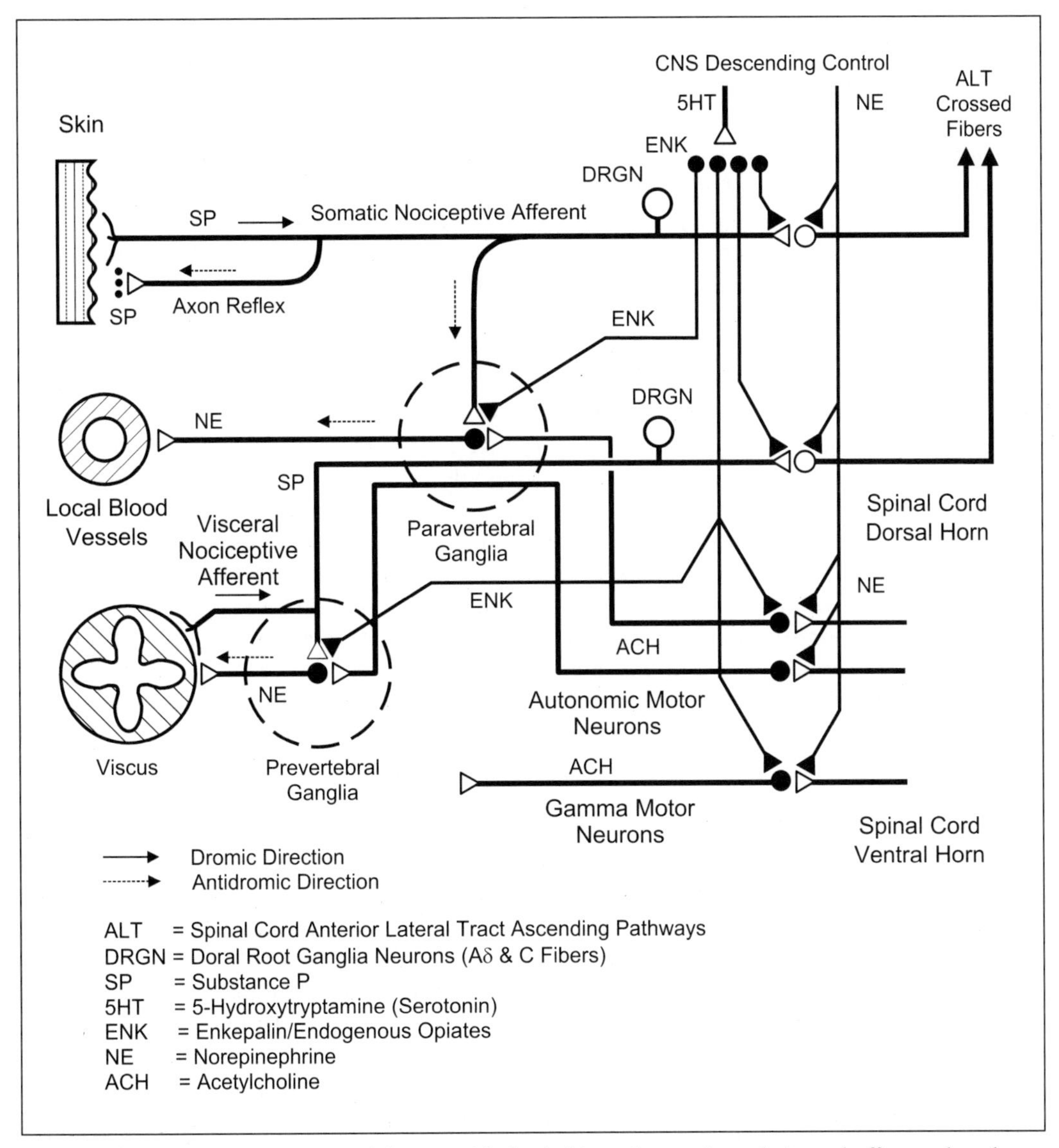

Figure 14.2 Schematic diagram of the possible branching of somatic and visceral afferent dorsal root neurons to produce axon reflexes, viscerosomatic communication, and referred pain, along with descending control pathways.

from the terminal branching fibers contributes to neurogenic inflammation by promoting vasodilatation of arterioles and capillaries, and dilatation of venules acting on NK1 receptors to promote plasma leakage at the needling site. Activation of the branching fiber to the paravertebral ganglia produces vasoconstriction contributing to upstream plasma leakage at the inflammatory site, and also restricts the reaction to the local area. Hence, neurogenic inflammation involves differential control of superficial and deep blood vessels where primary afferent neurons contribute to local inflammation surrounding the needle insertion site, and sympathetic vasoconstrictor neurons control veins related to the local area (Habler, Wasner, and Janig: 1997; Habler et. al.: 1998).

The formation of wheal and flare at the site of needle insertion is characteristic of neurogenic inflammation where plasma leakage is induced by dilatation of postcapillary and collecting venules through the action of substance P released from sensory neurons (Figure 14.2) acting on NK1 receptors on the endothelial cells of the venules (McDonald et. al.: 1996; Baluk: 1997). Evidence of substance P involvement is provided by the observation that venodilation is inhibited by the antagonist of NK1 receptors (Romerio, Linder, and Haefeli: 1999). Substance P also induces leukocytes to adhere to venular endothelium (Suzuki et. al.: 1995; Tominaga et. al.: 1999). Intra-arterial substance P infusion of the forearm produces vasodilatation that is attenuated by a dose-dependent antagonist of NK1 receptors, but which does not contribute to basal vascular tone (Newby et. al.: 1999). Other evidence of substance P acting on NK1 receptors is provided in the modulation of induced skin irritation and induction of itch-associated responses being inhibited by NK1 antagonists (Veronesi et. al.: 1995; Andoh et. al.: 1998).

One major role of substance P in local inflammation is the degranulation of local mast cells to release histamine and heparin, thereby contributing to plasma leakage. Initially, plasma leakage allows basophils attracted to the needling site to also degranulate histamine and heparin, which helps sustain the inflammatory reaction. Later, neutrophils and eosinophils are attracted, contributing to tissue healing. There may be a substance P-type neuropeptide that binds to receptors on monocytes and macrophages (Lucey et. al.: 1994), and cutaneous melanocytes may be associated with terminal endings of afferent fibers (Hara et. al.: 1996).

Spinal Integration Sites

The high-threshold substance P superficial afferent nociceptive Aδ and group III dorsal root neurons project to lamina I of the spinal cord dorsal horn, with collaterals to laminae III and IV, while the group IV and C neurons project to the outer region of lamina I. These neurons have substance P and NK1 autoreceptors in rats (Hu, Li, and Si: 1997; Von Banchet and Schaible: 1999) and activate NK1 receptors on nerve cells found in lamina I, laminae III and VI, the lateral spinal nucleus, and the area around the central canal (Littlewood et. al.: 1995; Ding et. al.: 1999). Some large cells in laminae III and IV have dendrites extending through lamina II and into lamina I. Substance P may not have any functional role on lamina II (substantia gelatinosa) neurons (Bleazard, Hill, and Morris: 1994). However, lamina II may be the site of second messenger systems involving the gamma isoform of protein kinase C (PKC gamma) that possibly lowers pain threshold (Basbaum: 1999). Substance P receptors (NK1) bearing nerve cells in laminae III and IV of rats receive monosynaptic input from myelinated (Aδ and group III fibers) primary afferents (Naim, Shehab, and Todd: 1998).

Lamina I neurons expressing NK1 receptors in rats seem to discriminate intensity of pain, while those in the deeper laminae (V–X) are involved in the detection and localization of particular nociceptive characteristics, principally joint and inflammatory pain (Doyle and Hunt: 1999). This latter feature would include the substance P afferent neuron participation in and response to neurogenic inflammation as a result of needling. Substance P receptor (NK1)–expressing neurons of the spinal cord dorsal horn have a major role in the generation and maintenance of chronic inflammatory and neuropathic pain (Nichols et. al.: 1999). Honor et.

al. (1999) observed acute inflammatory pain (> sixty minutes) in rats involving an ongoing release of substance P in lamina I; short-term inflammatory pain (three hours) with substance P released in lamina I, and laminae III and IV, due to both noxious and non-noxious somatosensory stimulation; and long-term pain of a similar pattern to short-term pain, except for a significant upregulation of substance P receptors in lamina I neurons.

The somatic substance P dorsal root ganglia (DRG) neurons travel with visceral afferent DRG neurons, and form communication links within the dorsal horn, giving rise to somatovisceral relationships. The somatic afferents also send signals to the ventral horn to stimulate group II static load neurons that provoke spinal reflexes, which give rise to PS. The DRG afferents also travel up and down in the tract of Lissauer and the DLF before synapsing on crossed ascending spinal pathways. The superficial fibers make connections along the DLF several spinal segmental levels above and below the primary site of entry. Branching at the cord entry is typical of afferent neurons and distributes the input signal to overlap with nociceptive fibers from superficial areas above and below the node being stimulated.

Ascending Pathways

Cutaneous and visceral nociceptive data is received in the dorsal horn of the spinal cord and conveyed to crossed neospinothalamic and paleospinothalamic neurons of the spinothalamic tract (STT), and neurons of the spinoreticular (SRT) and spinomesencephalic (SMT) tracts, all of which ascend via the anterior lateral tract (ALT). Only a small portion of the ALT that comprises the STT projects principally to the lateral portion of the ventral posterior lateral nucleus (VPL), central lateral intralaminar nucleus (CL), and medial posterior complex (POm) of the thalamus, which then send fibers to the sensory cortex. The major portion of the ALT comprises the SMT and SRT, which project to the midbrain, pons, and medulla. The neurons of origin of the SMT are concentrated in laminae I and V of the spinal cord dorsal horn, as are neurons of the STT. Some of the SMT neurons can be fired antidromically by electrical stimulation of the midbrain or thalamus, indicating some relationship with the STT. Neurons from the SMT and SRT project to areas of the reticular formation that runs the length of the brain stem, and then on to many specific regions within the midbrain, pons, and medulla. The brain stem is critical in mediating needling reaction, since it is the integration site of the somatic and visceral centers, including the nuclei of the vagus and other important cranial nerves.

Localization of substance P receptors in the CNS of rats shows a dense distribution to many brain nuclei, including the locus ceruleus, rostral half of the nucleus ambiguus, and the intermediolateral nucleus of the thoracic cord; moderate distribution is noted to nucleus raphe magnus, caudatoputamen, nucleus accumbens, laminae I and III of the caudal subnucleus of the spinal trigeminal nucleus, and lamina I of the spinal cord; and sparse distribution in the cerebral cortex, gigantocellular reticular nucleus, and lobules IX and X of the cerebellar vermis (Nakaya et. al.: 1994). Li et. al. (1998) also showed substance P receptor (NK1) neurons projecting to the periaqueductal gray from the lateral spinal nucleus, lamina I of the medullary and spinal dorsal horns, and laminae V and X of the spinal cord. Guan et. al. (1998) noted projections in rats to the nucleus of the solitary tract from lamina I of the medullary and spinal dorsal horns, lateral spinal nucleus, and lamina V of the spinal cord. Battaglia and Rustioni (1992) found that substance P neurons of origin in rats and cats by horseradish peroxidase (HRP) retrograde studies project from laminae I and V and the DLF via the STT to the somatosensory nuclei of the thalamus.

Substance P neurons also form synapses with noradrenergic neurons in the A7 catecholamine group (Proudfit and Monsen: 1999). Baulmann et. al. (2000) observed lower leg noxious stimulation response of NK1 receptor–bearing brain neurons located in the prefrontal cortex, hypothalamic ventromedial and dorsomedial nuclei, locus ceruleus, and the periaqueductal gray, involving nociception and central stress responses in rats. Bereiter et. al. (1998) observed that substance P receptors (NK1) are involved in corneal nociceptive transmission to brain stem neurons in the trigeminal subnucleus caudalis, and increased activity of the hypothalamic-pituitary axis of rats. These studies suggest that trigeminal and spinal substance P neurons, especially of lamina I, are involved in the transmission of somatic and visceral nociceptive information to key processing centers in the brain that potentially modulate pain.

Propriospinal Participation

There is a synergism between the nociceptive (somatic and visceral) and proprioceptive neurons: the latter are known to modulate pain, especially that of deep muscle tissue, and sometimes from visceral sources, typically presented in the clinical setting. The nociceptive neurons enhance and initiate propriospinal reflexes, and together they produce muscle flexion responses. These afferents from cutaneous and deep receptors typically mediate the defensive spinal reflex of ipsilateral flexion, accompanied by contralateral extension, such as that of jerking the hand away from a hot object or an encounter with a thorn. The study of flexor reflex in human tibialis anterior muscle indicates a possible convergence of mechanoreceptive and nociceptive inputs onto spinal reflex pathways (Ellrich and Treede: 1998). Visceral nociceptive afferents can stimulate propriospinal reflexes that result in either organ-referred pain or protective cramps overlying the inflamed area. Muscle reflexes also stimulate postganglionic sympathetic efferents innervating skeletal muscle vasculature (Hill, Adreani, and Kaufman: 1996).

Proprioceptive group II afferent neurons make widespread connections with the propriospinal system, sending terminal branches to all laminae of the dorsal horn, except lamina II, and ultimately synapsing on motor neurons. The muscle spindle afferents from the extremities send densely packed short branches up and down the tract of Lissauer and DLF over several segmental levels, while those of the axial muscles of the neck, back, shoulder girdle, and pelvic girdle send long branches, especially from the cervical segments, that may extend over the entire length of the spinal cord. Propriospinal neurons in C1–C2 spinal segments have been shown to project to L5–S1 segments of rat spinal cord (Miller et. al.: 1998).

Nociceptive (somatic and visceral) neurons and proprioceptive neurons synapse on neurons several segmental levels above and below their point of entry in the dorsal horn. These interconnections can give rise to the propagation of signals (PS) up and down the DLF from the spinal cord entry point of the afferent nociceptive nerve fibers that convey needling-reaction signals. Under certain threshold conditions, this propagated muscle reflex is felt to transmit along the superficial nodal pathways. The phenomenon of PS is important to the Chinese view of physiology and pathology, since impairment of this normal reflex leads to motor coordination disturbances, musculoskeletal problems, pain syndromes, and other disorders, including visceral problems. These conditions may be due to impairment of muscle spindle afferents that have a possible role in shaping and reinforcing motoneuron signals

(Windhorst and Kokkoroyiannis: 1991; Bergenheim, Johansson, and Pedersen: 1995). The clinical effectiveness of needling therapy is enhanced if PS is stimulated and directed to the affected area, even including to internal organs.

Importance of Muscle Spindle Afferents

The participation of the secondary muscle spindle static load afferents is needed to produce the PS stimulated by needling. These neurons are essential to normal muscle control by providing a feedback loop to the gamma-muscle spindle system. However, this feedback loop may also play a role in reflex-mediated muscle stiffness and dysfunction, since the activity of the primary muscle afferents is influenced by fusimotor reflexes from secondary muscle spindle afferents (Johansson, Djupsjobacka, and Sjolander: 1993). These associations also provide a means whereby stiffness, pain, and tenderness (*ahshi* and trigger points) can progressively develop from one muscle to the adjacent muscle along the longitudinal muscle distributions. The static load spindle afferents are also affected by local temperatures and pressures, providing a possible environmental influence on the development of muscle pain and dysfunction. Further, reduced blood circulation to muscles, as well as muscle contraction metabolic by-products, can activate group III and IV muscle afferents on the gamma-muscle spindles systems, stimulating primary and secondary muscle spindle afferents. Impaired regulation of microcirculation in the trapezius has been implicated in humans, with chronic neck pain presumably involving increased nociceptive activity, perhaps group III and IV muscle afferents (Larsson, Oberg, and Larsson: 1999).

Several key contraction metabolites and inflammatory agents, including bradykinin, arachidonic acid, potassium chloride (KCl), lactic acid, and 5-hydroxytryptamine (5HT), have been examined with respect to their influence on the muscle spindle system. Bradykinin has a function in glucose uptake by skeletal muscles, and B2 receptors are found on the plasma membranes of striated skeletal muscle cells in rats (Figueroa, Dietze, and Muller-Esterl: 1996). Intravenous (i.v.) injection of bradykinin actually inhibits nociceptive tail-flick reflex in rats, seemingly by inhibiting substance P visceral afferents from entering the spinal cord between C2 and T9 (Bauer, Meller, and Gebhart: 1992). However, intramuscular (i.m.) injection of bradykinin increases static fusimotor drive to muscle spindles (Pedersen et. al.: 1997; Wenngren et. al.: 1998). The possible influence of arterial injection of bradykinin and 5HT in one muscle on the primary and secondary muscle spindle afferents of the target and surrounding muscles was demonstrated in cats by Djupsjobacka et. al. (1995b). Close arterial, but not i.v., injection of arachidonic acid produced similar results of activating static load muscle spindle afferents (Djupsjobacka, Johansson, and Bergenheim: 1994). Close arterial, but not i.v., injection of KCl and lactic acid in one muscle influenced the primary and secondary muscle spindle afferents of the target and the surrounding muscles, predominantly activating static load muscle spindle afferents, while arterial injection of sodium chloride (NaCl) had no effect (Johansson, Djupsjobacka, and Sjolander: 1993; Djupsjobacka et. al.: 1995a).

Dorsal Root Potentials and Reflexes

Somatic and visceral nociceptive neurons and proprioceptive neurons give rise to dorsal root potentials (DRP) and dorsal root reflexes (DRR) that reflect up and down the tract of Lissauer and DLF of the spinal cord by firing the neurons above and below where they send branches.

Dorsal root potentials and reflexes (DRP/DRR) have a possible role in the mediation of afferent nociceptive inputs and supraspinal descending presynaptic inhibitions. They also have a possible role in peripheral inflammation with pathological consequences (Willis: 1999). Stimulation by needling therapy produces directed DRR to normalize pathological conditions. Somatic and visceral afferents mutually produce DRP in each other in areas where they converge in the spinal cord (Selzer and Spencer: 1969). These mechanisms are important to reflect information related to spinal reflexes and somatovisceral or viscerosomatic relationships. When threshold conditions are conducive and signal levels are high, DRP/DRR produce superficial muscle action potentials (MAP) that reflect as PS along the vessel and muscle distribution pathways. The intensity of the subjective experience of PS as a mild electrical sensation is proportional to the intensity of the MAP (Yan, Wang, and Hou: 1987). The importance of the tract of Lissauer and DLF of the spinal cord is to provide an integration pathway for spinal reflexes that are induced in somatic and visceral nociceptive afferent neurons.

Electroacupuncture produces DRP, and can expand the segmental spread of the potentials, as well as the amplitude of the potentials, indicating possible trans-segmental spread of afferent signals (Guo, Guan, and Wang: 1996). Electrical stimulation of the DLF below a transected level was found by Du and Zhao (1985) to produce weak inhibition of somatovisceral reflexes. This indicates that antidromic activation to produce somatovisceral and proprioceptive DRP reflexes possibly involves the DLF and the tract of Lissauer, and that supraspinal descending inhibition is mediated by the same region of the dorsal horn of the spinal cord. Foreman, Hammond, and Willis (1981) observed that both bradykinin injection into the heart and electrical stimulation of the vagus nerve of monkeys induced centrally mediated inhibition of somatovisceral reflexes only down to the segmental level that stimulation had been provided. Somatovisceral response, as evidenced by discharges in the vagus nerve resulting from needling Zusanli (ST 36) on the leg of rabbit, can be abolished by section of the ipsilateral lateral funiculus, including the DLF and tract of Lissauer (Chang et. al.: 1983). This also indicates that ascending stimulation of the DLF excites nuclei within the brain stem independent of nociceptive information transmitted along the anterior lateral tract (ALT). The ipsilateral nature of the needling-stimulated analgesia was also demonstrated by Yukizaki et. al. (1986), showing that electroacupuncture in human subjects increased tooth pain thresholds only on the treated side.

Propagated Sensation

The afferent group II neurons involved in PS are muscle spindle static or nuclear chain fibers that provide information on static tension, residual muscle tension, and length. Nociceptive needling reaction activates efferent proprioceptive neurons (gamma 1 and 2 fibers) at the same spinal segment that causes afferent proprioceptive group II nerves to fire. If muscle spindles are present in the underlying tissue at the node being needled, there is a greater likelihood that the subject will experience an immediate episode of PS. The conscious experience of PS generally follows the nodal pathways, and measures about 1–2 centimeters wide on the four extremities and about 10 centimeters wide on the trunk, with widespread branching in the head region. After travelling up the leg, PS branches out in a wide pathway on the trunk, showing the presence of extensive interconnections. PS may be felt to travel over one or two joints, but in sensitive individuals, the feeling can transmit along the entire nodal pathway being stimulated.

The incidence of PS, and the conscious awareness of it, is significantly higher in children than in adults (Yang et. al.: 1993). In most cases (65 to 75 percent of adult patients), needling sensation may be experienced without any subjective PS along the nodal pathway. This latent PS can be induced as a subjective experience, where the PS is felt immediately after needle insertion, by tapping directly along the course of the vessel or muscle pathway, demonstrating the involvement of intrafusal fibers (Yu et. al.: 1981; Zhu et. al.: 1981; Weng et. al.: 1990). Objective display of PS routes has been demonstrated by infrared imaging of the face and upper extremity (Liu et. al.: 1990a, 1990b). Stimulation and direction of PS, usually by appropriately applied finger pressure, to reach the affected area along a nodal or muscle pathway increases the effectiveness of acupuncture (You et. al.: 1987a) (Chapter 15).

Either subjective or latent PS can be blocked by mechanical pressure (approximately 500–800 gm/cm^2) applied perpendicularly and directly on the nodal pathway, but is not attenuated if the pressure is applied 1 centimeter laterally on either side of the pathway (Wu et. al.: 1993a, 1993b; Xu et. al.: 1993). PS recovers immediately after the pressure is removed. Voluntary contraction of the affected muscles along the course of PS also attenuates it. Heating the skin increases the rate of PS, but is difficult to achieve if the skin temperature is lower than 20° centigrade, and can be blocked by the local application of an ice pack on nodal locations (Wu and Hu: 1987). This finding is consistent with the static intrafusal muscle spindle behavior, which is inhibited when the temperature is lowered. Propagation rate of PS along the superficial body is about 1 centimeter per second, but occasionally can be as high as 10–20 centimeters per second (Hu et. al.: 1987). This velocity rate is considerably slower than the Aδ and C fibers, but is well within the range of the slow excitatory postsynaptic potentials (EPSP) attributed to the involved neurons (Katayama and Nishi: 1986). The slow rate of PS may also indicate the possible presence of numerous synaptic junctions in the propagation pathway, including participation with propriospinal neurons.

PS can be stimulated by needle insertion, moxibustion, pressure manipulation, vibration, acoustic stimulation, massage, chemical application, or electrostimulation. Percussed sound information can also be triggered to transmit along the vessel route, resulting in the generation of latent PS. PS is not affected or induced by strong suggestion or hint, and its rate of occurrence increases with frequency of treatment. Surgical procedures that cut through the vessel and muscle pathways attenuate or block PS, indicating that the integrity of the superficial tissue is necessary to the transmission of these signals. Scars that traverse the nodal distribution pathways are typically needled to reestablish PS communication routes. Cutting (transection) the spinal cord drastically reduces or completely abolishes PS, although it can be established in the upper extremities in some individuals with lower cord damage.

Propagated Sensation as Neural Reflex

The importance of stimulating DRR and subsequent PS is to ensure that a significant response is activated at the spinal segmental levels related to the specific somatic or visceral problem being treated. Also, the DRR signal may be essential to direct the supraspinal descending control processes to the segmental level of the spinal cord concerned. When conditions are right, needling produces high-threshold signals that simultaneously transmit as a DRR along related tracks in the DLF corresponding to the skin regions, vessels, and muscle distributions of the stimulated nodal pathway. Neuroelectrical recording of motoneurons and HRP retrograde transport studies in rats and cats by Xie, Li, and Xiao (1996) found that afferents from homonymous and synergistic muscles and skin overlying the muscles were involved in PS, and that motoneurons associated with a muscle distribution (Chapter 12) formed a discrete longitudinal column with definite boundaries in the spinal cord lateral ventral horn. Afferent impulses from stimulating PS along the large intestine nodal pathway can be recorded in the superficial nerves (Hu et. al.: 1993). PS stimulated by needling either Jiaxi (GB 43) or Hegu (LI 4) in sensitive responders produced short latent evoked potentials in the cortical somatosensory area I (SI).

The phenomenon of superficial PS appears to be the result of dromic/antidromic reflexes conducted up and down the DLF of the spinal cord that provoke group II static load muscle spindles (Figure 14.3). The incoming needle response can travel up and down the DLF, causing dorsal root neuron activation above and below the initiating spinal segment. If the stimulation is strong enough and the threshold conditions at the superficial regions on the skin are right (such as high temperature or low pressure), then the progressive interaction of each succeeding spinal segment possibly allows a vertical propagation of PS up and down the superficial routes on the body. For example, the needling sensation generated by stimulating one particular node (Figure 14.3, Node 1) is transmitted to the spinal cord to synapse on ascending crossed ALT fibers, and at the same time travels in the DLF to segmental levels above and below this entry site. If static load muscle spindles are present at the node being stimulated, then gamma efferents are fired, causing activation of the muscle spindle afferents. Meanwhile, the needling-induced nociceptive signal is simultaneously received at nodal entry levels above (Figure 14.3, Nodes 2 and 3) and below the initial node, which, either antidromically or dromically, fires nociceptive and proprioceptive neurons. This would then generate a progressive reaction that continues to stimulate nodal entry sites above and below the initial stimulated level until the entire cord is activated.

The DRR neural reflex up and down the DLF takes place due to the stimulation of a nodal site, but PS is not subjectively experienced unless a sufficient number of proprioceptive and nociceptive fibers are activated. Both the nociceptive and proprioceptive projection of spinal-to-spinal connections are ipsilateral in nature, with only a few connections being contralateral. Therefore PS along the nodal pathways is observed to be confined mainly to the same side of the body in which the needling reaction is being stimulated.

Somatovisceral Relationships

One of the most significant theories of Chinese medicine concerns somatovisceral relationships, where distribution vessels and their related neurovascular nodes, underlying skin zones, and muscle distributions are related to specific internal organs. Somatosomatic relationships are also recognized with respect to pain and dysfunction originating in one muscle being reflected to adjacent and other muscles along the muscle distributions. Viscerosomatic relationships are also recognized in terms of organ-referred pain reflecting in certain body regions, and in organ traction as noted during surgery. Viscerovisceral relationships occur as well, where the function or treatment stimulation of one particular organ produces autonomic reflexes that influence another organ.

Somatovisceral reflex response to stimulating cutaneous, muscle, and articular sensory afferents has been measured in several different internal organs and major vessels. Some of these reflexes display dominant sympathetic efferent participation, while others have

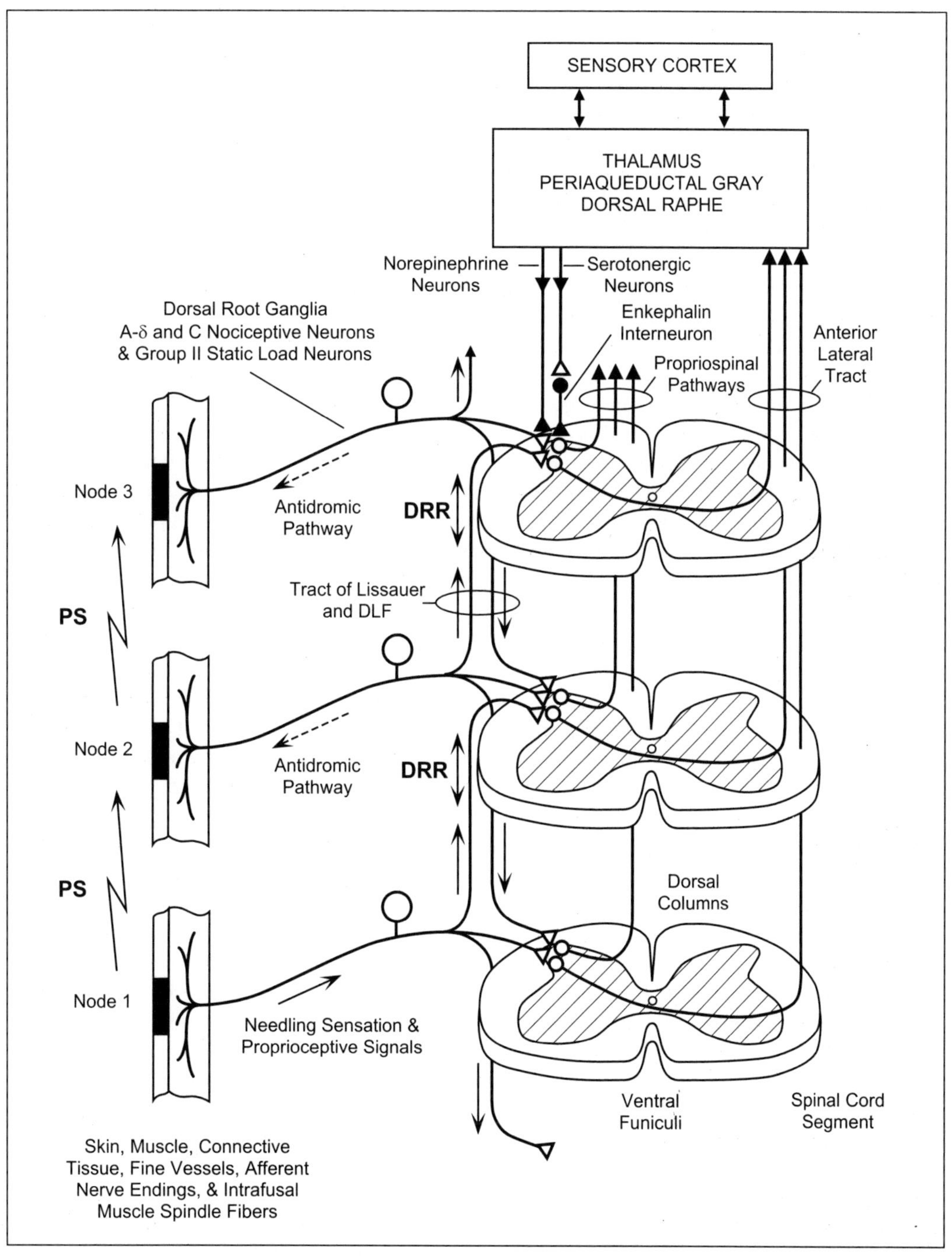

Figure 14.3 Schematic diagram of the possible mechanisms of producing PS along superficial pathways, initiated by somatic nociceptive afferents with proprioceptive afferent participation to produce DRR and supraspinal stimulation, providing descending control via serotonergic and norepinephrine pathways.

parasympathetic efferent attributes. Supraspinal and generalized characteristics are exhibited, and some reflexes demonstrate segmental and propriospinal features. The nature of somatovisceral reflexes depends on the specific internal organ, the particular location being stimulated, and the method of stimulation (Sato: 1992, 1995, 1997). The difference in somatovisceral reflex in each organ or sympathetic system is possibly a function of the spinal cord having functionally distinct reflex pathways unique to different aspects of the vascular system and each organ (Janig: 1996). These spinal circuits may be the basis for all homeostatic regulation involving the autonomic systems, which are represented in the brain stem and hypothalamus.

Somatovisceral neurons are reported to be located in laminae I and V of the dorsal horn and in the ventral horn of the spinal cord (Cervero: 1986; Light and Perl: 1979). The Aδ sympathetic visceral and superficial somatic Aδ neurons have similar distributions to lamina I and V, indicating they are most likely to give rise to somatovisceral relationships. Visceral inputs have been shown to converge with somatic inputs onto STT neurons of the ALT. Cervero (1986) reports that dorsal horn and other spinal cord neurons are either exclusively somatic, or neurons that require a visceral excitatory drive in addition to somatic input. Most nociceptive signals of visceral origin travel in afferent sympathetic nerves and can also be excited by noxious stimulation of their related somatic receptive fields, whereas parasympathetic visceral afferents are mainly concerned with non-sensory afferent visceral function (Cervero: 1985).

Common Somatic and Visceral Integration Sites

The convergence of somatic and visceral afferent neurons provides the main anatomical basis for nodal stimulation to influence the internal organs. A limited number of key nodes have been studied by injecting HRP into nodal sites and internal organs of test animals, then tracing the retrograde transport of this material in the nerves supplying the spinal cord. Results were reviewed to assess the possible overlap of somatic and visceral afferent neurons at their segmental entry level to the spinal cord. Some studies have examined the electrical activity of dorsal horn neurons in response to electroacupuncture on arm and leg nodes to determine a possible convergence in common spinal segments. Liu et. al. (1993) measured the response of afferent dorsal horn neurons at T2–T3 spinal segments in rabbits by electroacupuncture to either Neiguan (PC 6) or Zusanli (ST 36). Neurons that responded were mostly excited by Neiguan (PC 6) and inhibited by Zusanli (ST 36). Six fibers that responded to both nodes were all inhibited by Zusanli (ST 36), while five of the six were excited and one inhibited by Neiguan (PC 6), showing convergence of afferent neuron response, but with each node having different physiological effects. He et. al. (1995) showed that hind paw pain was inhibited in rats by electroacupuncture on Zusanli (ST 36) located on the leg, but was ineffective on node Xiaguan (ST 7) located on the face, showing a possible segmental effect.

Heart Afferents

Comparison of the afferent somatic projection levels by HRP retrograde from nodes Neiguan (PC 6) in rabbits and cats (Tao, Li, and Li: 1984; Wang, Zhao, and Wang: 1984; Wang et. al.: 1984a), and Shenmen (HT 7) (Tao, Li, and Dang: 1987) and Shaohai (HT 3) in cats (Tao, Dang, and Li: 1987), typically employed in treating heart conditions, show a corresponding overlap at the same spinal cord levels as the heart visceral afferents (Wang et. al.: 1984b). This information (Table 14.2) is consistent with the spinal level at which electrical potentials are induced in the dorsal root of the spinal cord by electrostimulation of Neiguan (PC 6) (Liu et. al.: 1984). The study of heart sympathetic afferent neuron projections to the spinal cord of cats by HRP retrograde analysis showed segmental distribution to C8–T9 for heart and cardiac nerves, and T1–T5 for medium and inferior cardiac nerves (Tao and Li: 1993). Labeled fibers were observed in laminae III to VII of the spinal cord.

Stomach Afferents

The node Zusanli (ST 36) is a commonly used site for stomach and other gastrointestinal problems. Retrograde transport analysis by injection of HRP into the cardia, pylorus, tunica serosa, and wall of rabbit stomach was compared with the Zusanli (ST 36) nodal site (Tao et. al.: 1984a, 1984b). The visceral afferents from various regions of the stomach show a range from C4–T12, indicating a small overlap with Zusanli (ST 36) on the lower end of the range (Table 14.3). However, stomach wall afferent projections to the spinal ganglia (T3–L4) show a very wide range of spinal levels and a good correspondence with Zusanli (ST 36). Unilateral injection of HRP into nodes Zusanli (ST 36) and Ruzhong (ST 17), respectively, in rats showed transport to neurons at L4–5 and T4–6 spinal segments (Xu et. al.: 1996). Electroacupuncture at Zusanli (ST 36) and Ruzhong (ST 17) caused increased uptake of HRP and the spreading of labeled cells to adjacent dorsal roots.

Table 14.2 Comparison of somatic afferent projections to the spinal cord from nodes Neiguan (PC 6), Shenmen (HT 7), and Shaohai (HT 3), with afferent projections from the heart.

Area Examined	*Electrostimulation*	*Spinal Integration Level*[1]
Neiguan (PC 6)	C4–T1, most at C5–C7	C5–T1, with 76% at C7–C8
Shenmen (HT 7)		C6–T1, with 90% at C8–T1
Shaohai (HT 3)		C5–T5, most at T1
Heart (Organ)		C5–T5, most at T1 in spinal cord T2–T6, in sympathetic trunk

1. HRP retrograde transport method.

Table 14.3 Comparison of somatic afferent projections to the spinal cord from node Zusanli (ST 36), with afferent projections from various parts of the stomach.

Area Examined	*Spinal Integration Level*[1]
Zusanli (ST 36)	T10–S3, with most at L4–S2
Stomach	
Cardia	C4–T12
Pylorus	T1–L4
Tunica Serosa	C4–L7, with most at T5–T12
Stomach Wall	T5–T9 of spinal cord T3–L3 of spinal ganglia

1. HRP retrograde transport method.

Projection sites to the brain stem by HRP injection into the anterior stomach wall reaches localized areas of the vagus center, including the dorsal motor nuclei (Li et. al.: 1984a; Li and Tao: 1984). Those found in the nodular ganglia of the vagus center mostly projected from the pylorus of the stomach and the least from the cardia (Xi and Tao: 1984). Afferent fiber projections by HRP retrograde from the nodal site Sibai (ST 2), located below the orbit of the eye, showed distribution to the semilunar ganglion of the trigeminal nerve, facial motor nerve nucleus, oculomotor nucleus, upper cervical ganglion, and motor nucleus of the trigeminal nerve (Tao, Xu, and Li: 1987).

Gallbladder Afferents

Segmental distribution of spinal sensory nerves supplying the nodes Ganshu (BL 18), Pishu (BL 20), Liangmen (ST 21), and Qimen (LV 14) often used in treating gallbladder problems, as well as afferent neurons supplying the gallbladder itself in a separate group of animals, were examined by HRP retrograde transport in guinea pigs (Tao, Jin, and Ren: 1991). A mutual overlap of five to seven spinal segments was observed between the four nodes and the gallbladder afferents.

Bladder Afferents

The distribution of visceral afferent neurons from the bladder in rabbits integrates in the spinal cord from T6 down to Cox 1, showing good correspondence with somatic afferent inputs from the peroneal and tibial nerves that serve bladder vessel nodes on the lower legs (Li et. al.: 1984b). This data shows a bimodal distribution of afferent neurons with one concentration between S2–S5, and another between L2–L4 (Wu et. al.: 1984) (Table 14.4). The concentration in the lower area corresponds with the bladder communication (*shu*, 输) node, Pangguanshu (BL 28) (Table 15.5), and parasympathetic function, while the upper group corresponds to the kidney communication node, Shenshu (BL 23), and sympathetic function. Historically, moxibustion is applied to the terminal node of the bladder vessel pathway Zhiyin (BL 67) to invert malpositioned fetuses. The study of this nodal site and the uterus by HRP methods in rabbits found afferent projections distributed from Zhiyin (BL 67) converging on the spinal cord between L2–S1 (Weng et. al.: 1984) (Table 14.4). Visceral afferent neurons from the uterus spread from T11–S3, showing an overlap with afferents of Zhiyin (BL 67). A randomized controlled study by Cardini and Huang (1998) using moxibustion on Zhiyin (BL 67) corrected the breech presentation in 98 of 130 fetuses (75.4 percent).

Table 14.4 Comparison of somatic afferent projections to the spinal cord from the peroneal and tibial nerves and node Zhiyin (BL 67), with afferent projections from the bladder and uterus.

Area Examined	*Spinal Integration Level*[1]
Peroneal and Tibial Nerves	L6–S3
Zhiyin (BL 67)	L2–S1
Bladder	T6–Cox 1 Bimodal distribution concentrated at S2–S5 and L2–L4
Uterus	T11–S3

1. HRP retrograde transport method.

Visceral Responses

Confirmation of somatovisceral relationships is provided by observing visceral reactions to needling the somatic body. Nodal locations have somewhat different effects, and some site locations may actually counteract the actions of other nodes used in a treatment protocol. Xu and Chen (1999) observed that electroacupuncture on often-used nodal sites such as Neiguan (PC 6), Pishu (BL 20), and Zusanli (ST 36) had little effect on gastrointestinal peristalsis in normal mice. Pishu (BL 20) was significantly antagonistic to Zusanli (ST 36) in normal mice. Electroacupuncture on Zusanli (ST 36) markedly decreased atropine-induced peristalsis, whereas Neiguan (PC 6) was significantly antagonistic to Pishu (BL 20) in atropine-treated mice. Yu et. al. (1996) observed an inhibition of sympathetic discharges of postganglionic fibers of the celiac ganglion in healthy rabbits due to electroacupuncture at Zusanli (ST 36) and Yanglingquan (GB 34), with Zusanli (ST 36) producing a greater inhibition of sympathetic discharges than Yanglingquan (GB 34). Needling stimulation to the abdomen and hind limb of rats elicited increased adrenal medullary hormones and adrenal nerve activity (Sato et. al.: 1996). Adrenal nerve activity was abolished by severing the nerves supplying the hind limb and abdomen.

Needling Zusanli (ST 36) decreases 5HT and muscarine receptor binding capacity in the cerebral cortex, hippocampus, striatum, spinal cord, and spleen in rats, while producing analgesia, whereas needling Taichong (LV 3) had no effect (Mo et. al.: 1994). Brain stem and medulla oblongata 5HT receptor binding decreased, but was unchanged in the thalamus, while muscarine receptors showed an opposite trend. Internal organs amenable to performance assessment in both human and animal subjects provide a means of confirming somatovisceral relationships. The following is a summary of studies comparing specific nodal sites with induced visceral activity, or in producing beneficial impact on the viscera.

Heart Disease and Function

Studies involving acute myocardial infarction, rheumatic valvular disease, angina pectoris, left ventricular function, heart microcirculation, and arrhythmia, especially tachycardia, show a significant decrease in symptoms, including pain of angina as well as improvement in heart function, as measured by electrocardiogram (ECG) and other means (Bi et. al.: 1984; Cheng et. al.: 1984; Gao et. al.: 1984a, 1984b; Li et. al.: 1984; Nanning Cardiovascular Research Group: 1984; Wang, Xu, and Wang: 1984). Nodal site Neiguan (PC 6) demonstrated the greatest statistical significance in treating heart problems. Other locations showing good response include Quze (PC 3), Geshu (BL 17), the communication node for the diaphragm and the special location for blood, the heart communication site Xinshu (BL 15), the communication node for the stomach Weishu (BL 21), and Zusanli (ST 36). Nodes on the arms such as Waiguan (SJ 5) and Lieque (LU 7), and leg locations Xuanzhong (GB 39), Zhongdu (LV 6), and Xiguan (LV 7) had no effect.

Stomach Function

The dual feature of needling stimulation on the activities of the stomach and the relationship of certain nodal sites shows that the basic electrical gastric rhythm is inhibited in most normal subjects by needling Zusanli (ST 36), but increases in a small percentage of subjects, and is unchanged in some (Xu and Wang: 1984). Inhibition is apparent in those individuals whose electrogastrogram (EGG) values were high before treatment; in contrast, EGG values rose in those with the lowest pretreatment levels. Needling therapy demonstrates either an inhibitory or excitatory function depending on the initial pretreatment condition. Treatment tends to normalize stomach function. Individuals with duodenal ulcer and other problems show higher pretreatment EGG values, which are reduced toward the normal range as a result of needling Zusanli (ST 36). Patients with superficial gastritis and gastric cancer have pretreatment EGG parameters below the normal range; these increase toward normal levels as a result of needling. Stimulation of the stomach communication node Weishu (BL 21), recruitment (*mu*, 募) node Zhongwan (RN 12), Zusanli (ST 36), Pishu (BL 20), and Liangmen (ST 21) show the greatest inhibition of EGG values. Nodal sites Touwei (ST 8) on the head and Yanglingquan (GB 34) on the leg are about one-half as effective. Lin et. al. (1997) also reported that electroacupuncture on Zusanli (ST 36) and Neiguan (PC 6) enhanced gastric myoelectrical activity in human subjects.

Noguchi and Hayashi (1996) observed a gastric acidity increase in rats by electroacupuncture to the hind limb that was abolished by severing the sciatic nerve, indicating somatic afferents as the stimulating pathway. No response to electroacupuncture was noted after vagotomy, while response was significantly enhanced after sympathectomy, demonstrating that branches of the vagus nerve to the stomach serve as the efferent pathway. Electroacupuncture on Zusanli (ST 36) was observed to regulate stomach hyperactivity induced by electrostimulation of the lateral hypothalamus in rabbits (Ma and Liu: 1994). Study of cat medulla oblongata showed inhibitory and excitatory sites for stomach muscle and electrical activity (Ouyang and Xu: 1984, 1987). Both excitatory and inhibitory areas were located in the nucleus raphe magnus, nucleus raphe pallidus, nucleus gigantocellularis, nucleus pontis centralis, nucleus trapezoidalis, and medial reticular formation. Inhibitory units were more prevalent that excitatory locations. Sectioning of the DLF spinal cord at T5, vagus nerve, or the splanchnic nerve attenuated either the needling effect or the action of electrical stimulation of the medulla oblongata, but did not abolish it entirely.

Small Intestine Motility

Needle insertion at Zusanli (ST 36) in rabbits with strong twirling produces a stronger inhibition of stomach motility than does simple insertion and retention with no manipulation (Liu et. al.: 1987). Insertion at nodal site Xiaohai (SI 8) inhibits the motility of the small intestine. Needle insertion with light twirling only slightly reduces small intestine motility, but has no measurable effect on its electrical activity. However, strong twirling manipulation produces greater inhibition of small intestine motility, with a subsequent change in electrical wave amplitude and frequency. Needling Zusanli (ST 36) with different twisting strengths in rabbits shows that strong needle stimulation causes reduced intestinal motility, while light manipulation results in increased motility (Yu et. al.: 1984). This possibly indicates that strong manipulation provokes sympathetic reaction, while light manipulation enhances parasympathetic function in the case of the intestine. Diarrhea in patients and induced hyperperistalsis in normal subjects was inhibited and small intestine function normalized by applying ultrasound for two minutes on nodal sites Zusanli (ST 36) on the leg and Tianshu (ST 25) overlying the small intestine (Jin et. al.: 1987).

Gallbladder Contractions and Ejecting Stones

Nodal sites on the leg, including Yanglingquan (GB 34), Dannang (extra), and Zusanli (ST 36), on the right side, can induce gallbladder contractions with measurable electrical muscle activity and contractions in the Oddi sphincter of the gallbladder, whereas Shousanli (LI 10) located on the arm has little effect (Sun, Cheng, and Liu: 1979; Yun, Kai, and Qiu: 1979; Zhang et. al.: 1983). Nodal sites Jujue (SP 16) and Burong (ST 19) located near the region overlying the gallbladder, along with the leg sites, promote contraction in the common bile duct (Yun, Kai, and Qiu: 1979). Stimulation of Qimen (LV 14) and Riyue (GB 24), overlying the region of the gallbladder itself, was necessary for the ejection of gallstones (Wendeng Central Hospital Cholelithiasis Treating Group: 1979).

Bladder Function

Needling either the skin or muscle tissue of the perineum produced reflex inhibition of urinary bladder micturition contractions in rats, whereas needling the face, neck, fore limb, chest, abdomen, back, and hind limb had no effect (Sato, Sato, and Suzuki: 1992). Needling of the muscle tissue produced a greater response than just needling the skin, and severing the pudendal nerve supplying the perineum abolished the reflex inhibition. Patients with residual urine problems and paraparesis (partial paralysis of the lower limbs) were effectively treated with nodal sites at the same spinal level as the bladder, using the communication node Pangguanshu (BL 28) and recruitment node Zhongji (RN 3) of the bladder, and Ciliao (BL 32) (Wu et. al.: 1984). However, distal node locations on the opposite side of the leg to the bladder vessel, including Sanyinjiao (SP 6), Yinlingquan (SP 9), and Yingu (KD 10), had no effect. Needling stimulation on bladder function in rabbits showed a decreasing order of effectiveness to produce bladder contractions (parasympathetic function) for nodal sites Pangguanshu (BL 28) and Ciliao (BL 32) in the sacral area, and Qugu (RN 2), Zhongji (RN 3), and Guanyuan (RN 4) located on the lower abdominal centerline.

Needling Pangguanshu (BL 28) produces bladder contractions and hence parasympathetic response. Needling Shenshu (BL 23) produces bladder relaxation, which is a sympathetic response. Strong electrostimulation to Shenshu (BL 23) was also observed to cause local muscle spasms, and bring on other sympathetic outflow characteristics, such as accelerated heart and increased respiration rates. Projection of bladder afferents shows a bimodal distribution that corresponds to Shenshu (BL 23) and Pangguanshu (BL 28) (Table 14.4).

Cortical Activation by Acupuncture Stimulation

Functional magnetic resonance imaging (fMRI) techniques permit visualization of minute changes in blood oxygenation in vascularized areas, such as in various regions of the brain. This provides in vivo anatomical details of the brain where increased functional activity occurs as a result of simple external stimulation, such as shining a light in the eyes to stimulate the visual cortex, or playing music to stimulate the auditory cortex. Cho et. al. (1998, 1999) needled nodes Zhiyin (BL 67) and Guangming (GB 37), which have visual-related indications, and Xiaxi (GB 43) and Waiguan (SJ 5), which have auditory-related indications. The fMRI images of the visual cortex as a result of needling Zhiyin (BL 67) compared well with that derived by shining a light in the eyes. Functional MRI images of the visual cortex resulting from needling Guangming (GB 37) also compared favorably with light stimulation, but were more laterally situated and showed some overlap with the auditory cortex. Needling Xiaxi (GB 43) produced fMRI auditory cortex images that correlated well with those obtained by playing music, but had some overlap with the visual cortex. Electroacupuncture applied to Waiguan (SJ 5) similarly obtained an auditory cortex response that was comparable to an fMRI image as a result of playing music. Needling non-node locations did not stimulate useful fMRI images.

Measurements in cortical regions of the brain while needling the four nodes Zhiyin (BL 67), Guangming (GB 37), Xiaxi (GB 43), and Waiguan (SJ 5) demonstrate one major property of nodes: the ability to produce effects that act afar from the location being stimulated. This would require somatic and autonomic reflexes along the spinal cord to influence vascular or neural centers in specific regions of the brain. The bladder distribution vessel includes the vertebral arteries that supply the visual cortex and other regions of the brain (Chapter 11). Hence, it would be expected that needling nodes along the bladder distribution vessel could mediate changes in the visual cortex. These distal effects are different from the common overlap of visceral and somatic neurons with reference to rotating malpositioned fetuses (see Bladder Afferents, page 276) using Zhiyin (BL 67). The gallbladder distribution vessel starts on the head and covers the lateral aspect of the head, partly overlapping the region of the visual cortex, before descending down the lateral aspect of the body. This distribution vessel also sends arterial branches to the internal ear (Chapter 11). Hence, it would be expected that needling nodes on the gallbladder distribution vessel could influence the auditory cortex and the lateral aspect of the visual cortex. The internal membrane (*sanjiao*, 三焦) distribution vessel is a vein that drains the same regions on the lateral head supplied by the gallbladder distribution vessel, including a vein from the internal ear (Chapter 11). Hence, it would be expected that some nodes along the internal membrane distribution vessel could influence the auditory cortex. The fMRI images may provide the first clues to the specific viscerosomatotopic organization of the nodal sites on the body and how it is reflected in the brain.

Longitudinal Organization and Nodal Indications

The preceding information lends credence to the concept of vertical organization along longitudinal body regions (yin-yang divisions) that contain the distribution vessels, nodal pathways, and muscle distributions. Nodal locations may represent unique somatotopic (body surface) sites in terms of their clinical utility. The early Chinese correlated the longitudinal pathways with specific internal organs (Chapters 3 and 11). Hence some locations on the body surface represent viscerosomatotopic sites as well. This suggests that some indicated uses of nodes are based solely on their location on the body surface. A review of traditional indications for nodes reveals a significant correlation between nodal site location and function. A parallel can be drawn between the somatotopic and viscerosomatotopic organization of the nodal pathway system, and the spinal segmental distribution of the autonomic visceral and coincident integration of superficial somatic nerves at the same spinal or overlapping segmental levels. This is especially true for vessel pathways that distribute over the body trunk (Chapter 11). A review of indications for the allowance (*ren*, 任) vessel node locations on the body centerline, as an example, shows that visceral and somatic indications correlate well with spinal nerve segmental levels (Table 14.5). An apparent linear relationship is demonstrated between the somatotopic location of the node and clinical manifestations related to the internal systems whose afferent neurons integrate near to or at the same spinal cord segment level as the somatic afferents from the nodal location.

Controlling Pathways

Using particular nodal sites to direct restorative responses to disordered areas of the external and internal body forms the foundation of needling therapy (Chapter 15). Clinical effects are

Table 14.5 Main indications of the twenty-four allowance (*ren*) vessel nodes (Figure 11.13) distributed down the anterior body centerline from RN 24 below the lower lip, continuing down the throat, chest, abdomen, and lower abdomen to RN 1, located at the perineum, showing their correspondence with the underlying internal organs and structures.

Main Indications	24	23	22	21	20	19	18	17	16	15	14	13	12	11	10	9	8	7	6	5	4	3	2	1
Mental Disorders	X									X	X													X
Deviation of Mouth and Eyes	X																							
Swollen Gums	X																							
Toothache	X																							
Facial Puffiness	X																							
Salivation	X	X																						
Subglossal Pain		X																						
Aphasia/Stiff Tongue		X																						
Sudden Hoarseness		X	X																					
Difficulty Swallowing		X	X					X			X													
Hiccup			X					X	X															
Sore/Dry Throat			X																					
Asthma, Cough			X	X	X	X	X	X											X					
Chest/Intercostal Pain				X	X	X	X	X																
Nausea									X	X	X	X	X											
Cardiac Pain										X	X													
Epilepsy										X	X	X												
Palpitation											X													
Vomiting											X	X	X	X	X									
Insomnia												X	X											
Abdominal Distension												X	X	X				X						
Abdominal Pain												X	X	X	X	X	X	X	X	X	X	X		
Jaundice													X											
Indigestion													X		X									
Diarrhea													X		X	X	X		X	X	X			
Edema														X		X		X	X	X				
Epigastric Pain															X									
Flaccid Apoplexy																	X		X		X			
Hernia																		X	X	X	X	X	X	
Leukorrhea																		X	X	X	X	X	X	
Irregular Menstruation																		X	X		X	X	X	X
Dysmenorrhea																			X		X	X	X	
Amenorrhea																			X	X				
Uterine Bleeding																			X	X	X	X		
Impotence																			X			X	X	
Nocturnal Emission																			X		X	X	X	X
Constipation																			X					
Enuresis																			X	X	X	X	X	X
Urine Retention																X					X			X
Anuria																				X				
Vaginitis																						X		X
Hemorrhoids																								X

mediated through its influence on several key nuclei in the brain stem to promote homeostasis and supply supraspinal pathways to specific spinal cord levels via the DLF and tract of Lissauer. Descending signals provide inhibition of somatic and visceral pain neurons, restore somatic motor function and reduce spasms, and promote homeostasis by restoring autonomic motor (viscera and blood vessel) function. Reflex activity of the spinal afferent system and subsequent supraspinal descending control stimulated by needling the superficial body are basically the same as those involved in the endogenous control of pain, visceral functional activities, and homeostasis. These processes are quite complex and not fully understood. Descending control can be influenced by the somatosensory cortex via the thalamus, and from nuclei within the limbic lobe or basal ganglia systems—but the most significant control of needling effects are mediated by centers in the brain stem, the most important of which involve the nucleus raphe magnus in the final pathway to the spinal cord. Both 5HT and norepinephrine nerve fibers are involved in the descending control via the DLF, and analgesia is only completely abolished when both sets of these neurons are destroyed (Hammond: 1986).

Multiple Descending Pain Control Pathways

One descending control pathway involves enkephalin-containing 5HT (serotonin) neurons, which appear to mediate endogenous pain and visceral homeostatic control processes (Figure 14.2). Needling therapy normally activates this pathway to treat disease and restore health. The other pathway, involving norepinephrine neurons, may be involved in stress analgesia, which can be quickly induced when external stimuli are potentially life threatening, as demonstrated by the fact that people generally feel no pain initially after suffering an accidental injury, including bone fractures. Needling-invoked and stress analgesia may only differ as a result of the magnitude of the applied stimulus to bring about the reaction. Stress analgesia is influenced by the intensity, or in the case of electrical stimulation, the amplitude and increased frequency, of the applied signal. He et. al. (1995) showed that afferent neurons at the T12–L1 spinal level activated by noxious stimuli applied to the hind paw of rats were inhibited by low-intensity electroacupuncture applied to Zusanli (ST 36) on the leg, but were not affected by electroacupuncture at Xiaguan (ST 7) on the face. However, high-intensity electroacupuncture at Xiaguan (ST 7) produced a significant analgesic effect on the T12–L1 neurons, which was negated by lesion of the nucleus raphe magnus. Some needling techniques that use strong manual stimulation of just one or two proximal or distal nodes may be producing their analgesic effect by bringing the descending norepinephrine pathway into play.

In normal needling analgesia, plasma cortisol levels show little change, and norepinephrine and cyclic adenosine monophosphate (cAMP) show significant decreases; while cortisol, norepinephrine, and cAMP all show a significant increase with stress analgesia (Xu et. al.: 1984; Zhou, Xuan, and Han 1985). Morphine also produces analgesia, and influences certain brain nuclei. A further complication in understanding the effects of needling is that repeated use can produce tolerance that can involve either 5HT or norepinephrine, and can show a cross-tolerance to morphine (Han, Li, and Tang: 1985; Zhou et. al.: 1985).

The most important nuclei involved in serotonergic (5HT) descending control pathways due to needling are the periaqueductal gray (Cao, Wang, and Jiang: 1984; Gu, Li , and Chen: 1984; Liu and Zhang: 1984), nucleus dorsal raphe, nucleus raphe magnus (Ammons, Blair, and Foreman: 1984; Shi and Zhu: 1984a, 1984b, 1984c; Chapman, Ammons, and Foreman: 1985; Holt, Akeyson, and Knuepfer: 1991), nucleus reticularis paragigantocellularis, and the arcuate nucleus of the hypothalamus (ARC). In addition to these nuclei, the noradrenergic (norepinephrine) supraspinal pathways also include the locus ceruleus, the lateral reticular nucleus, and descending norepinephrine fibers from cell groups A1 and A5. Electrical stimulation of these areas produces descending inhibition of afferent nociceptive signals and motor fibers; Jurna (1980) notes that stimulation of the periaqueductal gray inhibits both proprioceptive and C fiber afferents. Most of the above nuclei participate in mediating needling and electroacupuncture analgesia, stress analgesia, morphine analgesia, and tolerance. Stress analgesia mostly involves the nucleus dorsal raphe, locus ceruleus, and ARC (Di et. al.: 1984; Guo, Yin, and Yin: 1984; Yu, Gong, and Yin: 1984). Morphine analgesia involves the ARC as well (Guo, Yin, and Yin: 1984). The final descending control pathways to the trigeminal nucleus and the spinal cord involve both norepinephrine and 5HT.

Final Descending Pathways

The periaqueductal gray is a primary reception center for ascending nociceptive information, as well as receiving descending inhibition from the somatosensory cortex via circuits that distribute to the nucleus dorsal raphe. The nucleus raphe magnus is perhaps the most important final integration site for descending 5HT fibers, possibly involving 5HT1 receptors (el-Yassir and Fleetwood-Walker: 1990). Neurons in the periaqueductal gray or nucleus raphe magnus that respond to somatic or visceral noxious stimuli have significant ipsilateral projection fibers to the trigeminal nucleus and spinal cord via the DLF. Basbaum et. al. (1977) observed that analgesia produced by electrical stimulation of the periaqueductal gray is attenuated by ipsilateral lesion of the DLF. Many descending fibers are enkephalin-containing 5HT neurons, which synapse onto dorsal horn nociceptive inhibitory interneurons that have opiate receptors (Foreman, Hammond, and Willis: 1981; Gu, Li, and Chen: 1984), possibly inhibiting NK1 receptors on substance P neurons (Traftòn et. al.: 1999). Aicher et. al. (2000) indicate that antinociception by mu-opiate receptors may involve postsynaptic second-order nociceptive interneurons in the spinal trigeminal nuclei and spinal cord dorsal horns in rats. Iontophoretic application of naloxone or methysergide, antagonists of opiates and 5HT respectively, to dorsal horn neurons blocks the inhibitory effect of either needling or nucleus raphe magnus stimulation.

The lateral reticular nucleus also receives a large number of ascending ALT nociceptive neurons, which are somatotopically organized. Most of the norepinephrine neuron bodies of the medulla are scattered throughout the lateral reticular nucleus, and may be the source of the descending norepinephrine neurons that project to the spinal cord via the DLF. The norepinephrine neurons apparently act directly on spinal cord dorsal nociceptive neurons, gamma motoneurons, and the preganglionic sympathetic neurons, without the involvement of an interneuron (Figure 14.2). The late slow EPSP produced in the paravertebral and prevertebral ganglia by antidromic stimulation via branches of the primary nociceptive afferent neurons are presnaptically inhibited by descending pathways involving enkephalins (Dalsgaard et. al.: 1982; Dun and Jiang: 1982; Konishi, Tsunoo, and Otsuka: 1979; Konishi et. al.: 1980) (Figure 14.2). Possible inhibitory small intensely fluorescent (SIF) interneurons are also present in the autonomic ganglia that contain other neurotransmitters, including norepinephrine, involving alpha-adrenergic receptors (Christ and Dun: 1986). It has been shown that this pathway may respond to plasma levels of norepinephrine released by strong stimulation of the adrenal glands, as might be experienced in a stress reaction.

Summary of Overall Pathways

Communication pathways mediating the responses to needling are relatively complex. A highly simplified illustration is provided in Figure 14.4. Needling the superficial body provokes afferent nociceptive (pain) neurons that distribute to the dorsal horn of the spinal cord (1). These pain neuron signals then trigger gamma loop efferents in the ventral horn (4), and also activate neurons that cross over to the other side of the spinal cord to be transmitted up to the brain (3). Some of this information (3) travels to the sensory cortex, when the individual may consciously experience needling sensations. Most of the data travels to the brain stem regions.

Activation of the afferent muscle spindle static load proprioceptive neurons (2), either by the gamma loop (via 4 and 5), or possibly by bradykinin (B2) released during needling, transmits signals to the spinal cord dorsal horn. Both nociceptive and proprioceptive signals stimulate additional neurons that transmit signals to the ventral horn of the spinal cord (4), which activate somatic motor nerves (5) to muscles, and autonomic motor nerves to peripheral blood vessels (6) and to the internal organs (7).

Afferent proprioceptive information is also transmitted up and down the spinal cord producing muscle, nociceptive, and visceral reflexes along the cord remote from the spinal segmental level at which the stimulation is provided. The neurons associated with the muscle system comprise a pathway known as the gamma loop (2, 4, and 5), which is necessary for muscle function even though voluntary motor signals are provided by descending response

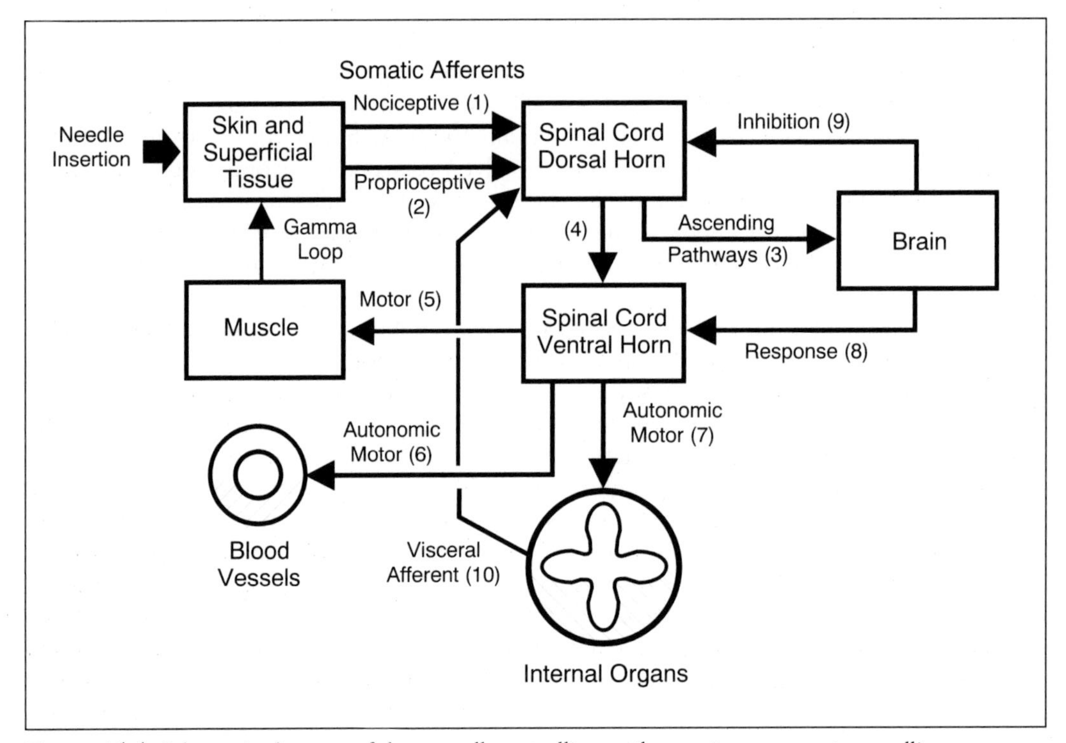

Figure 14.4 Schematic diagram of the overall controlling pathways in response to needling stimulation.

pathways (8) from the brain. Afferent muscle information is also transmitted to the brain via ascending pathways (3) in spinal tracts different from those carrying the pain signals.

Certain regions or nuclei within the brain stem, involving the periaqueductal gray and several raphe nuclei, including the nucleus raphe magnus, eventually activate supraspinal descending pathways in the spinal cord (9), which provide inhibition and control. These signals can inhibit pain, relieve muscle contractions, normalize vascular tone, and restore blood flow. Inhibition of autonomic motor fibers also normalizes organ activity. Descending control is only directed back down to spinal segmental levels that are stimulated by needling (Foreman, Hammond, and Willis: 1981; Foreman: 1986).

Internal organs, including blood vessels, also have afferent nociceptive neurons (10) that indicate pain and inflammation. These signals also transmit to the dorsal horn of the spinal cord. These signals cannot apparently be transmitted along the ascending pathway (3) without a corresponding input or associated somatic nociceptive receptive field neuron (1). This arrangement of afferent signals indicates that somatovisceral relationships are part of the basic organization of the neural communication and control systems (Cervero: 1985, 1986). If the pain signals from the viscera (10) exceed a certain threshold, then the neurons in the somatic nociceptive pathway (1) can be activated antidromically to produce referred pain in the related somatic receptive field. All nociceptive pathways can be antidromically stimulated. Afferent nociceptive visceral neurons (10) can also stimulate muscle reflexes (involving 4, 5, and 10).

15

Treatment Approaches

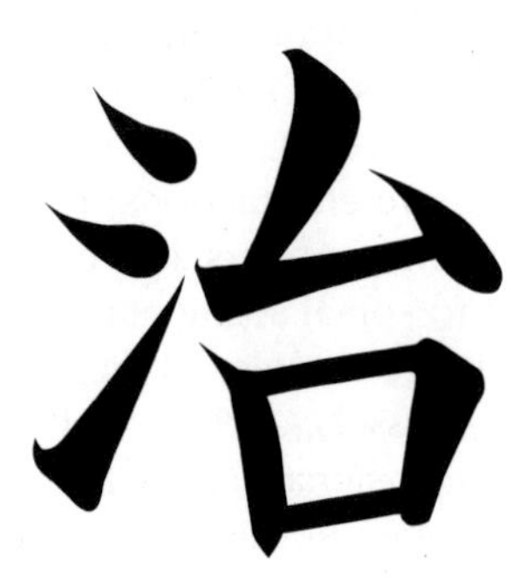

Zhi: To Treat

Altogether the principles of needling therapy start with the distribution vessels, the circulation routes of nutrients [ying], and understanding the vessel measurements. Needling is applied to the distribution vessels of the five viscera in the case of internal [deep] disorders. Needling is applied to the distribution vessels of the six bowels for external [superficial] conditions.

Yellow Emperor, *NJLS 48 (Obeying the Taboos)*

Herbal remedies, needling therapy, and moxibustion are the three most common methods of treatment in Chinese medicine. Other modes of care may be employed depending on the specific problem being treated (Chapter 5). Use of herbal medicine is straightforward, with remedies being selected for their properties, their affinity with a particular vessel and internal organ, and for their specific therapeutic effect. Needling is a more sophisticated therapeutic strategy that considers selection of nodes, stimulation technique, duration of needle insertion, and other factors. Needling is used to treat nearly all acute and chronic disorders, and many conditions respond only to this type of stimulation. Nutritional therapy is also essential, especially in cases of overconsumption, and also in addressing deficiencies. Herbs are also used in combination with nutritional therapy, as are other treatment approaches, including needling.

The unique Chinese physiological model, with its distribution vessels and related nerves providing communications pathways to the internal organs and giving rise to several hundred critical nodes, may appear to contain an overwhelming amount of information, causing possible confusion about where to start in treating specific disorders. Added to this is the fact that one disease may be treated using different approaches, and that the same treatment may be applied to more than one disorder. The *Neijing* recognizes potential problems in dealing with such a large amount of information, and discusses the need to summarize minute details into useful concepts (see quote from *NJLS 48*, in Chapter 1). The resulting principles of treatment provide a logical process for arriving at the best treatment strategy. Success in treatment relies on accurate diagnosis of the presenting complaint.

Treatment strategies generally address problems in terms of the three broad categories (Chapter 13): strengthening body resistance and eliminating pathogenic factors; regulating yin-substance and yang-function, including internal organ conditions and physiological balance; and restoring disturbances related to blood and vital substances (*ying*, 营; *wei*, 卫; *shenjing*, 神精; and *qi*, 气). Some of the specific therapeutic techniques include clearing heat, warming cold, and removing obstructions. Disease manifestations are usually addressed in terms of possible excess and deficiency conditions as a fundamental therapeutic concept. However, the primary and secondary manifestations of disease must be examined. Primary refers to the root (*ben*, 本) cause of the problem, which is often chronic in nature, while secondary refers to the superficial or outward (*biao*, 表) symptoms, and the acute presentation of a condition. Acute disorders are treated first, but the root cause of the problem is addressed as well. Therapies are applied to bring about specific reactions to address a particular diagnosis. Full details of the application of Chinese medical treatments are beyond the scope of this text, however a summary is provided to illustrate the basic concepts.

Principles of Treatment

Basic principles of treatment are summarized in *NJLS 48* (*Obeying the Taboos*). A student in ancient times had to be well trained in the fundamental concepts of Chinese physiology—including knowledge of internal organs, muscle distributions, distribution and collateral vessels, node locations related to the vessels, and diagnostic techniques—before being taught the principles of treatment. Students were also required to obey the taboos of not transmitting the theory and details of Chinese medicine to those who are lazy, selfish, and unwilling to serve others.

Therapeutic Considerations

The general principles of treatment are summarized by the Yellow Emperor in *NJLS 48* as follows:

> Altogether the principles of needling therapy start with the distribution vessels, the circulation routes of nutrients [ying], and understanding the vessel measurements. Needling is applied to the distribution vessels of the five viscera in the case of internal [deep] disorders. Needling is applied to the distribution vessels of the six bowels for external [superficial] conditions. The state of the defensive function must be examined with respect to the origins of all diseases. Hollowness [deficiency] and solidness [excess] are to be regulated to halt hollow [deficient] and solid [excess] disorders. Collateral vessels are to be drained off [reduced] by the letting of blood in the case of clots, and the patient will recover.

The Yellow Emperor then explains the importance of differentiating between the radial pulse at the wrist, which is symptomatic of the internal regions (five viscera), and the carotid pulse at the neck, which is symptomatic of the external regions (six bowels). A slow or intermittent pulse condition is to be treated by bloodletting of the collateral vessels to remove clots, combined with drinking herbal remedies. The Yellow Emperor also notes that taut muscle pain is to be treated by selecting nodes along the affected muscle distribution. In addition, it is necessary to examine the patient by palpating the areas of the origin and extremities of the symptoms, and scrutinizing areas of cold or heat, to determine whether the disease is internal or external in nature.

The Great Treatise

Different disease conditions require emphasis on a particular treatment approach. Most of the typical conditions are summarized in the *Great Treatise* presented in *NJLS 48*:

> Only when one has obtained an understanding of the conveyance of nutrients [ying] throughout the vessels can one be taught the *Great Treatise*, which states that flourishing [excess] conditions should only be treated by draining off [reducing] techniques; hollow [deficient] conditions should only be treated by mending [reinforcing] techniques; acute disorders should be treated with both needling and moxibustion, and by drinking herbal remedies; and depressed vessels [those that fail to pop up when pressed] should only be treated by the application of moxibustion therapy. Conditions that are neither flourishing nor hollow should be treated by selecting the affected distribution vessel. It is said to cure the affected distribution vessel the patient must drink herbal remedies, and receive moxibustion and needling therapy. Rapid pulse conditions should be treated by drawing out. Conditions with a big pulse and weak constitution should be treated by peace and calm [rest and relaxation], with no physical exertion permitted so as not to fatigue the patient.

Primary and Secondary Manifestations

Disease conditions usually manifest with primary (ben) and secondary (biao) symptoms (Table 15.1). During diagnosis it is important to distinguish between the root cause (primary manifestation) and the outward symptoms (secondary manifestation) of a disorder: these two aspects of a disease are also referred to as chronic and acute symptoms. Treatment of a chronic disorder while ignoring signs of an acute problem can result in the secondary condition becoming worse. Treatment of an acute disorder while ignoring an existing chronic condition can produce negative results. It is also important to determine if the condition being treated is mild or severe. In severe disorders it is then necessary to consider the stage of transformation of the disease, since improper treatment can be life threatening.

Differentiating Between Root Cause and Outward Signs

Primary and secondary conditions are discussed in *NJSW 65* (*Symptoms, Root Cause, and Transformation of Disease*), where Qibo notes:

Table 15.1 Comparison of primary and secondary characteristics of disease.

	Primary (Ben)	*Secondary* (Biao)
Pathogenesis	Antipathogenic Function	Pathogenic Factor
Etiology	Root Cause	Clinical Manifestation
Location	Internal Organs	Exterior Body
Duration	Chronic	Acute
Transformation	Original Disorder	Complication

> Ordinarily the methods of needling therapy must differentiate between yin and yang attributes, consider the correspondence between the initial and later conditions of the disease, determine the application of either direct or indirect needling, and determine the phase of the transformation between the secondary symptoms and root cause of the disorder. Therefore it is said that when the patient has outward symptoms, one must treat these secondary conditions. When the patient has manifestations of a primary condition, one must treat the root causes.
>
> Sometimes in a primary disorder, treatment is directed toward the secondary symptom, and sometimes a secondary disorder is treated by considering the primary root cause. Therefore in clinical treatment, the secondary conditions are sometimes selected to bring about a beneficial change, or the root cause is sometimes selected to bring about a beneficial change. Sometimes inverse needling is applied to bring about a change, or the direct method of needling is applied to bring about a beneficial change. Therefore, understanding the application of direct and indirect methods in a straightforward manner, without consulting others, as well as understanding the aspects of outward symptoms and root cause of disease, is paramount for the practitioner. Not understanding the outward symptoms and root cause of disease is called reckless practice [malpractice].

Diseases are clinically evaluated according to their primary and secondary aspects. The root cause and chronic nature of a disorder is distinguished from its outward (acute) symptoms. The root cause may be determined first, but presenting acute symptoms are treated first, particularly in serious situations, where the acute symptoms are treated first and the root cause is treated only after the acute symptoms are relieved. When the root cause and outward symptoms are both serious, both conditions can be addressed simultaneously. Some secondary conditions are resolved by treating the root cause. Conversely, treating secondary conditions sometimes resolves the root cause. The overall goal of treatment is to finally resolve the root cause of the disease.

Chronic and acute conditions can be compared in terms of their main features (Table 15.1). The pathogenesis of secondary conditions is related to the excess pathogenic factor, while that of the primary condition is related to the impaired state of physiological balance, antipathogenic function, or homeostasis. In terms of etiology the secondary condition is represented by the clinical manifestation, while the primary condition is the basic cause. The location of the secondary condition is in the exterior body, which includes all the muscle systems, while the primary cause is located in the internal organs. In terms of duration, the secondary condition is acute and the primary is chronic. The secondary condition represents a complication in terms of transformation of the disease, while the primary cause is the original disorder.

Treating Outward Symptoms First

Acute urgent conditions cannot be ignored and must be addressed before treating existing chronic disorders. The outward symptoms (biao) of exterior disease are treated before the chronic disease. When the secondary symptoms are resolved, treatment of the root cause (ben) is addressed. When no urgencies exist, treating the primary signs usually resolves the secondary symptoms. This is called "tracing the root for treating disease." In some situations, the secondary manifestations may be similar to the chronic symptoms, although their pathogenesis and etiology are different. Separate approaches are employed to treat the root cause and the secondary symptoms. This is called "treating the same disease with different methods." Usually the root cause and outward symptoms are treated at the same time. This is called "treating different diseases with the same method."

With respect to the clinical transformation of a disease, it is important to complete an early diagnosis of the condition before it is allowed to transform into a more serious stage (Chapter 13). In the treatment and prevention of disease, it is necessary to understand the rules by which a disease can internally transform. Generally, transformations follow the five-phase victorious route of transmission. If the transformations of a disease are ignored and left untreated, the disease can change into a more difficult, and sometimes even serious, disorder. After the disease starts to transform it may be difficult to determine its true source or original root cause.

Therapeutic Methods

Candidate treatment methods are selected, guided by the treating principles, to resolve the problem determined from the differentiation of presenting syndromes. The affected vessel, internal organ, muscle distribution, or physiological system are all taken into account. Specific critical nodes are selected to address the presenting complaints and the appropriate therapeutic method is applied. The fundamental goal of treatment is to strengthen body resistance and eliminate pathogenic factors; regulate autonomic balance (yin and yang); and restore the balance of blood and vital substances (ying, wei, shenjing, and qi). Any of the treatment methods (Chapter 5) that are effective for a specific problem can be applied, including the use of herbal medicine, moxibustion, and needling, keeping in mind restrictions on applying the latter two techniques to certain nodes.

Fundamental Scope of Treatment

General guidelines for treating disease as a result of attack by the six environmental factors (the six sky-airs) using either herbal remedies or needling, or both, or using heat to warm cold conditions, are detailed in *NJSW 74* (*Great Treatise on the Important Truth*):

> For treating victorious and revenging diseases: a cold disease is heated, and a hot disease is to be made cold; a warm disease is cleared, and a cool disease is warmed; a dispersing disease is gathered [constricted], and a restricted disease is dispersed; a dry disease is lubricated; an acute disease is calmed; a firm disease is softened, and a fragile disease is firmed; a declining disease is mended, and a strong disease is drained off. Each environmental factor will certainly be cleared and calmed, and the disease-causing factors will decline and depart. This is the fundamental guideline for treating disease.

Therapeutic methods are summarized in the six general categories of reinforcing, reducing, clearing heat, warming cold, and ascending and descending therapy. In some situations there may be opposing conditions, such as deficiency in an area of the body while another exhibits excess conditions, or heat and cold may be present at the same time. In this situation both conditions are treated simultaneously. Herbal remedies are selected for their specific therapeutic action, while needling techniques are applied to bring about certain physiological responses in the body. In either case, both herbal medicine and needling are applied consistent with the six therapeutic methods. Moxibustion is applied to warm cold, reinforce yang function, and strengthen defensive function, if no signs of heat are present.

Reinforcing Deficiency

Reinforcing methods are applied to strengthen body resistance, replenish vital substances (ying, wei, shenjing, and qi) and blood, restore yin-substance and yang-functional attributes, restore internal organ function, and restore the balance between internal and external vessels. Reinforcing therapy is not applied if the pathogenic factors are still strong and excessive. Reinforcing therapy is applied to address the main specific problem and the treatment approach can vary depending on the situation.

A number of different therapies can be used to reinforce deficiencies. Herbal remedies or needling locations are selected for their known replenishing effects on vital substances, blood, yin-substance, or yang-function, such as replenishing blood and vital substances with nodes Pishu (BL 20), Geshu (BL 17), Zusanli (ST 36), Sanyinjiao (SP 6), and Taichong (LV 3), or replenishing yin substance with Taixi (KD 3), Zhaohai (KD 6), and Zhishi (BL 52). When a particular organ distribution vessel is involved, nodes are selected in relation to the particular vessel, or for their reinforcing effect on the affected vessel, such as by needling one of the related source (*yuan*, 原) and communication (*shu*, 输) locations, or using communication sites to strengthen organ yang-function and recruitment (*mu*, 募) nodes to strengthen organ yin-substance: communication nodes are located on the back of the body; recruitment nodes on the front. Source (yuan) and collateral (*luo*, 络) nodes (Table 9.5) related to the internal-external terminal collateral vessels can be considered in using one yin-yang paired vessel to reinforce the other. Pain and musculoskeletal dysfunction can be reinforced by local, proximal, and distal sites selected along the affected muscle distribution(s).

Reducing Excess

Reducing methods are used to dissipate pathogenic factors, remove stagnation, and restore the body's resistance. Reducing excess syndromes is often easier and responds faster than does reinforcing deficiencies. Herbal remedies are considered to address specific conditions, while needling therapy can be employed as the main treatment approach, and can include bleeding to remove stagnation. Cupping therapy can also be applied to remove deep blockages or stagnation of blood and vital substances. Moxibustion can be used to restore the body's resistance and to dissipate cold.

Strategies for reducing excess include the following: excess vital substances (ying, wei, shenjing, and qi) are reduced by selecting nodes that have a direct effect on vital substances themselves; blood circulation is stimulated and stasis removed by pricking corresponding nodes in the affected area; and internal organ–related distribution vessels are reduced by employing the sea (*he*, 合) and recruitment locations related to the affected vessel. The accumulation (*xi*, 郗) and well (*jing*, 井) nodes can also be considered, such as in lung excess where reducing therapy is applied to either or both the sea node Chize (LU 5) and recruitment site Zhongfu (LU 1), or in the case of large intestine excess, which is reduced by using recruitment site Tianshu (ST 25), sea location Quchi (LI 11), and the lower sea site Shangjuxu (ST 37). Internal-external organ distribution vessels are reduced by using the source node of the affected excess vessel, along with the collateral node location of the yin-yang matched pair, providing this vessel itself is not excessive. Pain and musculoskeletal dysfunction is reduced by local, proximal, and distal locations selected along the affected muscle distributions, with additional nodes to dispel specific pathogenic factors.

Clearing Heat

Clearing heat methods are applied to reduce fevers and pathogenic heat for resuscitation, or to restore yin deficiency in the case of false heat. Heat syndromes are considered to be excess, internal, or deficient in nature: different treatment approaches are considered for each category. Excess heat is an exterior disorder as a result of external attack of cold or wind, and involves an active struggle between antipathogenic function and pathogenic factors. Internal heat results from transmission of external pathogenic factors to the interior, or is the result of internal hypofunction. Herbal remedies for clearing heat associated with affected organs and conditions are selected, based on the specific condition. Excess and internal heat are excess in nature and reducing therapy is applied. Needle stimulation may be stronger than average, but retention time is shorter (two minutes or less). Deficiency heat syndromes are the result of yin substance deficiency failing to control yang function: treatment for a yin deficiency involves mild stimulation and longer duration of needle retention.

Examples of clearing heat include dispelling excess pathogenic heat by the use of nodes Dazhui (DU 14), Quchi (LI 11), and Hegu (LI 4), using reducing methods with short retention times; and selecting well (*jing*, 井), spring (*rong*, 荥), and river (*jing*, 经) nodes along the associated distribution vessel to treat interior heat syndromes of the internal organs, such as treating a lung heat condition by reducing the sea node Chize (LU 5), accumulation node Kongzui (LU 6), river node Jingqu (LU 8), and the spring node Yuji (LU 10). For clearing heat and resuscitation, Renzhong (DU 26) and the well sites are both needled with reducing techniques, or bloodletting is applied; for fever or high fever due to vigorous heat in the nutrients, defensive substances, and vital air systems, sea sites of the related bowel are employed; and for deficient heat, the recruitment and communication locations, singular vessel confluent sites, and nodes known to reinforce yin, such as Zhaohai (KD 6), and Zhishi (BL 52) to strengthen kidney yin, are considered.

Warming Cold

Cold is due to invasion of the body by exterior cold, or is the result of interior deficiency in yang function. Cold syndromes are considered to be exterior, interior, or deficient in nature. Exterior cold is characterized by an accumulation of wind-cold on the surface of certain areas of the body, impairing defensive function (*weiqi*, 卫气). Interior cold is characterized by pathogenic cold penetrating to the interior, causing development of yin substance excess and yang function deficiency. Deficiency cold syndromes are often associated with chronic diseases that result in deficiency of both vital substances and yang function. Some cold syndromes can be complicated with signs of heat, such as exterior heat with internal cold, or heat in the upper body and cold in the lower body. Warming methods are used to dispel cold, remove obstructions, nourish yang function, and warm the abdominal cavity. Herbal remedies of a warming nature are considered. Needling with longer retention times can be employed to remove cold from vessels, and moxibustion is frequently used as well. Needles are stimulated more strongly, but retained for shorter periods in deficient cold syndromes due to yang function deficiency.

Approaches to warming cold include, for exterior cold, needling along the affected vessel and retaining needles for a longer period, and/or the application of moxibustion along vessel nodes; and for interior cold, needling and application of moxibustion to nodes that influence the affected internal organ, such as communication nodes and other sites selected to address specific cold symptoms. Warming deficient cold involves needling of a short duration to restore affected organ yang function, and moxibustion can be applied to Shenque (RN 8) with salt, and to Guanyuan (RN 4). Exterior heat with internal cold, often occurring in winter, is treated by selecting nodes from the internal membrane (*sanjiao*, 三焦), large intestine, and lung distribution vessels. Heat in the upper body with cold symptoms in the lower part of the body is treated by clearing heat from the upper body using nodes on the three yang vessels of the hand, and warming cold in the lower body by moxibustion on the legs of the three yin vessels of the foot.

Ascending Therapy

Vital substances of the spleen, kidneys, and liver normally ascend via the venous system; the functional activity of these organs is thought to ascend. When this upward venous flow is impaired, pure yang fails to ascend, causing the sinking of vital substances (ying, wei, shenjing, and qi) in the abdominal cavity (middle *jiao*). Herbal remedies are employed for their ascending properties to address specific conditions of the affected organ. Ascending therapy involves reinforcing needling methods and moxibustion used on local nodes, along with Baihui (DU 20), Qihai (RN 6), Guanyuan (RN 4), and Zusanli (ST 36). Ascending therapy is not considered in cases of yin substance deficiency or yang function hyperactivity.

Descending Therapy

Food and water in the stomach and bowels, and bile from the gallbladder, normally descend through the digestive tract; the functional activity of these organs is thought to descend. When the downward direction of flow is disturbed, this results in the upward perversion of stomach and gallbladder functional activity, causing possible disturbance to the liver as well. Herbal remedies are employed for their descending properties to address specific conditions of the affected organ. For stomach regulation, reinforcing needling therapy is applied to Tanzhong (RN 17), Zhongwan (RN 12), Neiguan (PC 6), and Zusanli (ST 36). If the liver is involved in upward disturbance, the nodes Fengchi (GB 20), Taichong (LV 3), and Yongquan (KD 1) are employed to soothe the liver and subdue liver yang functional activity. Descending therapy is not considered in cases of deficiency syndromes in the upper body or excess conditions in the lower body.

Needling Therapy

The insertion and manipulation of fine metal needles to bring about a therapeutic effect is unique to Chinese medicine. Needling (acupuncture) tends to restore homeostasis (*zheng*, 正) by normalizing sympathetic and parasympathetic outflow, which has an influence on restoring visceral function and blood circulation. Typically, sympathetic activities are reduced. Homeostasis is promoted by reducing pain, restoring blood flow, normalizing immune system balance, and restoring visceral balance. Needling therapy is a complex treatment approach that requires knowledge of the nodes and their selection, as well as how to manipulate the tissue reactions to enhance either the inflammatory or anti-inflammatory phase of the process. Factors considered by the practitioner include selection of appropriate nodes, strength of stimulation, method of manipulation, depth and duration of insertion, basic constitution of the patient, presenting exterior and interior conditions, and the therapeutic method to be employed. The defensive and reflex mechanisms activated by needling intervention are also activated by the application of other therapies including moxibustion, massage, pressure, cupping, and additional modalities. Needling manipulation techniques are applied consistent with the node function and desired tissue reaction.

Although inserting needles may be relatively simple, great skill is required to bring about a controlled response. Most contemporary treatments use the fine filiform needle. The *NJLS 3* (*Understanding the Fine Needle*) goes so far as to judge the competency of practitioners based on their skill in applying the fine needle:

> To say it is easy to apply the fine needle means that it is easy to talk about it. To say it is difficult to apply the fine needle means it is difficult to actually insert needles into a person. An unskilled practitioner is someone who is restricted to needling techniques based on observing or watching.
>
> A highly skilled physician observes the patient's vitality [spirit] and is able to observe the conditions of blood and vital substances to determine excess and deficiency, and apply reinforcing [mending] or reduction [draining off] as needed.
>
> Unskilled practitioners attend to the critical junctures, they restrict their application to nodes on the four extremities, and they have no understanding of the flow of blood and vital substances, or the dynamic interaction of homeostatic balance [zheng] and pathogenic factors [*xie*, 邪].

Depth of Needle Insertion

Each node that is suitable for needling has a nominal insertion depth at some particular angle to the skin relative to the patient's size, shape, and condition. Lin (1997) conducted an extensive study involving numerous live subjects and human cadavers, measuring electrical resistance and using computed tomography of the chest to verify safe depths of needling. He concluded that insertion depths indicated in the twentieth-century acupuncture texts are greater than the ancient documents. Lin verified that the length between the creases on the second joint of the middle finger while flexed is an acceptable standard *cun* (寸, Chinese inch) to apply to needle insertion depth for adults, but not for newborns. He also concluded that the safe depth to obtain needling reaction (*deqi*, 得气) corresponds to the patient's body thickness, and was not related to electrical resistance of the node.

Within the nominal safe range, needles can be inserted at a superficial, medium, or full depth. The various levels produce slightly different tissue reactions and stimulate different afferent nerve fibers. Needling is applied to eliminate pathogenic factors (xie), and to regulate yin substance and yang function attributes. The depth of insertion has an influence on the characteristics of the response: shallow insertion is applied to remove pathogenic factors, and promote the flow of blood and vital substances; medium insertion removes yin pathogenic factors; and deeper insertion elicits a nutrient-based reaction. Details about the depth of insertion are provided in *NJLS 6* (*Longevity, Premature Death, Firmness, and Softness*), *NJLS 7* (*Quality Needling*), and *NJLS 9* (*From Beginning to End*), collectively summarized as follows:

Shallow Insertion

Shallow insertion through the skin brings on a nutrient (ying) response to release blood and eliminate external (yang) pathogenic factors. This involves inserting the needle just below the skin to provoke responses to address external (yang) pathogenic assault, partly because the skin is related to the lungs—the lungs are usually affected initially in acute pathogenic attacks. It is also thought that shallow insertion has a preferential influence on provoking viscerosomatic responses.

Medium Insertion

Medium depth of insertion just into the skeletal muscles brings on a defensive (wei) response, releasing vital substances and removing internal (yin) pathogenic factors. Insertion at this level promotes a defensive reaction that has an influence on the lymphatics, and hence is used to resolve various yin disorders such as edema or swelling.

Deep Insertion

Deeper insertion into the skeletal muscles promotes the flow of nutrients, vital air, and other substances, causing internal heat generation to treat cold rheumatism. When nutrients are flowing freely, needling is stopped. The arrival of nutrients means that reinforcing (mending) treatment has brought about solidness, and reduction (draining off) has brought about hollowness. In the case of treating someone with a delicate constitution, or in a poor physical shape, cold rheumatism requires the addition of herbal heat packs. Insertion into muscles brings on a response that directly influences the muscle distributions. This insertion level is commonly employed in the treatment of musculoskeletal problems. In the case of cold rheumatism, it helps warm the muscles by restoring the flow of blood and vital substances to supply nutrients (ying) and oxygen from vital air (qi) to the muscle tissues.

Needle Manipulation

Needle manipulation refers to the strength of movement and motion of the needle once it is inserted. Various techniques are used to either reduce an excess or strengthen a deficiency (Table 15.2). Reducing (draining off) and reinforcing (mending) are generally applied to reduce excess external pathogenic factors and mend internal yin conditions. Treatment for cold conditions, for example, is generally viewed in terms of warming cold, but is not thought of in terms of reducing.

Strong manipulation of the needle produces more tissue-damage products at the site of insertion (Chapter 14). This enhances the inflammatory (yang) phase of the reaction, especially if the needle is not retained for more than two to four minutes. This technique is used in reducing (draining off) an excess, such as clearing heat. It is also applied to restore yang function in cases such as hypothyroidism or metabolic hypofunction due to excess yin substance subduing yang function. Strong stimulation of nodes can provoke visceral yang (sympathetic) effects, which usually inhibit the gastrointestinal system while increasing heart rate and blood pressure (Table 4.5).

Table 15.2 Reinforcing and reducing methods of needle manipulation.

Technique	*Reinforcing (Mending)*	*Reducing (Draining Off)*
Speed	Insert slowly and gently with little or no rotation, withdraw quickly.	Insert quickly and forcefully with more rotation, withdraw slowly and gently.
Lifting and Thrusting	Thrust firmly and quickly, and lift gently and slowly. Lift and thrust approximately three or four times in 10 seconds, with small amplitude of ¼ to ⅜ inch, depending on thickness of muscles and length of needle.	Thrust gently and slowly, and lift forcefully and quickly. Lift and thrust approximately six or seven times in 10 seconds, with greater amplitude of ⅜ to ½ inch, depending on thickness of muscles and length of needle.
Rotation	Slow and gentle rotation of approximately 180°. Perform five complete rotations in about 10 seconds.[1]	Rapid and forceful rotation up to 360°. Perform ten complete rotations in about 10 seconds.[1]
Direction of Vessel	Insert needle along the course of the vessel to stimulate and obtain *deqi* to propagate signal in the direction of insertion; or Lift needle to just under the skin after initial *deqi* and redirect along course of vessel.	Insert needle against the course of the vessel to stimulate and obtain *deqi* to propagate signal in the direction of insertion; or Lift needle to just under the skin after initial *deqi* and redirect against course of vessel.
Open or Closed	Press hole quickly after needle withdrawal to prevent vital substances from escaping.	Shake the needle while withdrawing it to enlarge hole and allow pathogenic factors to be dispelled.
Respiration	Insert needle when patient breathes in, and withdraw needle when patient breathes out.	Insert needle when patient breathes out, and withdraw needle when patient breathes in.

1. To rotate in the same direction can cause nerve and muscle fibers to wrap onto the needle, causing significant pain and discomfort.

There are many clinical conditions where strong stimulation is used with longer retention times, including for musculoskeletal problems where strong stimulation is needed to produce highly directed descending control signals and to activate proprioceptive and motor signals. This approach is used in treating obstructive (*bi*, 痹) and flaccid (*wei*, 痿) syndromes. The greater amount of tissue reactants produced by strong needle manipulation enhances the tissue repair phase, thereby promoting healing. The longer retention time helps restore blood flow to the muscle tissues.

Mild needle stimulation produces less tissue-damage products, and if the needle is retained for a longer time (fifteen to twenty-five minutes) it enhances the anti-inflammatory phase of the tissue reaction. This has the effect of strengthening yin substance and also provokes parasympathetic response. This technique is used to treat false heat and hypersensitivity problems caused by yin substance deficiency, and acts to normalize blood flow in the superficial and deep regions. Mild stimulation with long retention is not used in treating true heat conditions, especially heat in the blood.

Needle Retention Time

Retention time is the single most important factor in needling therapy, as it influences the tissue reactions in terms of either promoting inflammatory or anti-inflammatory responses. Strong stimulation with short retention time (two to four minutes) is used to enhance the inflammatory phase of the needling response to reduce an acute condition. Short retention with strong stimulation is also used to treat visceral function (yang) deficiency, as found in conditions such as hypothyroidism. Long insertion times (fifteen to twenty-five minutes) enhance the controlling phase of the tissue reaction, and produce anti-inflammatory responses to treat false heat due to visceral substance (yin) deficiency, and to promote tissue repair and reduce pain.

Manipulating Propagated Sensations

In some clinical situations it is beneficial to provoke or promote propagated sensations (PS) along a particular vessel or muscle pathway, notably in situations where the problem lies deep in the body and there may not be an obvious node to use. Promoting PS is also helpful in obstinate cases that are responding poorly. The PS can be propagated along vessel and muscle pathways, and is felt more easily in younger people (Yang et. al.: 1993). Since PS depends on the participation of static load muscle spindles, it can be enhanced by increasing local temperatures or lowering ambient pressure, such as by cupping. Finger pressure can be applied along the nodal pathway being stimulated to either redirect or inhibit PS (Wu et. al.: 1993a, 1993b; Xu et. al.: 1993). Clinical success is higher if PS travels to the affected area being treated, such as in regulating cardiac function (You et. al.: 1987b), promoting blood circulation to remove blood stasis (Cheng, Wu, and Qie: 1990), disease of the face (Liu et. al.: 1990b), vascular tension and obstruction in the neck (Qie, Cheng, and Cheng: 1991), coronary heart disease (You: 1992), and myopia in youngsters (Li et. al.: 1993). The primary significance of PS is to stimulate spinal afferent systems to bring about centrally mediated control over a broader range of spinal levels.

Use of Critical Nodes in Treatment Strategies

The application of specific nodes in clinical strategies derived by the early Chinese physicians is consistent with the physiological mechanisms that mediate reactions to needling the superficial body, including manipulating needle insertion in terms of both strength and duration to produce specific tissue reactions. The anatomical location of nodes and their influence on local, proximal, or distal regions, neuroanatomical relationships, internal organ relationships, affected vessel, or muscle distribution are all considered in the selection and use of nodes. The two most important features taken into account are the spinal segmental relationships between certain body regions and the internal organs, and the contribution of propriospinal pathways to activate centrally mediated effects. Segmental relationships are considered when influencing a particular internal organ, vascular structure, or muscle distribution through the selection of local and adjacent nodes. Propriospinal influence is considered in the case of spreading the centrally mediated descending control over a wider course of the spinal cord and body through the use of nodes that are proximal and distal to the problem area.

The ancient Chinese physicians established the relationships between the internal organs (Chapter 3), distribution vessels (Chapter 11), and the muscle pathways (Chapter 12). Once a diagnosis indicates the involvement of a particular internal organ, vessel pathway, or muscle distribution, nodes are selected on the distribution vessel that supplies the affected area. Nodes that have indications for visceral problems show definite somatovisceral relationships over particular body regions that are generally consistent with the same spinal segmental levels of autonomic nerves serving the internal organs. This information provides a guide to selecting the local and adjacent candidate nodes for treatment. Selection of appropriate proximal and distal nodes on the target distribution vessel then completes a typical treatment protocol. The term proximal refers to nodes that are closest to the spinal cord, such as nodes located on the back, or those located at the highest spinal segment level. Distal locations are usually on the arms or hands, or the legs and feet. The therapeutic method employed dictates how the nodes are to be manipulated. Additional nodes may also be included in the treatment plan, selected for certain special relationships as exhibited by recruitment, communication, confluent, and five-phase nodes, as well as those chosen for their known special effects or special meeting locations.

Visceral Normalization

With respect to visceral function, needle stimulation tends to restore homeostasis by promoting sympathetic and parasympathetic balance. This is equivalent to restoring yang function and yin substance. Somatic afferents activated by needling then provoke visceral afferents. Descending control mechanisms inhibit or normalize visceral motor signals, and disinhibit the controlling pathways of somatic afferents affecting the viscera at the paravertebral ganglia levels (Figure 14.2). Node selection includes choosing sites at the same spinal nerve integration level as afferent visceral neurons to assure the greatest effect on local and adjacent nodes. Proximal and distal nodes are selected on the same distribution vessel related to the problem, or may involve related communication nodes and distal locations known to affect the particular organ involved. Treatment may bring about local effects, such as restoring blood flow, as well as central effects of normalizing autonomic balance.

For example, Chen (1997) successfully treated anovulatory patients (non-ovulating females) with electroacupuncture using nodes Zhongji (RN 3), Guanyuan (RN 4), and Zigong (extra node: uterus) as local and adjacent sites. These nodes all have an influence on the uterus and on the vessels supplying the uterus, as does Sanyinjiao (SP 6), which can be used as a distal node. Chen confirmed through rat studies that the treatments normalized the hypothalamic-pituitary-ovarian axis, showing a normalization of the autonomic nervous system. Another study by Stener-Victorin et. al. (1996) used only proximal and distal nodes to reduce the blood flow resistance in the uterine arteries of infertile women. Electroacupuncture at 100 Hz was applied to proximal nodes Shenshu (BL 23) and Pangguanshu (BL 28), which share overlapping regions with sympathetic neurons from the uterus. Using electroacupuncture at 100 Hz is known to stimulate segmental-related inhibition. In addition, 2 Hz electroacupuncture was applied to distal nodes Sanyinjiao (SP 6) and Chengshan (BL 57).

Pain and Musculoskeletal Disorders

The main benefits of needling-induced mechanisms related to the treatment of musculoskeletal problems are the promotion of pain inhibition, reducing contractions and spasms of muscles, restoring proprioceptive and motor function, and restoring blood flow to the muscles. Clinical effectiveness is assured when node selections are consistent with the muscle distributions involved in the problem. This follows the same logic of using local and adjacent nodes located where the problem exists, along with proximal and distal nodes. The key to successfully treating musculoskeletal problems is to select nodes that lie mostly within the affected muscle distribution (Chapter 12). As an example, an elbow problem manifesting in the large intestine muscle distribution is treated using Quchi (LI 11), Chize (LU 5), and Tianjing (SJ 10) as local and adjacent nodes, with Hegu (LI 4) as a distal node, and Dazhu (BL 11) and Feishu (BL 13) as proximal candidates. These latter two nodes are used to address the superficial rhomboid muscles between the spine and the scapula that are assigned to the large intestine muscle distribution. Without applying the proximal and distal nodes, clinical success in treating the elbow is limited.

Logic of Needling Treatment Formulas

The spinal afferent processing system, dominated by nociceptive and proprioceptive information, transmits needling-induced (deqi) afferent signals that stimulate higher levels in the central nervous system (CNS). This initiates CNS-mediated processes to provide a directed descending control for the inhibition of pain, autonomic motor (vascular and visceral), and somatic motor (muscle) signals down to the same spinal segment level as the afferent input (deqi) signal. These inhibitory or normalizing control signals from the brain stem restore autonomic nervous system balance, inhibit the pain neurons, restore vascular and visceral tone, and relax muscle tissue in the needle insertion area.

Specific regions of the body are affected depending on the particular nodes selected and the manner in which these sites are stimulated. These relationships are the result of the longitudinal organization of the spinal cord, the vessels, and the muscle systems. From these observations, the Chinese noted that clinical efficiency is greater when directing the descending control over a range of nodal levels. Basically, this involves the use of nodes in the local and adjacent areas of the problem to assure that restorative signals are directed to the main area of concern. Proximal nodes located closest to the appropriate spinal nerve entry point to the spinal segmental level are selected to assure that descending control is focused at the correct spinal level. Use of communication nodes is a common example. Finally, sites are often selected that are distal to the condition being treated (Figure 15.1). Collectively, the use of local and adjacent, proximal, and distal points assures the best coverage to bring about a controlled therapeutic response. If PS can be stimulated to reach the affected area, it results in spreading a high-threshold signal between the proximal and distal nodes, thus providing broad descending control response affecting a wide range of the spinal cord.

The use of nodes along the distribution vessels is the basic treatment approach. However, many of these nodes are also viewed in terms of particular categories or classifications that have special properties, anatomical features, and physiological relationships. Hence, supplementary nodes are often included in the treatment protocol, in addition to the local and adjacent, proximal, and distal candidates. The most common special grouping of nodes includes the following categories:

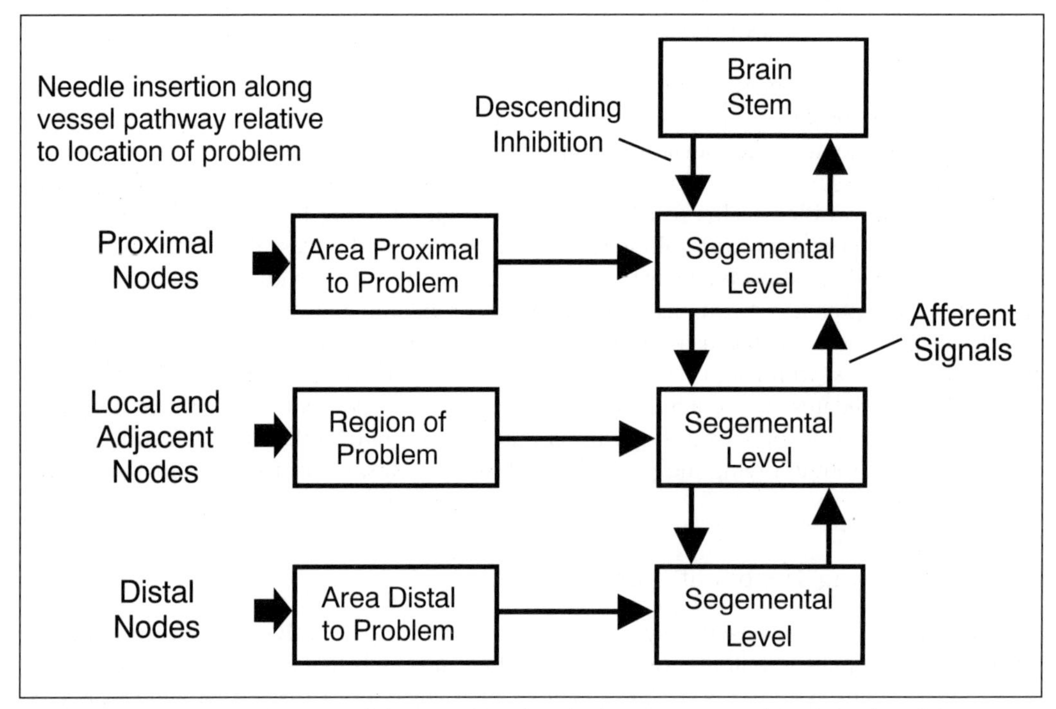

Figure 15.1 Schematic diagram of the use of local and adjacent, proximal, and distal nodal sites to bring about a directed descending control for the effective treatment of particular problems.

Lower Sea Nodes
Lower sea (he) nodes described in the *Neijing* provide a means whereby the three yang vessels of the hand communicate with the three yang vessels of the foot (Table 15.3). Here, the large intestine vessel communicates with the stomach, the small intestine with the gallbladder, and the internal membrane (sanjiao) with the bladder. These lower sea nodes are used in the treatment of problems specific to the bowel that they are related to, and can be applied as distal sites on the legs for the three bowel-related vessels of the arm. This provides the means of directing descending control signals, activated by needling the lower sea locations, down to spinal levels that affect the related bowel. The treatment of large intestine problems, for example, would typically involve the use of nodes on the large intestine distribution vessel, located on either the hand or arm, to serve as proximal nodes. Other nodes would be selected on the abdominal region to serve as local and adjacent nodes segmentally associated with the large intestine. Communication or recruitment nodes could also be selected. Finally, the lower sea node for the large intestine, Shangjuxu (ST 37), is selected as the distal node to direct descending control over the spinal region that influences the large intestine. Propriospinal reflexes can also be initiated by needling large intestine–related nodes on the hand, arm, and abdomen; these then travel to lower levels of the spinal cord and thereby direct descending control to the large intestine.

Eight Influential Nodes
The eight influential nodes are special sites that have long been observed to promote responses beneficial to specific regions, organs, or tissues of the body (Table 15.4). Influential nodes are

Table 15.3 Lower sea (*he*) nodes related to the six bowels (*fu* organs).

Six Bowels	*Lower Sea (*He*) Node*
Stomach	Zusanli (ST 36)
Large Intestine	Shangjuxu (ST 37)
Small Intestine	Xiajuxu (ST 39)
Gallbladder	Yanglingquan (GB 34)
Bladder	Weizhong (BL 40)
Internal Membrane (*Sanjiao*)	Weiyang (BL 39)

Table 15.4 Eight influential nodes related to the internal organs, vital air, blood, and body tissues.

Area of Influence	*Node*
Viscera (*Zang* Organs)	Zhangmen (LV 13)
Bowels (*Fu* Organs)	Zhongwan (RN 12)
Vital Air (*Qi*)	Tanzhong (RN 17)
Blood (*Xue*)	Geshu (BL 17)
Muscles (*Jin*)	Yanglingquan (GB 34)
Vessels (*Mai*)	Taiyuan (LU 9)
Bones (*Gu*)	Dazhu (BL 11)
Marrow (*Sui*)[1]	Xuanzhong (GB 39)

1. Also refers to brain neural tissue and the spinal cord.

usually added to a treatment formula when treating conditions in one of the eight categories: viscera, bowels, vital air, blood, muscles, vessels, bones, and marrow. Zhangmen (LV 13), the influential node for the viscera, is located on the lateral sides of the abdomen just below the tip of the eleventh rib. This node is also the recruitment node for the spleen, which has an influence on the viscera as well. The relationship between this node and the viscera may be the result of its location and spinal segment level where its afferent neurons integrate in the spinal cord, overlapping afferent neurons from the viscera. The equivalent influential node for the bowels, Zhongwan (RN 12), is located on the centerline of the abdomen situated over the middle of the abdominal cavity. This location, which provides a local and adjacent site for the bowels and a proximal node for the stomach, is used in treating most stomach and digestive problems. Tanzhong (RN 17), the influential node for vital air (qi), is located in the middle of the chest and has a demonstrated effect on lung activity and breathing.

Recruitment and Communication Nodes

These special communication nodes have a clear correlation with their spinal afferent neuron integration levels and their assigned organs (Table 15.5). Recruitment sites are located on the anterior trunk of the body and are used to address problems with yin substance of the organs. The communication nodes are located on the back of the trunk, and the locations correspond with bladder distribution vessel nodes. Communication nodes are used in addressing problems of yang functional activity. Nominal spinal segmental integration levels are also included in Table 15.5.

Table 15.5 Recruitment (*mu*) and communication (*shu*) nodes on the anterior and posterior trunk regions, related to specific viscera and nominal spinal afferent segmental levels.

Organ	*Recruitment (Mu) Node*	*Nominal Spinal Nerve Level*	*Communication (Shu) Node*	*Nominal Spinal Nerve Level*
Lungs	Zhongfu (LU 1)	T2	Feishu (BL 13)	T3–4
Pericardium	Tanzhong (RN 17)	T4	Jueyinshu (BL 14)	T4–5
Heart	Juque (RN 14)	T6	Xinshu (BL 15)	T5–6
Diaphragm			Geshu (BL 17)	T7–8
Lower Esophagus			Weiguanxiashu (Extra)	T8–9
Liver	Qimen (LV 14)	T5	Ganshu (BL 18)	T9–10
Gallbladder	Riyue (GB 24)	T6	Danshu (BL 19)	T10–11
Spleen	Zhangmen (LV 13)	T8	Pishu (BL 20)	T11–12
Stomach	Zhongwan (RN 12)	T7	Weishu (BL 21)	T12
Internal Membrane	Shimen (RN 5)	T11	Sanjiaoshu (BL 22)	T12–L1
Kidneys	Jingmen (GB 25)	T10	Shenshu (BL 23)	L2
Intestinal Content			Qihaishu (BL 24)	L3
Large Intestine	Tianshu (ST 25)	T9–10	Dachangshu (BL 25)	L4
Jejunum–Ileum Transition			Guanyuanshu (BL 26)	L5
Small Intestine	Guanyuan (RN 4)	T11–12	Xiaochangshu (BL 27)	S1
Urinary Bladder	Zhongji (RN 3)	T12	Pangguanshu (BL 28)	S2
Anus			Baihuanshu (BL 30)	S4

Collateral and Source Nodes

Collateral (luo) and source (yuan) nodes (Table 9.5) are extremely important since these are the only sites used to influence the relative blood flow between yin and yang matched organ-paired distribution vessels, affecting refined substances and vital air (qi) from one vessel to the next (Figure 9.3). The collateral nodes are also employed to treat indications of the collateral vessels (Table 9.4).

To reinforce a deficient organ (zangfu) vessel using the internal-external relationship of the paired yin and yang organs, the collateral node is considered in conjunction with a source node. The collateral node should always draw from the paired source node. This approach can only be used when the paired organ vessel is not deficient, otherwise to draw upon a deficient vessel will only cause a deeper deficiency in that particular organ.

An excess condition of a zangfu vessel can also be reduced using the internal-external relationship of the paired yin-yang organs. Here, the source node of the excess vessel is selected along with the collateral node of the paired vessel. As in the case of deficiency, the collateral location always draws from the paired source node. When dealing with reducing an excess, this approach can only be used when the paired organ vessel itself is not in excess, otherwise to draw upon its paired excess vessel will only cause a greater problem in the vessel organ system.

Accumulation Nodes

Accumulation (xi) nodes (Table 9.5) are important locations of influence on the extremities. A store of vital substances from each distribution vessel is thought to accumulate at these locations. Application of these nodes in conjunction with the five-phase nodes is appropriate when these stores of vital substances need to be drawn upon. This situation usually occurs in acute disorders affecting a particular vessel or organ. For this reason, accumulation nodes are often indicated in the treatment of acute conditions.

Eight Singular Vessel Nodes

The confluent nodes of the eight singular vessels are used to treat disorders in the indicated regions represented by the connections with their regulated vessels (Table 9.3). The eight sites are considered important in clinical practice and may be used independently. They are applied in the case of an internal disorder that is causing the main distribution vessels to overflow, when it is necessary to drain off the surplus to restore balance. For example, problems in the allowance (*ren*, 任) vessel, as reflected by the confluent regions of its regulated (lung) vessel, can be treated using Lieque (LU 7). Disorders in the medial lifting (*yinqiao*, 阴蹺) vessel can be treated using Zhaohai (KD 6), which could also be combined with its couple node Lieque (LU 7) on the upper extremity. In the case of treating lung yin substance deficiency, the confluent node of the allowance and medial lifting vessels, Lieque (LU 7) and Zhaohai (KD 6), are also selected because they are confluent with the lungs, throat, and diaphragm. They function to clear the throat, eliminate dryness, nourish yin substance, and cause lung air (qi) to descend. Likewise, Houxi (SI 3) and Shenmai (BL 62) could be combined to treat conditions involving regions of the inner canthus, neck, ear, shoulder, and back. Neiguan (PC 6) and Gongsun (SP 4) can be combined to treat disorders of the heart, chest, and stomach.

Communication Nodes on the Extremities

Needling sites on the extremities are possibly more reactive than other locations because of the greater number of sensory nerves and the dense distribution of motor nerves and blood vessels. Each of the distribution vessels of the viscera has five communication nodes located between the terminus of the extremity and the elbow or knee (Table 15.6). The bowels have five such nodes (Table 15.7), plus one source node not included with the five (Table 9.5). The source nodes for the viscera (Table 9.5) are coincident with the stream or soil phase nodes. The two sets of five nodes on the yin and yang vessels are described in terms of water flowing from smaller to ever-enlarging streams, as a corollary of blood, refined substances, and vital air (qi) flowing through the vessels.

The first nodal sites are named well (jing) at the terminal end of a toe or finger, usually located at the corner of the digital nail. The flow of vital substances at the well nodes is shallow and slight. These sites are needled and sometimes bled for diseases of the viscera, especially internal heat, and afflictions in the region below the heart. The next points in line are spring (rong) nodes, located on the digital, palmar, and plantar regions. The flow of vital substances is slightly greater at the spring nodes, and these are indicated for diseases associated with changes in coloration, and also fevers. Next are the stream (shu) nodes where vital substance flow is profuse, located around the ankle and wrist joints. Stream nodes are indicated for intermittent illnesses, and for heaviness of the body and joints. River (jing) nodes are then located at the wrists, ankles, knees, and arms, and vital substances are in constant motion. These nodes are used for illnesses that affect the voice, including dyspnea, coughs, chills, and fevers. The last are sea (he) nodes, located at the elbow and knee joints, where vital substances are deep and plentiful. Sea nodes are indicated for ailments of the stomach, especially due to overeating; for an upsurge of vital function; and diarrhea.

Table 15.6 The five communication (*shu*) and earth-phase neurovascular nodes of each yin distribution vessel.

Phase	*Wood*	*Fire*	*Soil*	*Metal*	*Water*
Vessel	*Well* (Jing)	*Spring* (Rong)	*Stream* (Shu)	*River* (Jing)	*Sea* (He)
Lung	Shaoshang (LU 11)	Yuji (LU 10)	Taiyuan (LU 9)	Jingqu (LU 8)	Chize (LU 5)
Spleen	Yinbai (SP 1)	Dadu (SP 2)	Taibai (SP 3)	Shangqiu (SP 5)	Yinglingquan (SP 9)
Heart	Shaochong (HT 9)	Shaofu (HT 8)	Shenmen (HT 7)	Lingdao (HT 4)	Shaohai (HT 3)
Kidney	Yongquan (KD 1)	Rangu (KD 2)	Taixi (KD 3)	Fuliu (KD 7)	Yingu (KD 10)
Pericardium	Zhongchong (PC 9)	Laogong (PC 8)	Daling (PC 7)	Jianshi (PC 5)	Quze (PC 3)
Liver	Dadun (LV 1)	Xingjian (LV 2)	Taichong (LV 3)	Zhongfeng (LV 4)	Ququan (LV 8)

Table 15.7 The five communication (*shu*) and earth-phase neurovascular nodes of each yang distribution vessel.

Phase	*Metal*	*Water*	*Wood*	*Fire*	*Soil*
Vessel	*Well* (Jing)	*Spring* (Rong)	*Stream* (Shu)	*River* (Jing)	*Sea* (He)
Large Intestine	Shangyang (LI 1)	Erjian (LI 2)	Sanjian (LI 3)	Yangxi (LI 5)	Quchi (LI 11)
Stomach	Lidui (ST 45)	Neiting (ST 44)	Xiangu (ST 43)	Jiexi (ST 41)	Zusanli (ST 36)
Small Intestine	Shaoze (SI 1)	Qiangu (SI 2)	Houxi (SI 3)	Yanggu (SI 5)	Xiaohai (SI 8)
Bladder	Zhiyin (BL 67)	Zutonggu (BL 66)	Shugu (BL 65)	Kunlun (BL 60)	Weizhong (BL 40)
Internal Membrane	Guanchong (SJ 1)	Yemen (SJ 2)	Zhongzhu (SJ 3)	Zhigou (SJ 6)	Tianjing (SJ 10)
Gallbladder	Zuqiaoyin (GB 44)	Xiaxi (GB 43)	Zulinqi (GB 41)	Yangfu (GB 38)	Yanglingquan (GB 34)

Five-Phase Nodes
The five communication nodes are also assigned to the five earth phases, and are sometimes referred to as "command nodes" (Tables 15.6 and 15.7). The treatment application of five-phase nodes is particularly useful in addressing internal organ imbalances and emotional problems. Non-five-phase nodes are often included in the treatment plan as well. Some practitioners emphasize the use of the five-phase treatment schemes, although the ancient Chinese physicians recognized a potential problem in terms of the skill of a practitioner by concentrating only on nodes in the extremities (see quote from *NJLS 3* in Needling Therapy, page 294). A summary of the five-phase treatment approach is provided below.

Five-phase internal organ relationships provide patterns of physiological influence mediated through the birth (*sheng*, 生), victorious or control (*sheng*, 胜, or *ke*, 克), or insulting (*wu*, 侮) modes (Figure 3.2). Theoretically the communication sites permit manipulation of the phases through these three unique modes of control. The actual function of the internal organs may interact in terms of the five-phase relationships, but only those in the creation cycle provide any practical treatment benefits. The association of one phase with the next in a clockwise direction is viewed in terms of a mother-son relationship (Figure 3.2). Mother and son relationships are applied when treating deficiency (hollow) or excess (solid) conditions. Appropriate nodes (Table 15.8) are usually applied to either reinforce the mother phase to strengthen the son in the case of deficiency, or to reduce the son phase to sedate the mother in the case of an excess condition.

Frequency and Number of Treatments

Needle stimulation produces profound restorative effects, especially in treating acute disorders. Many problems are resolved with just one or two treatments; in chronic and intractable cases, a series of treatments may be necessary to incrementally resolve the condition. Treatment is most effective if in the early phases it is relatively frequent, such as every other day, with the occurrence decreasing as the condition improves. If treatments are not maintained relatively

Table 15.8 Mother and son nodes for reinforcing and reducing in the five-phase arrangement.

Vessel	*Mother (Reinforcing)*	*Son (Reducing)*
Lung	Taiyuan (LU 9)	Chize (LU 5)
Large Intestine	Quchi (LI 11)	Erjian (LI 2)
Stomach	Jiexi (ST 41)	Lidui (ST 45)
Spleen	Dadu (SP 2)	Shangqiu (SP 5)
Heart	Shaochong (HT 9)	Shenmen (HT 7)
Small Intestine	Houxi (SI 3)	Xiaohai (SI 8)
Bladder	Zhiyin (BL 67)	Shugu (BL 65)
Kidney	Fuliu (KD 7)	Yongquan (KD 1)
Pericardium	Zhongchong (PC 9)	Daling (PC 7)
Internal Membrane	Zhongzhu (SJ 3)	Tianjing (SJ 10)
Gallbladder	Xiaxi (GB 43)	Yangfu (GB 38)
Liver	Ququan (LV 8)	Xingjian (LV 2)

often in the early phases, positive effects can be negated. In treating substance use, treatments may be provided on a daily basis for a week or more to address withdrawal symptoms.

The number and frequency of treatments recommended for each disease is based on demonstrated clinical results. However, each case is unique unto itself and every problem is analyzed on its own merits. Once a problem is diagnosed, the patient is advised on what to expect in the course of treatment. Acute problems usually respond more quickly; chronic problems require more treatments. The number of treatments for a given disorder depends mostly on how long the person has had the problem, whether only external factors are involved, or whether the problem is complicated by internal factors (emotional, substance use, and dietary factors). Practitioners of ancient times faced the same difficulty of estimating how many treatments it would take to resolve a particular problem.

Successive Order of Treatments

Some general guidelines are provided in the *Neijing* on treating acute and chronic disorders. The first reference is provided in *NJLS 6*, where Bogao states:

> Wind and cold harm the body; while worry, fear, and anger harm functional activity. Impaired vital function harms the viscera, and visceral disease results. When cold injures the body, the body is diseased; when wind harms the muscles and vessels, the muscles and vessels become diseased. This is the successive order in which the body and vital functions are affected by external and internal causes.
>
> A disease of nine days' duration should be given three needling treatments. A disease of one month's duration should be given ten needling treatments. These guidelines can be proportionately applied to all diseases. In the case of chronic and persistent rheumatism in the body, examine the collateral veins primarily for bloodletting to relieve the condition.
>
> If a disease of the body of one month's duration has not yet affected the internal organs, the needling treatments are reduced by half [five treatments]. If a disease of the body of one month's duration is preceded by a visceral condition, then the number of treatments should be doubled [twenty treatments].

Additional guidelines on treatment schedules for chronic problems where pathogenic factors have penetrated into the body are provided in *NJLS 9*:

> In the case of a chronic ailment where the pathogenic factor has penetrated deep into the body, it should be treated with needling by deep insertion and prolonged retention of the needle. Treatments are applied every other day until recovery. First, it is necessary to regulate both the left and right sides of the body [since vessels are distributed on each side] to remove the pathogenic factor from the blood vessels. This is a fundamental principle of treatment.

Typical Treatment Schedules

These guidelines on treatment schedules in the *Neijing*, along with the observation that duration of symptoms is a good predictor of response to treatment, are reasonably consistent with present-day clinical experience. Uncomplicated acute disorders of less than nine days' duration usually respond in three to five treatments; those of one month or less usually respond in five to ten treatments. Conditions lasting one month or less that involve internal factors are usually resolved in ten to twenty treatments. In general, up to three treatments per week for one or two weeks is typical early in the case. Treatment frequency then progressively declines until the problem is fully resolved or improved to its maximum recovery potential.

In a typical case that is expected to require up to twenty treatments the schedule could cover a ten-week period as follows: three treatments for each of the first two weeks, followed by two treatments per week for the next six weeks, and finally one treatment per week for the last two weeks. The clinical response is evaluated each time the patient returns for the next treatment. If improvement is greater than anticipated, the number and frequency of treatments is correspondingly decreased. Conversely, a poor response may indicate the need to spread the treatments over a longer period of time.

Chronic disorders, often of long duration, or those involving significant trauma or involving CNS complications usually require more treatments spread out over a longer time period. The ancient Chinese noted that, in treating those suffering from stroke, if patients had lost the ability to speak along with paralysis, full recovery was unlikely; for those whose speech was unaffected, recovery was possible. In either case, needling is applied to bring about significant therapeutic benefit.

Standards of Practice

Early Chinese doctors set high standards for students and practitioners alike. The study of medicine was restricted to those who had high ethical principles, were not lazy, and who demonstrated a desire to help others. Books were written to maintain a consistent technical base, and care was taken to adhere to the fundamental concepts. Despite all this, there were potential problems with inconsistent training and students not fully comprehending their lessons. Some were apparently distracted by false schools, only to be led astray by unsound and confusing information gathered along the way. These individuals sometimes had doubts about their teachers and even the validity of Chinese medicine itself. The most grievous errors were failing to grasp the complexities of blood and nutrient circulation, incorrect diagnoses, and inappropriate treatment of patients, any of which were considered malpractice. These concerns are summarized in *NJSW 78* (*Committing the Four Mistakes in Clinical Practice*), where the Yellow Emperor discusses the "four mistakes" in clinical practice:

> The twelve distribution vessels and the 365 collateral vessels [one at each critical juncture] are a [physiological] feature that all human beings possess. This is perfectly understood. Physicians put this knowledge to good use. Therefore, the reason for an inaccurate diagnosis is that the physician's mind cannot focus on one thing. Their will [*zhi*, 志] and intentions [*yi*, 意] are not logical, causing the mutual interrelationship between the external and internal to be lost. This in turn causes the practitioner to experience dangerous disbelief and doubt, and leads to the four mistakes as follows:

First Mistake

> To examine a patient without understanding the nature of yin and yang characteristics, and without understanding the logic of upstream [venous] and downstream [arterial] flow of circulation.

Second Mistake

To receive instruction from teachers and quit before one's training is complete, to learn confused medical skills from false schools and workshops, to erroneously advertise and exaggerate one's medical skills, to recklessly use the stone needles to cause punishment to the patient's body [overtreatment].

Third Mistake

Failure to consider the patient's social status [worker or nobleperson] and whether they are poor or wealthy, whether they live in an expensive or low-cost residence, and whether they are classified as being either fat or skinny, and if their bodies are either cold or warm, as well as failure to consider whether their eating and drinking habits are suitable, and whether the patient is courageous or nervous. Not understanding this fully will cause mental confusion on the part of the physician and the diagnosis will not be self-evident.

Fourth Mistake

To examine a sick patient without asking about the beginning of the illness, and whether worry and anxiety or general sufferings, as well as drinking and eating habits, have compromised their moral integrity, and if there are excessive habits in their daily lives or if they have been harmed by the use of toxic drugs or narcotics. Not to ask about these matters before completing the pulse diagnosis at the wrist to determine what disease is causing the internal symptoms is to foolishly give a name to the disorder through gross negligence, instead of applying careful diagnosis.

In Summary

Therefore, a physician may become well known by the common people through word of mouth, spreading as far away as a thousand miles. However, physicians will not be considered good practitioners if they do not understand the principles of complete pulse diagnosis [nine pulse indications in the three regions, Table 10.1], or if they perform examination and diagnosis without inquiry into the state of human affairs of the patient. The principles of treatment follow established rules that are easy to nurture. To hold only to the pulse diagnosis at the wrist and not consider the pulses of the five viscera, and not consider the origins of all disease, physicians may start to blame themselves [for poor success] or blame their teachers for not providing complete or adequate training.

Therefore it is said that providing treatment without following established logic, but instead to discard medical skills, is to treat the patient recklessly, even though once in a while it may produce a cure. It is foolish to be content with accidental success.

Ah regretfully! The principles of treatment are so deeply profound that one must know their theories intimately. The way of these principles is so vast that it can be compared to the size of sky and earth, or matched with the expanse of the four seas. If one does not comprehend one's training and instruction in these matters, reception of the bright principles of treatment will be obscured.

Notes

Chapter 1

1. The *Yellow Emperor's Internal Classic* (*Huangdi Neijing*) is divided into the *Suwen* and *Lingshu* volumes. The initials *NJSW* for the *Huangdi Neijing Suwen*, and *NJLS* for the *Huangdi Neijing Lingshu*, are used throughout this text in citations to specific treatises, followed by the number of the treatise being referenced. The title of each treatise is also given in its first citation in each chapter.

2. The term acupuncture—derived from the Latin word *acus*, meaning needle, and *puntura*, meaning to puncture—was coined by the early Jesuits at a time when all Western scholarly and medical writings were in Latin.

3. One of the meanings of the character *luo* (络) is collateral vessel, as clearly defined in the *Neijing*. Mathews (1931) defines luo as unreeled silk, hemp, cotton fiber, a cord, to spin silk, to connect, continuous, and blood vessels.

4. The original pictograph of the character *jing* (经), used for longitudinal or distribution vessels, shows rivers flowing underground, with a man standing on the ground examining the underlying veins (Wieger: 1965). Later the radical *mi* (糸), related to textile materials or tissue, was added. Jing is applied to things that run lengthwise, such as classic scrolls comprising bound longitudinal strips of bamboo, distribution vessels, arteries and veins, the warp of a fabric, and navigational meridians. Jing also means to pass through (hence distribution), pass by, to experience, constant, recurring, standard of conduct, invariable rule, and to regulate (Mathews: 1931).

5. The term acupoint is a 1980s contraction of acupuncture point, and means needle point, suggesting that the critical junctures or nodes are restricted to needling alone. This is possibly restrictive or misleading, since some nodal sites cannot be needled, and therapeutic means other than needling can be applied to most nodal locations.

6. References to specific nodes (acupoints) throughout this text give the node's pinyin Chinese name, followed by a two-letter abbreviation for its distribution vessel (Table 9.1), and its corresponding number along the nodal pathway (Figures 11.1 to 11.14).

7. Dao means the way, or path, and is generally understood as the correct or true way. Dao also refers to the laws of nature, and more specifically, can mean ditch, as in irrigation ditch or gutter. It is spelled *tao* in the Wade–Giles system of romanization, but still pronounced dao.

Chapter 2

1. The concept of virtue (*de*, 德), probably dating back to the earliest times of Chinese culture, was accorded great importance during the Zhou period and is the other major topic of the *Dao De Jing*. Virtue for the Chinese has a moral connotation, but the emphasis is on fulfilling one's full potential. Virtue is discussed in the *Great Norm*, contained in the Zhou *Mandate of Heaven*, which was supposedly written around 1111 BCE. Here, the virtue of respectfulness is applied to appearance, agreement for speech, clarity for seeing, definition for hearing, and exploration for thinking. Respectfulness leads to concern, agreement leads to orderliness, clarity leads to wisdom, definition leads to reasoning, and exploration leads to intelligence.

2. The five earth phases of wood, fire, soil, metal, and water, and the six sky-airs of *jueyin* (厥阴), *shaoyin* (少阴), *taiyin* (太阴), *shaoyang* (少阳), *yangming* (阳明), and *taiyang* (太阳), are first mentioned in the nine categories of the *Great Norm*, contained in the Zhou *Mandate of Heaven*.

3. The names of the six sky-airs of wind, heat, damp, fire, dry, and cold are used interchangeably with the name of their respective body regions of jueyin, shaoyin, taiyin, shaoyang, yangming, and taiyang, as defined in Chinese anatomical notation in the yin-yang system. When any of the six sky-airs become pathogenic, they preferentially attack their associated body region.

4. The time of Laozi (or Lao-tsu, as his name was spelled under the older Wade–Giles system of romanization) is not known for certain. Some Chinese scholars place him about twenty years senior to Kong Fuzi (Confucius). Unconfirmed reports suggest the two met in 517 BCE. If Laozi was the person in charge of the Zhou archives, that would place him there at about 374 BCE.

Chapter 3

1. During the Han dynasty (206 BCE–220 CE) the *cun* (寸) was equal to 0.902 U.S. inches (2.30 centimeters). If the measurements during the Zhou and Han periods were the same, 1 Chinese foot (*chi*, 尺), which consists of 10 cun, would be equal to 9 inches in U.S. measurements. An individual who was 8-Chinese-feet tall in ancient China would be equivalent to 6-feet tall. One *zhang* (丈) is 10 Chinese feet, which in ancient times was equal to 7.5 feet in U.S. terms.

2. The internal membrane system (*sanjiao*, 三焦) consists of the serous membranes in the pleura and the peritoneum. The parietal peritoneum lines the abdominal walls and undersurface of the diaphragm, while the parietal pleura tissues cover the walls of the thorax and upper surface of the diaphragm, as well as the pericardium. The visceral peritoneum envelops the abdominal organs, except for the kidneys, while the visceral pleura tissue enfolds the lungs. The parietal and visceral membranes are separated by serous fluids to reduce friction.

3. The Chinese character used to denote extraordinary in this case can either be pronounced *ji*, which means single, odd, surplus, or remainder; or pronounced *qi*, meaning strange, wonderful, extraordinary, marvelous, or rare (Mathews: 1931; Wieger: 1965). Hence, special *fu* (府) organs could be described as either singular (ji) or extraordinary (qi), depending on the pronunciation used.

4. One *sheng* (升) is equal to about 0.222 U.S. gallons (1 liter).

5. One *jin* (斤) is equal to about 1.1 U.S. pounds (0.5 kilogram).

6. Most ancient cultures developed an appreciation for the importance of maintaining daily habits with respect to diurnal periods of light and dark, as well as to monthly and seasonal periods. The Chinese were the first to systematically associate specific periods of the day with each internal organ, and to develop what is now known as chronobiology. Each organ is thought to either dominate or perform a critical function during its assigned two-hour period, and is also associated with a specific monthly and seasonal period. Hence, certain types of disorder could predominate during certain times of the day, month, or year. Diseases were noted to improve during some time periods and get worse at others. For maximum effectiveness, a treatment approach therefore had to take into account the time of day, as well as in which time period or season the patient would be most likely to recover.

7. The brain is referred to as the sea of marrow (*suihai*, 髓海), where the character *sui* (髓) means marrow when used in relation to bones, but spinal marrow or spinal cord when used with respect to the brain and the back, such as in *jisui* (脊髓) or spinal cord. The character *hai* (海) means sea. Hence, suihai can be interpreted as sea of neural tissue. The term spinal marrow was still being used in the West during the nineteenth and twentieth centuries to indicate the spinal cord. Other evidence that the character sui refers to the spinal cord is that beef spinal cord, a highly appreciated food item, is called *niusui* (牛髓).

Chapter 5

1. The Chinese believed that wind, being the main carrier of environmental factors, could steal or deplete one's vital substances, and hence was referred to as "stealing wind." Examples of the way in which wind acts as a "thief" are the wind chill factor in winter and heat wave in summer.

2. Despite throwing off the old superstitions of the Shang dynasty, the Zhou and several subsequent dynasties maintained an official divination department.

3. Regulating tissues refers to reducing inflammation, addressing *ahshi* (阿是) (sensitive locations), and promoting healing.

Chapter 7

1. Pensiveness, related to the spleen and intent, involves thinking too much, and can also be called contemplation or meditation.

2. The influence of thyroid hormones on respiration may be the result of increasing protein synthesis in the mitochondria of the cells. Here the effect may be to increase adenosine triphosphate (ATP) utilization, resulting in heat production and increased oxygen uptake.

3. Lipolysis is the process of breaking down stored fat for conversion in the liver to useful energy products.

Chapter 8

1. Blood consists of plasma and cellular components that are mostly red blood cells. The total blood volume represents about 8 percent of body weight, with five-eighths attributed to the plasma, and three-eighths to blood cells. The volume of red blood cells, referred to as the hematocrit, represents approximately 47 percent of the total blood volume in males, and about 42 percent in females. The hematocrit reflects the blood's viscosity and oxygen-carrying capability. A variation in the total cellular content of blood can be detected in the pulses.

Chapter 9

1. The Chinese character *ji* means single, odd (as applied to a number), surplus, or remainder (Mathews: 1931; Wieger: 1965), which seems to adequately describe the nature of these vessels, with single and hence "singular" being the best fit. This character can also be pronounced *qi*, which means strange, wonderful, extraordinary, marvelous, or rare. Consequently, the terms "extraordinary" and "extra" are commonly used for the singular vessels. This is similar to the way the singular or extraordinary *fu* organs are described.

2. The Chinese character *chong* means to dash against, to clash with (because of the presence of a strong pulse), to pour out, or to infuse (Mathews: 1931; Wieger: 1965). Chong also means thoroughfare, which best describes this vessel.

3. The character *ren* means to allow, appoint, tolerate, or bear, as in bear responsibility. Ren is also a term for an official position or office, or means to employ or put in office (Mathews: 1931; Wieger: 1965). Most of these terms fail to adequately describe the ren vessel. The word "allowance" may come close to the capacitance nature of the *renmai*.

4. The word *du* means to oversee, superintend, direct, or reprove. It also means governor, and hence "governing" is a common translation for this term. The term governing makes most sense because the du vessels influence all of the internal organs. Du also refers to the center of the back seam in a coat, which is analogous to this vessel's position on the body (Mathews: 1931; Wieger: 1965).

5. The character *qiao* means to lift up (such as lifting a leg), hold up (such as a finger), on tiptoe, or on stilts. It could also refer to crossing the legs, in which case one can observe these vessels. None of these definitions give a clue to what the ancient Chinese had in mind when they named the qiao vessels. The word "lifting" has been selected in this book as the closest translation, with medial lifting applied to the *yinqiao*, and lateral lifting to the *yangqiao* vessel.

6. The character *wei* (维) means to hold together, hold fast, tie up, maintain, or safeguard. The superficial veins form networks, with numerous connections to other veins, hence the idea of holding together or holding fast makes sense. In this book, medial holding has been selected as the most appropriate translation for the *yinwei* vessel, while lateral holding is used for the *yangwei* vessel. This same character (wei) is also used to describe the vascular and neural connections to the eyes and the heart.

Chapter 10

1. A *ke* is a Chinese time period equal to one-hundredth of a day. There are 1,440 minutes in each twenty-four-hour period; 1 ke is equal to 14.4 minutes. Ke-zero is taken to start at midnight, and ke-fifty occurs at noontime.

2. The Chinese understood that speech was the result of air breathed out of the lungs, and consequently a decrease in lung functional activity affects the ability to speak.

3. Dividing the 1,440 minutes in each twenty-four-hour period by twenty-eight constellations yields an average constellation period of 51.4 minutes. Dividing 51.4 minutes by the 28.8-minute (2 *ke*) defensive substance circulation time calculates to approximately one-and-eight-tenths of a cycle per average constellation period.

4. This treatise of the *Neijing* notes an average of one-and-eight-tenths defensive substance cycles for each constellation, not quite two complete cycles.

Chapter 11

1. The Chinese word *shou* for hand also means arm, or upper extremity; *zu* used for foot also means leg, or lower extremity.

2. This refers to the vessel pathway up to Yingxiang (LI 20) on the same side, but is frequently interpreted to mean that the vessel crosses over to the other side of the mouth.

Chapter 12

1. The Chinese character *jin* refers to skeletal muscle, including tendons, fascia, and muscle tissue. Some interpretations refer to jin as tendinomuscular structures.

2. This refers to motor impairment on the right side due to cerebral damage on the left, consistent with the motor cortex for muscles on the right being in the left part of the brain.

Chapter 14

1. Mast cells are located in tissue sites, including adjacent to blood vessels, and release histamine, heparin, and other substances into the local area of needle insertion, producing a vasodilatory inflammatory condition in response to the minute tissue damage caused by needling. Mast cell plasma counterparts are the basophils attracted to the site of needle insertion.

2. This superficial reaction is referred to as the "triple response," and was first described by Sir Thomas Lewis in 1937 as part of a nocifensor system that responds to tissue damage (Lembeck: 1985). Suspected mediators were considered to be slow-reacting substances of anaphylaxis (SRS-A). Major contributors to the inflammatory reaction are identified as leukotrienes, histamine, and platelet activating factors (PAF).

3. The immune complement system is mediated by plasma proteins that respond to pathogenic agents or, in the case of the alternative pathway, to tissue damage. These complement proteins, designated by the letter C followed by a number, interact in a certain sequence causing mast cells to degranulate and attracting immune cells to the site of damage (or needle insertion) to mount a defensive response.

4. Important aspects of the controlling process include the histamine released from mast cells and basophils, causing the adrenal glands to release epinephrine, which in turn inhibits the release of histamine. Eosinophils release the enzyme histaminase, which breaks down histamine, and also releases arylsulfatase B, which breaks down leukotrienes. Plasmin degrades Hageman Factor XIIa. Aggregated platelets release endoglucuronidase to degrade heparin and heparan sulfate. Corticosteroids stabilize the cell membrane and inhibit the formation of arachidonic acid.

5. All the somatic and visceral afferent nerves, including those of the anterior lateral tract (ATL), can be fired in the reverse direction (antidromic) when stimulated at their terminal end, causing the nerve fiber to be activated as if it had been stimulated at its sensory end. Most interactions between nerve fibers that give rise to dorsal root potentials (DRP), muscle action potentials (MAP), propagated sensations (PS) along the vessel and muscle routes, and viscerosomatic responses involve some antidromic activity.

List of Tables

References

Agren, H. "Treatise on Acupuncture Academic Thesis for the Degree of Medicinae Doctor at Uppsala University 16 May 1829 by Gustaf Landgren." *Comparative Medicine East and West* 5 (3–4) (1977): 199–210.

Aicher, S. A., S. Sharma, P. Y. Cheng, L. Y. Liu-Chen, and V. M. Pickel. "Dual Ultrastructural Localization of Mu-Opiate Receptors and Substance P in the Dorsal Horn." *Synapse* 36 (l) (April 2000): 12–20.

Ammons, W. S., R. W. Blair, and R. D. Foreman. "Raphe Magnus Inhibition of Primate T1–T4 Spinothalamic Cells with Cardiopulmonary Visceral Input." *Pain* 20 (3) (November 1984): 247–60.

Andoh T., T. Nagasawa, M. Satoh, and Y. Kuraishi. "Substance P Induction of Itch-Associated Response Mediated by Cutaneous NK l Tachykinin Receptors in Mice." *Journal of Pharmacology and Experimental Therapeutics* 286 (3) (September 1998): 1,140–5.

Ansel, J. C., C. A. Armstrong, I. Song, K. L. Quinlan, J. E. Olerud, S. W. Caughman, and N. W. Bunnett. "Interactions of the Skin and Nervous System." *Journal of Investigative Dermatology, Symposium Proceedings* 2 (1) (August 1997): 23–6.

Baldry, P. E. *Acupuncture, Trigger Points and Musculoskeletal Pain.* London: Churchill Livingstone, 1989.

Baldry, P. E. *Acupuncture, Trigger Points and Musculoskeletal Pain: A Scientific Approach to Acupuncture for use by Doctors and Physiotherapists in the Diagnosis and Management of Myofascial Pain.* Edinburgh, New York: Churchill Livingstone, 1993.

Baluk, P. "Neurogenic Inflammation in Skin and Airways." *Journal of Investigative Dermatology, Symposium Proceedings* 2 (1) (August 1997): 76–81.

Basbaum, A. I. "Spinal Mechanisms of Acute and Persistent Pain." *Regional Anesthesia and Pain Medicine* 24 (1) (January–February 1999): 59–67.

Basbaum, A. I., N. J. Marley, J. O'Keefe, and C. H. Clanton. "Reversal of Morphine and Stimulus Produced Analgesia by Subtotal Spinal Cord Lesions." *Pain* 3 (1977): 43–56.

Battaglia, G., and A. Rustioni. "Substance P Innervation of the Rat and Cat Thalamus II: Cells of Origin in the Spinal Cord." *Journal of Comparative Neurology* 315 (4) (January 1992): 473–86.

Bauer, M. B., S. T. Meller, and G. F. Gebhart. "Bradykinin Modulation of a Spinal Nociceptive Reflex in the Rat." *Brain Research* 578 (1–2) (April 24, 1992): 186–96.

Baulmann, J., H. Spitznagel, T. Herdegen, T. Unger, and J. Culman. "Tachykinin Receptor Inhibition and C-Fos Expression in the Rat Brain Following Formalin-Induced Pain." *Neuroscience* 95 (3) (2000): 813–20.

Beck, William S., ed. "Leukocytes I. Physiology." *Hematology* 2nd ed. Cambridge, Mass.: The MIT Press, 1979, 337–359.

Benacerraf, Baruj, and Emil R. Unanue. *Textbook of Immunology.* Baltimore/London: Williams and Wilkins, 1979.

Bensky, Dan, and Randall Barolet. *Chinese Herbal Medicine: Formulas and Strategies.* Seattle: Eastland Press, 1990.

Bensky, Dan, and Andrew Gamble. *Chinese Herbal Medicine: Materia Medica.* Seattle: Eastland Press, 1986.

Berczi, I., I. M. Chalmers, E. Nagy, and R. J. Warrington. "The Immune Effects of Neuropeptides." *Bailliere's Clinical Rheumatology* 10 (2) (May 1996): 227–57.

Bereiter, D. A., D. F. Bereiter, B. H. Tonnessen, and D. B. Maclean. "Selective Blockade of Substance P or Neurokinin A Receptors Reduces the Expression of C-Fos in Trigeminal Subnucleus Caudalis after Corneal Stimulation in the Rat." *Neuroscience* 83 (2) (March 1998): 525–34.

Bergenheim, M., H. Johansson, and J. Pedersen. "The Role of the Gamma-System for Improving Information Transmission in Populations of Ia Afferents." *Neuroscience Research* 23 (2) (September 1995): 207–15.

Bernard, Claude *An Introduction to the Study of Experimental Medicine.* Paris: 1865 (First English edition, translated by Henry Copley Greene, New York: The Macmillan Company, 1927).

Bernstein, J. E., R. M. Swift, K. Soltani, and A. L. Lorincz. "Inhibition of Axon Reflex Vasodilatation by Topically Applied Capsaicin." *Journal of Investigative Dermatology* 76 (5) (May 1981): 394–5.

Bhoola, K. D. "Translocation of the Neutrophil Kinin Moiety and Changes in the Regulation of Kinin Receptors in Inflammation." *Immunopharmacology* 33 (1–3) (June 1996): 247–56.

Bhoola, K. D., C. D. Figueroa, and K. Worthy. "Bioregulation of Kinins: Kallikreins, Kininogens, and Kininases." *Pharmacology Review* 44 (1992): 1–80.

Bi Lige, Li Chuanjie, Zhu Baijun, and Wang Jia'en. "Treatment of Angina Pectoris by Acupuncture: An Observation on 140 Cases." *The Second National Symposium on Acupuncture and Moxibustion and Acupuncture Anesthesia,* Beijing: Foreign Languages Printing House, 1984, 5.

Bi Yongsun, Sun Hua, Guo Yi, Cao Zhenhua, Zhang Mingqin, and Zhang Bohua, *Chinese Qigong.* Zhang Enqin, ed. Shanghai: Publishing House of Shanghai College of Traditional Chinese Medicine, 1990.

Bjerring, P. L., and L. Arendt-Nielsen. "Inhibition of Histamine Skin Flare Reaction Following Repeated Topical Applications of Capsaicin." *Allergy* 45 (2) (February 1990): 121–5.

Bleazard, L., R., G. Hill, and R. Morris. "The Correlation Between the Distribution of the NK1 Receptor and the Actions of Tachykinin Agonists in the Dorsal Horn of the Rat Indicates that Substance P Does Not Have a Functional Role on Substantia Gelatinosa (Lamina II) Neurons." *Journal of Neuroscience* 14 (12) (December 1994): 7,655–64.

Bondt, Jakob de, Physician. *An Account of the Diseases, Natural History, and Medicines of the East Indies.* Translated from the Latin of James Bontius, London: T. Noteman, 1769.

Bowers, J. Z. "Englebert Kaempfer: Physician, Explorer, Scholar and Author." *Journal of the History of Medicine and Allied Sciences* 21 (July 1966): 237–259.

Bowers, J. Z., and R. W. Carrubba. "The Doctoral Thesis of Englebert Kaempfer on Tropical Diseases, Oriental Medicine and Exotic Natural Phenomena." *Journal of the History of Medicine and Allied Sciences* 25 (1970): 270–310.

Breivik, J. "Acupuncture and other Religions." *Tidsskrift for den Norske Laegeforening* 118 (22) (September 20, 1998): 3,491–2. (Norwegian)

Broffman, M., and M. McCullock. "Instrument-Assisted Pulse Evaluation in the Acupuncture Practice." *American Journal of Acupuncture* 14 (3) (1986): 255–259.

Brown, M. L., G. A. Ulett, and J. A. Stern. "Acupuncture Loci: Techniques for Location." *American Journal of Chinese Medicine* 2 (1974): 67–74.

Bunker, C. B., R. Cerio, H. A. Bull, J. Evans, P. M. Dowd, and J. C. Foreman. "The Effect of Capsaicin Application on Mast Cells in Normal Human Skin." *Agents and Actions* 33 (1–2) (May 1991): 195–6.

Cai Jingfeng. "Achievements in Ancient Chinese Pharmacology." In *Ancient China's Technology and Science.* Beijing: Foreign Languages Press, 1983, 352–357.

Cai Jingfeng. *Eating Your Way to Health: Dietotherapy in TCM.* Beijing: Foreign Languages Press, 1988.

Cannon, Walter B. "The Emergency Function of the Adrenal Medulla in Pain and Major Emotions." *American Journal of Physiology* 33 (1914): 356–372.

Cannon, Walter B. *The Wisdom of the Body.* New York: W.W. Norton & Co., 1932.

Cao, L. Q., and T. Wang. "The Change of the Concentration of Substance P in the Rats 'Channel' 'Point' Skin and Plasma in the Acupuncture Analgesia." *Zhen Ci Yan Jiu* [*Acupuncture Research*] 14 (4) (1989): 452–62. (Chinese)

Cao Xiaoding, Wang Miaozhen, and Jiang Jianwei. "Effects of Electroacupuncture and Iontophoresis of Etorphine and Noradrenaline on Neuronal Activity in Rabbits' Periaqueductal Gray Matter (PAG)." *The Second National Symposium on Acupuncture and Moxibustion and Acupuncture Anesthesia,* Beijing: Foreign Languages Printing House, 1984, 358–359.

Cardini, F., and W. X. Huang. "Moxibustion for Correction of Breech Presentation: A Randomized Controlled Study." *Journal of the American Medical Association* 280 (18) (November 11, 1998): 1,580–4.

Carrubba R. W., and J. Z. Bowers. "The Western World's First Detailed Treatise on Acupuncture: Willem ten Rhijne's De Acupunctura." *Journal of the History of Medicine and Allied Sciences* 29 (4) (October 1974): 371–398.

Cassedy, J. H. "Early Use of Acupuncture in the United States." *Bulletin of the New York Academy of Medicine* 50 (8) (1974): 892–896.

Ceniceros, S., and G. R. Brown. "Acupuncture: A Review of its History, Theories, and Indications." *Southern Medical Journal* 91 (12) (December 1998): 1,121–5.

Cerney, J. V. *Acupressure: Acupuncture Without Needles.* New York: Cornerstone Library, 1974.

Cervero, Fernando. "Visceral Nociception: Peripheral and Central Aspects of Visceral Nociceptive Systems." *Philosophical Transactions of the Royal Society of London, Series B: Biological Sciences* 308 (1, 136) (February 19, 1985): 325–37.

Cervero, Fernando. "Dorsal Horn Neurons and Their Sensory Inputs." In *Spinal Afferent Processing.* Tony L. Yaksh, ed. New York: Plenum Press, 1986, 197–216.

Chang, H. C., Y. K. Xie, Y. Y. Wen, S. Y. Zhang, J. H. Qu, and W. J. Lu. "Further Investigation on the Hypothesis of Meridian-Cortex-Viscera Interrelationship." *American Journal of Chinese Medicine* 11 (1983): 5–13.

Chapman, C. D., W. S. Ammons, and R. D. Foreman. "Raphe Magnus Inhibition of Feline T1–T4 Spinoreticular Tract Cell Responses to Visceral and Somatic Inputs." *Journal of Neurophysiology* 53 (3) (March 1985): 773–85.

Chapman, C. R., and C. Benedetti. "Analgesia Following Transcutaneous Electrical Stimulation and its Partial Reversal by a Morphine Antagonist." *Life Sciences* 21 (1977): 1,645–8.

Chapman, C. R., Y. M. Colpitts, C. Benedetti, R. Kitaeff, and J. D. Gehrig. "Evoked Potential Assessment of Acupunctural Analgesia: Attempted Reversal with Naloxone." *Pain* 9 (2) (October 1980): 183–97.

Chen, B. Y. "Acupuncture Normalizes Dysfunction of the Hypothalamic-Pituitary-Ovarian Axis." *Acupuncture and Electro-therapeutics Research* 22 (2) (1997): 97–108.

Chen, H. "Medical Exchanges Among China and Asian Countries." *Zhonghua Yi Shi Za Zhi* [*Chinese Medical Journal*] 26 (1) (1996): 43–9. (Chinese)

Chen Longshun, Fan Xiaoli, Tang Jingshi, Liu Xinzhong, and Hou Songlian. "Influence of Naloxone on the Analgesic Effects of Small-Sized Fibers." *Acupuncture Research*, Beijing: Foreign Languages Printing House, 1985, 86–87.

Cheng Baihua, Pan Cuiqin, Zhu Siling, Zhang Huizhen, Zhang Manli, and Chen Dazhong. "A Study on the 'Stabilizing and Tranquilizing' Effects of Neiguan Acupuncture." *The Second National Symposium on Acupuncture and Moxibustion and Acupuncture Anesthesia*, Beijing: Foreign Languages Printing House, 1984, 10.

Cheng, L., K. Wu, and Z. Qie. "Role of Qi in Reaching Affected Area Using Acupuncture in Promoting Blood Circulation to Remove Blood Stasis." *Zhong Xi Yi Jie He Za Zhi* [*Journal of Integrated Chinese and Western Medicine*] 10 (4) (April 1990): 209–11. (Chinese)

Cheng Xinnong. *Chinese Acupuncture and Moxibustion.* Beijing: Foreign Languages Press, 1987.

China Sports Magazine. *The Wonders of Qigong.* Los Angeles: Wayfarer Publications, 1985.

Cho, Z. H., S. C. Chung, J. P. Jones, J. B. Park, H. J. Park, H. J. Lee, E. K. Wong, and B. I. Min. "New Findings of the Correlation Between Acupoints and Corresponding Brain Cortices Using Functional MRI." *Proceedings of the National Academy of Science USA* 95 (5) (March 3, 1998): 2,670–3.

Cho, Z. H., S. H. Lee, I. K. Hong, E. K. Wong, and C. S. Na. "Further Evidence for the Correlation Between Acupuncture Stimulation and Cortical Activation." *Proceedings of the International Workshop, Society for Acupuncture Research*, University of California at Irvine, May 22, 1999.

Christ, Daryl D., and Nae J. Dun. "Endogenous Substances with Ganglionic Depressant Actions." In *Autonomic and Enteric Ganglia: Transmission and Its Pharmacology.* Alexander G. Karczmar, Kyozo Koketsu, and Syogoro Nishi, eds. New York: Plenum Press, 1986, 253–267.

Chuang, Y. M. *Historical Review of the Development of Chinese Acupuncture.* Taipei, Taiwan: 1978.

Cooper, Neal R. "The Complement System." In *Basic and Clinical Immunology,* 4th ed. Daniel P. Stites, John D. Stobo, H. Hugh Fudenberg, and J. Vivian Wells, eds. Los Altos, Calif.: Lange Medical Publications, 1982, 124–135.

Cowdry, E.V. "A Comparison of Ancient Chinese Anatomical Charts with the 'Funfbilderserie' of Sudhoffs." *Anatomical Records* 22 (1921a): 1–25.

Cowdry, E. V. "Taoist Ideas of Anatomy, the Basis of Chinese Medicine." *Annals of Medical History* 3 (4) (Winter 1921b): 301–309.

da Camino, F. S. *Sulla agopuntua con alcuni cenni sulla puntura electrica.* Venice: Antonelli, 1834.

da Camino, F. S. *Dell'agopuntua e della galvano-puntura.* Venice: Osservazioni, 1837.

Dalsgaard, C. J., T. Hökfelt, L. G. Elfin, L. Skirboll, and P. Emson. "Substance P–Containing Primary Sensory Neurons Projecting to the Inferior Mesenteric Ganglion: Evidence From Combined Retrograde Tracing and Immunohistochemistry." *Neuroscience* 7 (1982): 647–654.

Davis, C. L., S. Naeem, S. B. Phagoo, E. A. Campbell, L. Urban, and G. M. Burgess. "B1 Bradykinin Receptors and Sensory Neurons." *British Journal of Pharmacology* 118 (6) (July 1996): 1,469–76.

Dawson, P. M. "Su-Wen, the Basis of Chinese Medicine." *Annals of Medical History* 7 (1925): 59–64.

Deng, Y., Z. Fu, H. Dong, Q. Wu, and X. Guan. "Effects of Electroacupuncture on the Subcutaneous Mast Cells of Zusanli Acupoint in Rat with Unilateral Sciatic Nerve Transection." *Zhen Ci Yan Jiu [Acupuncture Research]* 21 (3) (1996a): 46–9. (Chinese)

Deng, Y., T. Zeng, Y. Zhou, and X. Guan. "The Influence of Electroacupuncture on the Mast Cells in the Acupoints of the Stomach Meridian." *Zhen Ci Yan Jiu [Acupuncture Research]* 21 (3) (1996b): 68–70. (Chinese)

Di Shi, Yin Weiping, Gong Shan, and Yin Qizhang. "Effects of Microinjection of Kainic Acid into Locus Coeruleus on Acupuncture, Stress and Morphine Analgesia." *The Second National Symposium on Acupuncture and Moxibustion and Acupuncture Anesthesia,* Beijing: Foreign Languages Printing House, 1984, 435–436.

Ding, Y. Q., H. X. Zheng, D. S. Wang, J. Q. Xu, L. W. Gong, Y. Lu, B. Z. Qin, J. Shi, H. L. Li, J. S. Li, R. Shigemoto, T. Kaneko, and N. Mizuno, "The Distribution of Substance P Receptor (NK1)-Like Immunoreactive Neurons in the Newborn and Adult Human Spinal Cord." *Neuroscience Letters* 266 (2) (May 7, 1999): 133–6.

Djupsjobacka, M., H. Johansson, and M. Bergenheim. "Influences on the Gamma-Muscle-Spindle System from Muscle Afferents Stimulated by Increased Intramuscular Concentrations of Arachidonic Acid." *Brain Research* 663 (2) (November 14, 1994): 293–302.

Djupsjobacka, M., H. Johansson, M. Bergenheim, and P. Sjolander. "Influences on the Gamma-Muscle-Spindle System from Contralateral Muscle Afferents Stimulated by KCl and Lactic Acid." *Neuroscience Research* 21 (4) (February 1995a): 301–9.

Djupsjobacka, M., H. Johansson, M. Bergenheim, and B. I. Wenngren. "Influences on the Gamma-Muscle-Spindle System from Muscle Afferents Stimulated by Increased Intramuscular Concentrations of Bradykinin and 5-HT." *Neuroscience Research* 22 (3) (June 1995b): 325–33.

Dong, Quansheng, and Zhang Rongtang. "The Relationship Between the Acupuncture Analgesia and the Afferent Fibers of Groups III and IV." In *Acupuncture Research.* Beijing, China: Foreign Languages Printing House, 1985, 84–85.

Dosch, Mathias. *Illustrated Atlas of the Techniques of Neural Therapy with Local Anesthetics.* Heidelberg: First English edition, Karl F. Haug Publishers, 1985.

Doyle, C. A., and S. P. Hunt. "Substance P Receptor (Neurokinin-1)–Expressing Neurons in Lamina I of the Spinal Cord Encode for the Intensity of Noxious Stimulation: A C-Fos Study in Rat." *Neuroscience* 89 (1) (March 1999): 17–28.

Du Huanji, and Zhao Yanfang. "Partial Antagonism of Naloxone Against the Inhibition of Viscerosomatic Reflex Induced by Brain or Peripheral Nerve Stimulation." In *Acupuncture Research.* Beijing: Foreign Languages Printing House, 1985, 105.

Dun, N. J., and Z. G. Jiang. "Noncholinergic Excitatory Transmission in the Inferior Mesenteric Ganglia of the Guinea Pig: Possible Mediation by Substance P." *Journal of Physiology* (London) 325 (1982): 145–159.

Eisenberg, D. M., R. B. Davis, S. L. Ettner, S. Appel, S. Wilkey, M. Van Rompay, and R. C. Kessler. "Trends in Alternative Medicine Use in the United States, 1990–1997: Results of a Follow-up National Survey." *Journal of the American Medical Association* 280 (18) (Nov 11, 1998): 1,569–75.

Eisenberg, D. M., R. C. Kessler, C. Foster, F. E. Norlock, D. R. Calkins, and T. L. Delbanco. "Unconventional Medicine in the United States: Prevalence, Costs, and Patterns of use." *New England Journal of Medicine* 328 (4) (January 28, 1993): 246–252.

Ellrich, J., and R. D. Treede. "Convergence of Nociceptive and Non-Nociceptive Inputs onto Spinal Reflex Pathways to the Tibialis Anterior Muscle in Humans." *Acta Physiologica Scandinvica* 163 (4) (August 1998): 391–401.

el-Yassir, N., and S. M. Fleetwood-Walker. "A 5-HT1-Type Receptor Mediates the Antinociceptive Effect of Nucleus Raphe Magnus Stimulation in the Rat." *Brain Research* 523 (1) (July 16, 1990): 92–9.

Ernst, E. "Acupuncture—How Effective is it Really?" *Fortschritte Medizin* 116 (1–2) (January 20, 1998): 20–6.

Fan, Warner J-W. *A Manual of Chinese Herbal Medicine—Principles & Practice for Easy Reference.* Boston, London: Shambhala, 1996.

Fang, B., and J. C. Hayes. "Functional MRI Explores Mysteries of Acupuncture." *Diagnostic Imaging* (San Francisco) 21 (7) (July 1999): 19–21.

Figueroa, C. D., G. Dietze, and W. Muller-Esterl. "Immunolocalization of Bradykinin B2 Receptors on Skeletal Muscle Cells." *Diabetes* 45 (January 1996) Supplement 1: S24–8.

Filshie, Jacqueline, and Adrian White, eds. *Medical Acupuncture: A Western Scientific Approach.* London: Churchill Livingstone, 1998.

Fleming, D. "Walter B. Cannon and Homeostasis." *Social Research* (New York) 51 (3) (1984): 609–40.

Floyer, Sir John. *The Physician's Pulse Watch: or, An Essay to Explain the Old Art of Feeling the Pulse, and to Improve it by the Help of a Pulse-Watch.* London, 1707.

Foreign Languages Press. *An Outline of Chinese Acupuncture.* Beijing: 1975.

Foreign Languages Press. *The Essentials of Chinese Acupuncture.* Beijing: Beijing, Nanjing and Shanghai Colleges of TCM, 1980.

Foreman, Robert D. "Spinal Substrates of Visceral Pain." In *Spinal Afferent Processing.* Tony L. Yaksh, ed. New York: Plenum Press, 1986, 217–242.

Foreman, Robert D., M. B. Hammond, and William D. Willis Jr. "Responses of Spinothalamic Tract Cells in the Thoracic Spinal Cord of the Monkey to Cutaneous and Viscera Inputs." *Pain* 11 (1981): 149–162.

Frank, B. L. "Neural Therapy." *Physical Medicine and Rehabilitation Clinics of North America* 10 (3) (August 1999): 573–82.

Fratkin, Jake Paul. *Chinese Herbal Patent Medicines: The Clinical Desk Reference.* Boulder, Colorado: Shya Publications, 2001.

Fraust, S. "For an Updated Acupuncture." *Revue Medicale de Bruxelles* 19 (4) (September 1998): A290–5. (French)

Frick, Oscar L. "Immediate Hypersensitivity." In *Basic and Clinical Immunology* 4th ed. Daniel P. Stites, John D. Stobo, H. Hugh Fudenberg, and J. Vivian Wells, eds. Los Altos, California: Lange Medical Publications, 1982, 250–276.

Gao Zhenwu, Yu Xianzhen, Shen Aixue, Qiu Jihua, Bao Li'en, Hu Zhonggen, and Lin Xiuchun. "Clinical Observation on Acupuncture for Treatment of Arrhythmia in 160 cases." *The Second National Symposium on Acupuncture and Moxibustion and Acupuncture Anesthesia,* Beijing: Foreign Languages Printing House, 1984a, 3.

Gao Zhenwu, Yu Xiaozhen, Wang Zhanglian, Sheng Aixue, Qiu Jihua, Bao Li'en, Lin Xiuchun, and Hu Zhonggen. "Study of Interrelation Between Regular Point and Heart." *The Second National Symposium on Acupuncture and Moxibustion and Acupuncture Anesthesia*, Beijing: Foreign Languages Printing House, 1984b, 7.

Gecse, A., B. Kis, Z. Mezei, and G. Telegdy. "The Effect of Bradykinin and Substance P on the Arachidonate Cascade of Platelets." *Immunopharmacology* 33 (1–3) (June 1996): 167–70.

Geng Junying, Huang Wenquan, Ren Tianchi, and Ma Xiufeng. *Practical Traditional Chinese Medicine & Pharmacology: Medicinal Herbs*. Beijing: New World Press, 1991a.

Geng Junying, Huang Wenquan, Ren Tianchi, and Ma Xiufeng. *Practical Traditional Chinese Medicine & Pharmacology: Herbal Formulas*. Beijing: New World Press, 1991b.

Gu Yuliang, Li Zhongsi, and Chen Peinan. "Effect of Electrical Stimulation of PAG on the Visceralgia Response Induced by Splanchnic Nerve Stimulation in Cats." *The Second National Symposium on Acupuncture and Moxibustion and Acupuncture Anesthesia*, Beijing: Foreign Languages Printing House, 1984, 363.

Guan, Z. L., Y. Q. Ding, J. L. Li, and B. Z. Lu. "Substance P Receptor–Expressing Neurons in the Medullary and Spinal Dorsal Horns Projecting to the Nucleus of the Solitary Tract in the Rat." *Neuroscience Research* 30 (3) (March 1998): 213–8.

Guo, D., X. Guan, and C. Wang. "Segmental Influence of Dorsal Root Action Potentials Evoked by Stimulating the Acupoints after Acupuncture along Meridians." *Zhen Ci Yan Jiu [Acupuncture Research]* 21 (2) (1996): 52–6. (Chinese)

Guo Shiyu, Yin Weiping, and Yin Qizhang. "Effects of Neonatal Administration of Monosodium Glutamate on Acupuncture Analgesia, Stress Analgesia and Morphine Analgesia in Adult Rats." *The Second National Symposium on Acupuncture and Moxibustion and Acupuncture Anesthesia*, Beijing: Foreign Languages Printing House, 1984, 431–432.

Habler, H. J., J. U. Stegmann, L. Timmermann, and W. Janig. "Functional Evidence for the Differential Control of Superficial and Deep Blood Vessels by Sympathetic Vasoconstrictor and Primary Afferent Vasodilator Fibers in Rat Hairless Skin." *Experimental Brain Research* 118 (2) (January 1998): 230–4.

Habler, H. J., G. Wasner, and W. Janig. "Interaction of Sympathetic Vasoconstriction and Antidromic Vasodilatation in the Control of Skin Blood Flow." *Experimental Brain Research* 113 (3) (March 1997): 402–10.

Hall, J. M. "Bradykinin Receptors." *General Pharmacology* 28 (1) (January 1997): 1–6.

Hammond, Donna L. "Control Systems for Nociceptive Afferent Processing: The Descending Inhibitory Pathways." In *Spinal Afferent Processing*. Tony L. Yaksh, ed. New York: Plenum Press, 1986, 363–390.

Han, Jisheng, and L. Terenius. "Neurochemical Basis of Acupuncture Analgesia." *Annual Review of Pharmacology and Toxicology* 22 (1982): 193–220.

Han Jisheng, Li Sijia, and Tang Jian. "Tolerance to Electroacupuncture and its Cross Tolerance to Morphine in the Rat." In *Acupuncture Research*, Beijing: China: Foreign Languages Printing House, 1985, 129.

Han Jisheng, J. Tang, M. F. Ren, Z. F. Zhu, S. G. Fan, and X. C. Qiu. "Central Neurotransmitters and Acupuncture Analgesia." *American Journal of Chinese Medicine* 8 (1980): 331–348.

Hara, M., M. Toyoda, M. Yaar, J. Bhawan, E. M. Avila, I. R. Penner, and B. A. Gilchrest. "Innervation of Melanocytes in Human Skin." *Journal of Experimental Medicine* 184 (4) (October 1, 1996): 1, 385–95.

Harvey, William. *Exercitatio Anatomica de Motu Cordis et Sanguinis in Animalibus*. Francofurti (Frankfurt): 1628. The first English text, *Anatomical Exercises on the Motion of the Heart and Blood in Animals*, translated and edited by Geoffrey Keynes, London: 1653.

He, X. L., X. Liu, B. Zhu, W. D. Xu, and S. X. Zhang. "Central Mechanism of An Extensive Analgesic Effect Due to Strong Electroacupuncture of Acupoint on Spinal Dorsal Horn Neurons." *Sheng Li Xue Bao [Acta Physiologica Sinica]* 47 (6) (December 1995): 605–9. (Chinese)

He, Z., D. Chen, X. Zou, and J. Zhou. "Role of Musculocutaneous Nerve in the Relationship Between 'Chutse' Acupoint and Heart." *Zhen Ci Yan Jiu [Acupuncture Research]* 18 (3) (1993): 236–9. (Chinese)

Head, William H. "On Disturbances of Sensation with Special Reference to the Pain of Visceral Disease." *Brain* 16 (1893): 1–133.

Heavey, D. J., R. Richmond, N. C. Turner, A. Kobza-Black, G. W. Taylor, C. G. Chappell, and C. T. Dollery. "Measurements of Leukotrienes C4 and D4 in Inflammatory Fluids." In *The Leukotrienes: Their Biological Significance.* Priscilla J. Piper, ed. New York: Raven Press, 1986, 185–198.

Helms, J. M. "An Overview of Medical Acupuncture." *Alternative Therapies in Health and Medicine* 4 (3) (May 1998): 35–45.

Hendricks, Robert G. *Lao-Tzu Te-Tao Ching: A New Translation Based on the Recently Discovered Ma-Wang-Tui Texts.* New York: Ballantine Books, 1989.

Herbert, M. K., and P. Holzer. "Interleukin-1 Beta Enhances Capsaicin-Induced Neurogenic Vasodilatation in the Rat Skin." *British Journal of Pharmacology* 111 (3) (March 1994): 681–6.

Higgs, G. A. "Source of Leukotrienes in Inflammation and Their Effect on Vascular Permeability." In *The Leukotrienes: Their Biological Significance.* Priscilla J. Piper, ed. New York: Raven Press, 1986, 135–140.

Hill, J.M., C. M. Adreani, and M. P. Kaufman. "Muscle Reflex Stimulates Sympathetic Postganglionic Efferents Innervating Triceps Surae Muscles of Cats." *American Journal of Physiology* 271 (1 Pt 2) (July 1996): H38–43.

Holt, I. L., E. W. Akeyson, and M. M. Knuepfer. "Medial Medullary Contribution to Tonic Descending Inhibition of Visceral Input." *American Journal of Physiology* 261 (3 Pt 2) (September 1991): R727–37.

Honor, P., P. M. Menning, S. D. Rogers, M. L. Nichols, A. I. Basbaum, J. M. Besson, and P. W. Mantyh. "Spinal Substance P Receptor Expression and Internalization in Acute, Short-Term, and Long-Term Inflammatory Pain States." *Journal of Neuroscience* 19 (17) (September 1, 1999): 7,670–8.

Hsu, Hong-Yen, and William G. Peacher, trans. *Shang Han Lun.* Long Beach, California: Oriental Healing Arts Institute, 1981.

Hu, H. Z., Z. W. Li, and J. Q. Si. "Evidence for the Existence of Substance P Autoreceptors in the Membrane of Rat Dorsal Root Ganglion Neurons." *Neuroscience* 77 (2) (March 1997): 535–41.

Hu, X. L., B. H. Wu, Z. M. Cai, W. F. Li, Z. Q. You, D. L. Chen, B. J. Li, S. H. Gong, and Q. R. Gao. "Observation on the Velocity of Propagated Sensation Along Channels." *Zhen Ci Yan Jiu [Acupuncture Research]* 12 Supplement 2 (1987): 39–44. (Chinese)

Hu, X., B. Wu, X. Huang, J. Xu, B. Yang, S. Gong, and B. Li. "Evidence for the Appearance of Peripheral Activator During the Advance of PSM." *Zhen Ci Yan Jiu [Acupuncture Research]* 18 (2) (1993): 115–22. (Chinese)

Hua, X. Y., S. M. Back, and E. K. Tam. "Substance P Enhances Electrical Field Stimulation-Induced Mast Cell Degranulation in Rat Trachea." *American Journal of Physiology* 270 (6 Pt 1) (June 1996): L985–91.

Huard, Pierre, and Ming Wong. *Chinese Medicine* (Translated from the French by Bernard Fielding). New York, Toronto: World University Library, McGraw-Hill Book Co., 1968.

Huneke, F., and W. Huneke. "Unfamiliar Remote Effects of Local Anesthetics." *Die Medizinische Welt* 27 (1928). (German)

Hwang, Y. C. "Anatomy and Classification of Acupoints." *Problems in Veterinary Medicine* 4 (1) (March 1992): 12–5.

Inoue, A., K. Ikoma, N. Morioka, K. Kumagai, T. Hashimoto, I. Hide, and Y. Nakata. "Interleukin-l Beta Induces Substance P Release from Primary Afferent Neurons Through the Cyclooxygenase-2 System." *Journal of Neurochemistry* 73 (5) (November 1999): 2,206–13.

Inoue, H., N. Nagata, and Y. Koshihara. "Involvement of Substance P as a Mediator in Capsaicin-Induced Mouse Ear Oedema." *Inflammation Research* 44 (11) (November 1995): 470–4.

Jancso, G., E. Kiraly, and A. Jancso-Gabor. "Direct Evidence for an Axonal Site of Action of Capsaicin." *Naunyn-Schmiedeberg's Archives of Pharmacology* 313 (1) (August 1980): 91–4.

Janig,W. "Spinal Cord Reflex Organization of Sympathetic Systems." *Progress in Brain Research* 107 (1996): 43–77.

Jin Wancheng, Wan Shaoying, Dai Dongyuan, Wang Hongshin, and Li Weili. "Experimental Study on Effects of Ultrasound Acupuncture at Zusanli and Tianshu on Intestinal Function." *Selections from Article Abstracts on Acupuncture and Moxibustion*, Beijing: November 22–26, 1987, 599.

Johansson, H., Djupsjobacka M, and Sjolander P. "Influences on the Gamma-Muscle-Spindle System from Muscle Afferents Stimulated by KCl and Lactic Acid." *Neuroscience Research* 16 (1) (January 1993): 49–57.

Jurna, I. "Effect of Stimulation in the Periaqueductal Grey Matter on Activity in Ascending Axons of the Rat Spinal Cord: Selective Inhibition of Activity Evoked by Afferent A Gamma and C Fiber Stimulation and Failure of Naloxone to Reduce Inhibition." *Brain Research* 196 (1980): 33–42.

Katayama, Y., and Syogoro Nishi. "Peptidergic Transmission." In *Autonomic and Enteric Ganglia: Transmission and Its Pharmacology.* Alexander G. Karczmar, Kyozo Koketsu, and Syogoro Nishi, eds. New York: Plenum Press, 1986, 181–196.

Kemme, M., D. Podlich, D. M. Raidoo, C. Snyman, S. Naidoo, and K. D. Bhoola. "Identification of Immunoreactive Tissue Prokallikrein on the Surface Membrane of Human Neutrophils." *Biological Chemistry* 380 (11) (November 1999): 1,321–8.

Kendall, D. E. "A Scientific Model for Acupuncture, Parts I and II." *American Journal of Acupuncture* 17 (3–4) (1989): 251–68, 343–60.

Khoe, W. H. "Ultrasound Acupuncture Used in Treatment of Low Back Pain and Sciatic Neuralgia Caused by Piriformis Muscle Spasm." *American Journal of Acupuncture* 1 (3) (1975): 53–7.

Khoe, W. H. "Ultrasound Acupuncture: Effective Treatment Modality for Various Diseases." *American Journal of Acupuncture* 5 (1) (1977): 31–4.

Kimura, M., K. Tohya, K. Kuroiwa, H. Oda, E. C. Gorawski, Z. X. Hua, S. Toda, M. Ohnishi, and E. Noguchi. "Electron Microscopical and Immunohistochemical Studies on the Induction of 'Qi' Employing Needling Manipulation." *American Journal of Chinese Medicine* 20 (1) (1992): 25–35.

Kong, Y. C., and D. S. Chen. "Elucidation of Islamic Drugs in Hui Hui Fang: A Linguistic and Pharmaceutical Approach." *Journal of Ethnopharmacology* 54 (2–3) (November 1996): 85–102.

Konishi, S., A. Tsunoo, and M. Otsuka. "Enkephalins Presynaptically Inhibit Noncholinergic Transmission in Sympathetic Ganglia." *Nature* (London) 282 (1979): 515–516.

Konishi, S., A. Tsunoo, N. Yanaihara, and M. Otsuka. "Peptidergic Excitatory and Inhibitory Synapses in Mammalian Sympathetic Ganglia: Roles of Substance P and Enkephalin." *Biomedical Research.* 1 (1980): 528–536.

Krstew, E., B. Jarrott, and A. J. Lawrence. "Bradykinin B2 Receptors in Nodose Ganglia of Rat and Human." *European Journal of Pharmacology* 348 (2–3) (May 8, 1998): 175–80.

Laakso, M. L., T. Porkka-Heiskanen, A. Alila, D. Stenberg, and G. Johansson. "Twenty-Four-Hour Rhythms in Relation to the Natural Photoperiod: A Field Study in Humans." *Journal of Biological Rhythms* 9 (3–4) (Winter 1994): 283–93.

Lam, F. Y., and W. R. Ferrell. "Capsaicin Suppresses Substance P–Induced Joint Inflammation in the Rat." *Neuroscience Letters* 105 (1–2) (October 23, 1989): 155–8.

Langevin, H. M., and P. D. Villancourt. "Acupuncture: Does it Work and, if so, How?" *Seminars in Clinical Neuropsychiatry* 4 (3) (July 1999): 167–75.

Larkin, S. W., L. Fraser, H. J. Showell, T. J. Williams, and J. B. Warren. "Prolonged Microvascular Vasodilation Induced by Leukotriene B4 in Human Skin is Cyclooxygenase Independent." *Journal of Pharmacological Experimental Therapy* 272 (1) (January 1995): 392–8.

Larsson, R., P. A. Oberg, and S. E. Larsson. "Changes of Trapezius Muscle Blood Flow and Electromyography in Chronic Neck Pain Due to Trapezius Myalgia." *Pain* 79 (1) (January 1999): 45–50.

Laufer, H. *Beitrage sur Kenntnis der Tibetanischen Medisin.* Berlin: Harrassowitz, 1900 Bd. 1, S. 1–41; Leipzig: Harrassowitz, 1900 Bd. 2, S. 43–90. (German)

Lee, Jane F., and C. S. Cheung. *Current Acupuncture Therapy.* Hong Kong: Medical Interflow Publishing House, 1978.

Lembeck, F. "Sir Thomas Lewis's Nocifensor System, Histamine and Substance P Containing Primary Afferent Nerves." In *Neurotransmitters in Action.* D. Bousfield, ed. Amsterdam, New York and Oxford: Elsevier Biomedical Press, 1985, 173–179.

Li, B. L. Li, J. Chen, L. Chen, W. Xu, R. Gao, B. Yang, W. Li, B. Wu, et. al. "Observation on the Relation Between Propagated Sensation Along Meridians and the Therapeutic Effect of Acupuncture on Myopia of Youngsters." *Zhen Ci Yan Jiu [Acupuncture Research]* 18 (2) (1993): 154–8. (Chinese)

Li Chuanjie, Bi Lige, Zhu Baijun, Lu Zhuoshan, and Bai Xihe. "Influence of Acupuncture on the Left Heart, Micro-Circulation and Plasma cAMP and cGAMP of the Patients Suffering from Acute Myocardial Infarction." *The Second National Symposium on Acupuncture and Moxibustion and Acupuncture Anesthesia*, Beijing: Foreign Languages Printing House, 1984, 8.

Li Dongqin, Shi Lanhua, Gao Yi, and Jiang Jingxian. *Prescriptions of Traditional Chinese Medicine.* Zhang Enqin, ed. Shanghai: Publishing House of Shanghai College of Traditional Chinese Medicine, 1990.

Li, H. "Research on Plasma TXA2, PGI2 Levels, Blood Stasis Syndrome and Promoting Blood Circulation." *Zhongguo Zhong Xi Yi Jie He Za Zhi [Chinese Journal of Integrated Chinese and Western Medicine]* 15 (11) (November 1995): 701–4. (Chinese)

Li, J. L., Y. Q. Ding, K. H. Xiong, J. S. Li, R. Shigemoto, and N. Mizuno. "Substance P Receptor (NK1)-Immunoreactive Neurons Projecting to the Periaqueductal Gray: Distribution in the Spinal Trigeminal Nucleus and the Spinal Cord of the Rat." *Neuroscience Research* 30 (3) (March 1998): 219–25.

Li Jishuo, Li Huimin, Qin Bingzhi, and Dou Hong. "The Innervation of the Anterior Wall of the Stomach in the Rabbit: A Study with the HRP Method." *The Second National Symposium on Acupuncture and Moxibustion and Acupuncture Anesthesia*, Beijing: Foreign Languages Printing House, 1984a, 487.

Li Jishuo, Qin Bingzhi, Li Huimin, and Lu Shaowen. "The Segmental Distribution of Visceral (Urinary Bladder) and Somatic (Sciatic Nerve) Afferent Fibers and the Relation Between Their Terminal Distributions in Spinal Cord of Rabbit—A Study with HRP Retrograde and Transganglionic Tracing Techniques." *The Second National Symposium on Acupuncture and Moxibustion and Acupuncture Anesthesia*, Beijing: Foreign Languages Printing House, 1984b, 484.

Li Ruiwu, and Tao Zhili. "The Original Nuclei of the Parasympathetic Preganglia Fibers of Stomach (HRP Method)." *The Second National Symposium on Acupuncture and Moxibustion and Acupuncture Anesthesia*, Beijing: Foreign Languages Printing House, 1984, 488.

Li, Y. K., and S. Z. Zhong. "Spinal Manipulation in China." *Journal of Manipulative and Physiological Therapeutics* 21 (6) (July–August 1998): 399–401.

Light, A. R., and E. R. Perl. "Spinal Termination of Functionally Identified Primary Afferent Neurones with Slowly Conducting Myelinated Fibers." *Journal of Comparative Neurology* 186 (1979): 133–150.

Lin, J. G. "Studies of Needling Depth in Acupuncture Treatment." *Chinese Medicine Journal* (England) 110 (2) (February 1997): 154–6.

Lin, W. H., M. H. Xu, J. D. Dai, G. M. Chen, J. Y. Shen, and S. M. Chen. "Relation Between Human Needling Sensation and Acupoint Structure Comparison of Needling Sensation Between Manual and Electroacupuncture." *Selections from Shanghai Journal of Acupuncture and Moxibustion, 1982–1984.* Shanghai: Shanghai Institute of Acupuncture and Meridian, 1985, 141–145.

Lin, X., J. Liang, J. Ren, F. Mu, M. Zhang, and J. D. Chen. "Electrical Stimulation of Acupuncture Points Enhances Gastric Myoelectrical Activity in Humans." *American Journal of Gastroenterology* 92 (9) (September 1997): 1,527–30.

Ling Yeou-ruenn. *A New Compendium of Materia Medica (Pharmaceutical Botany & Chinese Medicinal Plants)*. Beijing, New York: Science Press, 1995.

Littlewood, N. K., A. J. Todd, R. C. Spike, C. Watt, and S. A. Shehab. "The Types of Neuron in Spinal Dorsal Horn which Possess Neurokinin-1 Receptors." *Neuroscience* 66 (3) (June 1995): 597–608.

Liu, J., Z. Han, S. Chen, and Q. Cao. "Influence of Electroacupuncture on Electrical Activity of Dorsal Horn Neurons of the Thoracic Spinal Cord in the Rabbit." *Zhen Ci Yan Jiu [Acupuncture Research]* 18 (4) (1993): 267–70. (Chinese)

Liu, R., D. Zhuang, X. Yang, Y. Li, D. Zhang, B. Wen, and R. Zhang. "Objective Display on Phenomena of Propagated Sensation Along Channels (PSC)—Changes on the Infrared Thermal Image Channels Pathway of Upper Extremity." *Zhen Ci Yan Jiu [Acupuncture Research]* 15 (3) (1990a): 239–44. (Chinese)

Liu, R., D. Zhuang, X. Yang, Y. Li, D. Zhang, B. Wen, and R. Zhang. "Objective Observation on Phenomena of Sensation Along Channels (PSC) and QI Reaching to Affects Area (QIRA)—The Influence of Acupuncture Points on Infrared Thermal Image of Face." *Zhen Ci Yan Jiu [Acupuncture Research]* 15 (3) (1990b) 245–9. (Chinese)

Liu Ruiting, Xu Huiren, Fu Weixing, and Meng Jingbi. "An Afferent Pathway of Point 'Neiguan' in Cats—Observation on Evoked Potential of Dorsal Roots of Spinal Cord." *The Second National Symposium on Acupuncture and Moxibustion and Acupuncture Anesthesia*, Beijing: Foreign Languages Printing House, 1984, 384.

Liu Xiang, and Zhang Shouxin. "The Influence of Injection or Microinjection of Naloxone into PAG upon the Effect of Electroacupuncture on NRM Neurons." *The Second National Symposium on Acupuncture and Moxibustion and Acupuncture Anesthesia*, Beijing: Foreign Languages Printing House, 1984, 372.

Liu Zhiming, Jiang Songlin, Yu Yaocai, Sun Shentian, Yu Zhisun, and Li Juan. "Experimental Studies on the Effects of the Acupuncture Manipulation Upon Gastrointestinal Motility and Electricity." *Selections from Article Abstracts on Acupuncture and Moxibustion*, Beijing, November 22–26, 1987, 439.

Lotti, T., G. Hautmann, and E. Panconesi. "Neuropeptides in Skin." *Journal of American Academy of Dermatology* 33 (3) (September 1995): 482–96.

Lu, Gwei-Djen, and Joseph Needham. *Celestial Lancets: A History and Rationale of Acupuncture and Moxa.* Cambridge: Cambridge University Press, 1980.

Lucey, D. R., J. M. Novak, V. R. Polonis, Y. Liu, and S. Gartner. "Characterization of Substance P Binding to Human Monocytes/Macrophages." *Clinical and Diagnostic Laboratory Immunology* 1 (3) (May 1994): 330–5.

Luger, T. A., and T. Lotti. "Neuropeptides: Role in Inflammatory Skin Diseases." *Journal of European Academy of Dermatology and Venereology* 10 (3) (May 1998): 207–11.

Luger, T. A., R. S. Bhardwaj, S. Grabbe, and T. Schwarz. "Regulation of the Immune Response by Epidermal Cytokines and Neurohormones." *Journal of Dermatological Science* 13 (1) (October 1996): 5–10.

Luo Xiwen, trans. *Synopsis of Prescriptions of the Golden Chamber (Jin Gui Yao Lue Fang Lun)*. Beijing: New World Press, 1987.

Luo Xiwen, and Shi Jizhao, trans. *Treatise on Febrile Diseases Caused by Cold.* Beijing: New World Press, 1986.

Ma Jixing. "Acupuncture and Moxibustion." In *Ancient China's Technology and Science.* Beijing: Foreign Languages Press, 1983, 345–351.

Ma Kanwen. "Diagnosis by Pulse Feeling in Chinese Traditional Medicine." In *Ancient China's Technology and Science.* Beijing: Foreign Languages Press, 1983, 358–368.

Ma, C., and Z. Liu. "Regulative Effects of Electroacupuncture on Gastric Hyperfunction Induced by Electrostimulation of the Lateral Hypothalamus area of Rabbits." *Zhen Ci Yan Jiu [Acupuncture Research]* 19 (2) (1994): 42–6. (Chinese)

Magerl, W., J. Szolcsanyi, R. A. Westerman, and H. O. Handwerker. "Laser Doppler Measurements of Skin Vasodilation Elicited by Percutaneous Electrical Stimulation of Nociceptors in Humans." *Neuroscience Letters* 82 (3) (December 4, 1987): 349–54.

Mann, Felix. *Acupuncture: The Ancient Chinese Art of Healing and How It Works Scientifically.* London: William Heinemann Medical Books Ltd., 1962.

Mann, Felix. *The Meridians of Acupuncture.* London: William Heinemann Medical Books Ltd., 1964.

Mann, Felix. *Reinventing Acupuncture.* Oxford: Butterworth-Heinemann (Published in German by M.M.I. Verlag, Giessen; published in Italian by Editore Marrapese, Rome), 1992.

Mann, Felix. "A New System of Acupuncture." In *Medical Acupuncture: A Western Scientific Approach.* Jacqueline Filshie and Adrian White, eds. London: Churchill Livingstone, 1998, 61–66.

Mathews, R. H. *Mathews' Chinese–English Dictionary.* Shanghai: China Inland Mission and Presbyterian Mission Press, 1931.

Matsuda, H., K. Kawakita, Y. Kiso, T. Nakano, and Y. Kitamura. "Substance P Induces Granulocyte Infiltration Through Degranulation of Mast Cells." *Journal of Immunology* 142 (3) (February 1, 1989): 927–31.

Mayer, D. J., D. D. Price, and A. Rafii. "Antagonism of Acupuncture Analgesia in Man by the Narcotic Antagonist Naloxone." *Brain Research* 121 (214) (1977): 368–372.

Mayer, D. J., D. D. Price, J. Barber, and A. Rafii. "Acupuncture Analgesia: Evidence for Activation of a Pain Inhibitory System as a Mechanism of Action." *Advances in Pain Research and Therapy* (August 12, 1977): 751–4.

McCarroll, G. D., and B. A. Rowley. "An Investigation of the Existence of Electrically Located Acupuncture Points." *IEEE Transactions of Biomedical Engineering* 26 (3) (1979): 177–181.

McDonald, D. M., J. J. Bowden, P. Baluk, and N. W. Bunnett. "Neurogenic Inflammation. A Model for Studying Efferent Actions of Sensory Nerves." *Advancements in Experimental Medicine and Biology* 410 (1996): 453–62.

Michel, W. "Early Western Observations of Moxibustion and Acupuncture." *Sudhoffs Archiv Zeitschrift fur Wissenschaftsgeschichte* 77 (2) (1993): 193–222. (German)

Miller, K. E., V. D. Douglas, A. B. Richards, M. J. Chandler, and R. D. Foreman. "Propriospinal Neurons in the CI–C2 Spinal Segments Project to the L5–S1 Segments of the Rat Spinal Cord." *Brain Research Bulletin* 47 (1) (September 1, 1998): 43–7.

Misery, L. "Neuro-Immuno-Cutaneous System." *Pathologie-Biologie* 44 (10) (December 1996): 867–74. (French)

Misery, L. "Skin, Immunity and the Nervous System." *British Journal of Dermatology* 137 (6) (December 1997): 843–50.

Misery, L. "Langerhans Cells in the Neuro-Immuno-Cutaneous System." *Journal of Neuroimmunology* 89 (1–2) (August 14, 1998): 83–7.

Miyakawa, K. "An Examination of the Cunzhun Huan Zhong Tu." *Nippon Ishigaku Zasshi [Journal of Japanese History of Medicine]* 42 (1) (March 1996): 77–86. (Japanese)

Mo, Q., B. Gong, J. Fang, J. Li, J. Huang, K. Chen, X. Kuang, and J. Wang. "Influence of Acupuncture at Zusanli Point on Function of 5-HT and M Receptor in Rat's Brain and Spleen." *Zhen Ci Yan Jiu [Acupuncture Research]* 19 (1) (1994): 33–6. (Chinese)

Mohammad, S. Fazal, Reginald G. Mason, Ernst J. Eichwald , and John A. Shively. "Healthy and Impaired Vascular Endothelium." In *Blood Platelet Function and Medicinal Chemistry.* Andrew Lasslo, ed. New York: Elsevier Science Publishing Co., 1984, 129–173.

Moroz, A. "Issues in Acupuncture Research: The Failure of Quantitative Methodologies and the Possibilities for Viable, Alternative Solutions." *American Journal of Acupuncture.* 27 (1–2) (1999): 95–103.

Murakami, M., T. Kambe, S. Shimbara, and I. Kudo. "Functional Coupling Between Various Phospholipase A2s and Cyclooxygenases in Immediate and Delayed Prostanoid Biosynthetic Pathways." *Journal of Biological Chemistry* 274 (5) (January 29, 1999): 3,103–15.

Naidoo, Y., C. Snyman, D. M. Raidoo, K. D. Bhoola, M. Kemme, and W. Muller-Esterl. "Cellular Visualization of Tissue Prokallikrein in Human Neutrophils and Myelocytes." *British Journal of Haematology* 105 (3) (June 1999): 599–612.

Naim, M. M., S. A. Shehab, and A. J. Todd. "Cells in Laminae III and IV of the Rat Spinal Cord which Possess the Neurokinin-1 Receptor Receive Monosynaptic Input from Myelinated Primary Afferents." *European Journal of Neuroscience* 10 (9) (September 1998): 3,012–9.

Nakaya, Y., T. Kaneko, R. Shigemoto, S. Nakanishi, and N. Mizuno. "Immunohistochemical Localization of Substance P Receptor in the Central Nervous System of the Adult Rat." *Journal of Comparative Neurology* 347 (2) (September 8, 1994): 249–74.

Nanning Cardiovascular Research Group. "An Observation on the Difference of the Clinical Effects and the Main Points in the Treatment of Coronary Disease with Acupuncture." *The Second National Symposium on Acupuncture and Moxibustion and Acupuncture Anesthesia*, Beijing: Foreign Languages Printing House, 1984, 7.

Newby, D. E., D. G. Sciberras, C. J. Ferro, B. J. Gertz, D. Sommerville, A. Majumdar, R. C. Lowry, and D. J. Webb. "Substance P-Induced Vasodilatation is Mediated by the Neurokinin Type l Receptor but does not Contribute to Basal Vascular Tone in Man." *British Journal of Clinical Pharmacology* 48 (3) (September 1999): 336–44.

Nichols, M. L., B. J. Allen, S. D. Rogers, J. R. Ghilardi, P. Honore, N. M. Luger, M. P. Finke, J. Li, D. A. Lappi, D. A. Simone, and P. W. Mantyh. "Transmission of Chronic Nociception by Spinal Neurons Expressing the Substance P Receptor." *Science* 286 (5,444) (November 19, 1999): 1,558–61.

NIH Consensus Statement. *Acupuncture* 15 (5) (November 3–5, 1997): 1–34.

Noguchi, E., and H. Hayashi. "Increases in Gastric Acidity in Response to Electroacupuncture Stimulation of the Hindlimb of Anesthetized Rats." *Japanese Journal of Physiology* 46 (1) (February 1996): 53–8.

Nunn, John F. *Ancient Egyptian Medicine.* Norman, Oklahoma: University of Oklahoma Press, 1996.

O'Connor, John, and Dan Bensky. *Acupuncture: A Comprehensive Text.* Chicago: Eastland Press, 1981.

Osler, Sir William. *The Principles and Practice of Medicine* 8th ed. New York: Appleton, 1912.

Ouyang Shou, and Xu Guansun. "Activated Stereotaxic Structure Affecting on Gastroelectrical Activity by Point Acupuncture in Cat's Medulla Oblongata." *The Second National Symposium on Acupuncture and Moxibustion and Acupuncture Anesthesia*, Beijing: Foreign Languages Printing House, 1984, 530.

Ouyang Shou, and Xu Guansun. "Role of Formatio Reticularis of Medulla Oblongata in the Acupuncture Regulation of Gastroelectrical Activity in Cats." *Selections from Article Abstracts on Acupuncture and Moxibustion*, Beijing: November 22–26, 1987, 441.

Oyle, I. "Ultrasound Acupuncture: Theoretical Considerations and Possibilities in Family Practice." *American Journal of Acupuncture*, 2 (4) (1974): 275–77.

Packham, Marian A., and J. Fraser Mustard. "Normal and Abnormal Platelet Activity." In *Blood Platelet Function and Medicinal Chemistry.* Andrew Lasslo, ed. New York: Elsevier Science Publishing Co., 1984, 61–128.

Palos, Stephan *The Chinese Art of Healing.* Munich: 1963; English edition, Herder and Herder, 1971; Bantam Books, 1972.

Panuncio, A. L., S. De La Pena, G. Gualco, and N. Reissenweber. "Adrenergic Innervation in Reactive Human Lymph Nodes." *Journal of Anatomy* 194 (Pt 1) (January 1999): 143–6.

Pedersen, J., P. Sjolander, B. I. Wenngren, and H. Johansson. "Increased Intramuscular Concentration of Bradykinin Increases the Static Fusimotor Dive to Muscle Spindles in Neck Muscles of the Cat. *Pain* 70 (1) (March 1997): 3–91.

Pomeranz, Bruce, and Gabriel Stux, eds. *Scientific Bases of Acupuncture.* Berlin and Heidelberg: Springer-Verlag, 1988.

Proudfit, H. K., and M. Monsen. "Ultrastructural Evidence that Substance P Neurons Form Synapses with Noradrenergic Neurons in the A7 Catecholamine Cell Group that Modulate Nociception." *Neuroscience* 91 (4) (1999): 1,499–513.

Qie, Z. W., F. K. Cheng, and L. H. Cheng. "Blood Flow Capacity of the Vertebra and Cervical Artery Affected by Propagated Sensation with Acupuncture Excitation." *Zhong Xi Yi Jie He Za Zhi [Journal of Integrated Chinese and Western Medicine]* 11 (1) (January 1991): 31–35. (Chinese)

Qin, J., M. H. Jin, and J. H. Deng. "Clinical Study of Eliminating Dampness and Removing Blood Stasis in Treating Coronary Heart Disease—The Summary about Serial Study of Blood Stasis due to Dampness." *Zhongguo Zhong Xi Yi Jie He Za Zhi [Chinese Journal of Integrated Chinese and Western Medicine]* 17 (9) (September 1997): 519–22. (Chinese)

Qu Jingfeng, Zhang Shaohua, and Xie Rong. *The Chinese Materia Medica.* Zhang Enqin, ed. Shanghai: Publishing House of Shanghai College of Traditional Chinese Medicine, 1990.

Raidoo, D. M., and K. D. Bhoola. "Pathophysiology of the Kallikrein-Kinin System in Mammalian Nervous Tissue." *Pharmacology & Therapeutics* 79 (2) (August 1998): 105–27.

Regoli, D., S. Nsa Allogho, A. Rizzi, and F. J. Gobeil. "Bradykinin Receptors and their Antagonists." *European Journal of Pharmacology* 348 (1) (May 1, 1998): 1–10.

Reichmanis, M., A. A. Marino, and R. O. Becker. "Electrical Correlates of Acupuncture Points." *IEEE Transactions on Biomedical Engineering* 22 (1975): 533–535.

Reiter, R. J. "The Melatonin Rhythm: Both a Clock and a Calendar." *Experientia* 49 (8) (August 15, 1993): 654–64.

Roccia, L. "Chinese Acupuncture in Italy." *American Journal of Chinese Medicine* 2 (1) (January 1974): 49–52.

Romerio, S. C., L. Linder, and W. E. Haefeli. "Neurokinin-l Receptor Antagonist R116301 Inhibits Substance P–Induced Venodilation." *Clinical Pharmacology and Therapeutics* 66 (5) (November 1999): 522–7.

Rosenburg, D. B. "Wilhelm Ten Rhyne's De Acupunctura: An 1826 Translation." *Journal of the History of Medicine and Allied Sciences* 34 (1) (January 1979): 81–4.

Rosenburg, R. D. "Hemorrhagic Disorders I. Protein Interactions in the Clotting Mechanism." In *Hematology* 2nd ed. William S. Beck, ed. Cambridge, Mass.: The MIT Press, 1979, 485–515.

Rossi, R., and O. Johansson. "Cutaneous Innervation and the Role of Neuronal Peptides in Cutaneous Inflammation: A Minireview." *European Journal of Dermatology* 8 (5) (July–August, 1998): 299–306.

Ryan, D. "Toward Improving the Reliability of Clinical Acupuncture Trials: Arguments Against the Validity of 'Sham Acupuncture' as Controls." *American Journal of Acupuncture* 27 (1–2) (1999): 105–9.

Sarlandiere le Chevalier, J. B. *Memories sur l'Electropuncture.* Paris: Private publication, 1825.

Sato, A. "The Reflex Effects of Spinal Somatic Nerve Stimulation on Visceral Function." *Journal of Manipulative and Physiological Therapeutics* 15 (1) (January 1992): 57–61.

Sato, A. "Somatovisceral Reflexes." *Journal of Manipulative and Physiological Therapeutics* 18 (9) (November–December 1995): 597–602.

Sato, A. "Neural Mechanisms of Autonomic Responses Elicited by Somatic Sensory Stimulation." *Neuroscience and Behavioral Physiology* 27 (5) (September–October, 1997): 610–21.

Sato, A., Y. Sato, and A. Suzuki. "Mechanism of the Reflex Inhibition of Micturition Contractions of the Urinary Bladder Elicited by Acupuncture-Like Stimulation in Anesthetized Rats." *Neuroscience Research* 15 (3) (November 1992): 189–98.

Sato, A., Y. Sato, A. Suzuki, and S. Uchida. "Reflex Modulation of Catecholamine Secretion and Adrenal Sympathetic Nerve Activity by Acupuncture-Like Stimulation in Anesthetized Rat." *Japan Journal of Physiology,* 46 (5) (October 1996): 411–21.

Saunders, M. A., M. G. Belvisi, G. Cirino, P. J. Barnes, T. D. Warner, and J. A. Mitchell. "Mechanisms of Prostaglandin E2 Release by Intact Cells Expressing Cyclooxygenase-2: Evidence for a 'Two-Component' Model." *Journal of Pharmacology and Experimental Therapeutics* 288 (3) (March 1999): 1,101–6.

Schnorrenberger, C. C. "Morphological Foundations of Acupuncture: An Anatomical Nomenclature of Acupuncture Structures." *BMAS Acupuncture in Medicine* 14 (3) (November 1996): 89–103.

Scholzen, T., C. A. Armstrong, N. W. Bunnett, T. A. Luger, J. E. Olerud, and J. C. Ansel. "Neuropeptides in the Skin: Interactions Between the Neuroendocrine and the Skin Immune Systems." *Experimental Dermatology* 7 (2–3) (April–June 1998): 81–96.

Schott, G. D. "Visceral Afferents: Their Contribution to 'Sympathetic Dependent' Pain." *Brain* 117 (Pt 2) (April 1994): 397–413.

Schultz, W. *Shiatsu: Japanese Finger Pressure Therapy.* New York: Bell Publishing Co., 1976.

Schulze, E., M. Witt, T. Fink, A. Hofer, and R. H. Funk. "Immunohistochemical Detection of Human Skin Nerve Fibers." *Acta Histochemia* 99 (3) (August 1997): 301–9.

Selzer, M., and W. A. Spencer. "Convergence of Visceral and Cutaneous Afferent Pathways in the Lumbar Spinal Cord." *Brain Research* 14 (1969): 331–348.

Shi Qingyao, and Zhu Lixia. "The Effect of Electroacupuncture and Iontophoretic Enkephalin on the Neuronal Activity in Nucleus Raphe Magnus (NRM)." *The Second National Symposium on Acupuncture and Moxibustion and Acupuncture Anesthesia*, Beijing: Foreign Languages Printing House, 1984a, 369.

Shi Qingyao, and Zhu Lixia. "The Effect of Iontophoretic 5-HT and Electroacupuncture on the Activities of NRM Neurons." *The Second National Symposium on Acupuncture and Moxibustion and Acupuncture Anesthesia*, Beijing: Foreign Languages Printing House, 1984b, 370.

Shi Qingyao, and Zhu Lixia. "The Influence of Iontophoretic Naloxone Upon Acupuncture Effect on the Nucleus Raphe Magnus (NRM)." *The Second National Symposium on Acupuncture and Moxibustion and Acupuncture Anesthesia*, Beijing: Foreign Languages Printing House, 1984c, 368.

Soulié de Morant, Georges. *L'Acuponcture Chinoise.* Three volumes, Paris, 1957. (French)

Stener-Victorin, E., U. Waldenstrom, S. A. Andersson, and M. Wikland. "Reduction of Blood Flow Impedance in the Uterine Arteries of Infertile Women with Electro-Acupuncture." *Human Reproduction* (Oxford England) 11 (6) (June 1996): 1,314–7.

Stillings, D. "A Survey of the History of Electrical Stimulation for Pain to 1900." *Medical Instrumentation* 9 (6) (November–December 1975): 255–9.

Streilein, J. W., P. Alard, and H. Niizeki. "A New Concept of Skin-Associated Lymphoid Tissue (SALT): UVB Light Impaired Cutaneous Immunity Reveals a Prominent Role for Cutaneous Nerves." *Keio Journal of Medicine* 48 (1) (March 1999): 22–7.

Stucky, C. L., S. A. Thayer, and V. S. Seybold. "Prostaglandin E2 Increases the Proportion of Neonatal Rat Dorsal Root Ganglion Neurons that Respond to Bradykinin." *Neuroscience* 74 (4) (October 1996): 1,111–23.

Sun Fuling, Cheng Lianhu, and Liu Wenming. "Gustatory Phenomenon of the Spleen Channel." *Advances in Acupuncture and Acupuncture Anesthesia*, Beijing: Foreign Languages Printing House, June 1–5, 1979, 272.

Sun Guanren, Liu Zhaochun, Li Hongbo, Yang Suqin, and Chong Guiqin. *Health Preservation and Rehabilitation.* Zhang Enqin, ed. Shanghai: Publishing House of Shanghai College of Traditional Chinese Medicine, 1990.

Suzuki, H., S. Miura, Y. Y. Liu, M. Tsuchiya, and H. Ishii. "Substance P Induces Degranulation of Mast Cells and Leukocyte Adhesion to Venular Endothelium." *Peptides* 16 (8) (1995): 1,447–52.

Tailleux, P. "Louis Berlioz, Pionnier de l'Acupuncture." *Histoire des Sciences Medicales* 1986; 20 (2): 145–51. (French)

Tao Zhili, Dang Ruishau, and Li Qun. "The Segmental Distribution of the Afferent and Efferent Neurons in the Region of 'Shaohai' Point." *Selections from Article Abstracts on Acupuncture and Moxibustion*, Beijing: November 22–26, 1987, 480.

Tao Zhili, Li Ruiwu, and Dang Ruishan. "The Segmental Distribution of the Afferent and Efferent Neurons in the Region of 'Shenmen' Point." *Selections from Article Abstracts on Acupuncture and Moxibustion,* Beijing: November 22–26, 1987, 479.

Tao Zhili, Li Ruiwu, and Li Cuihong. "The Segmental Distribution of the Afferent Neurons of the 'Neiguan' Point." *The Second National Symposium on Acupuncture and Moxibustion and Acupuncture Anesthesia*, Beijing: Foreign Languages Printing House, 1984, 491.

Tao Zhili, Wang Liangpei, Li Ruiwu, Zhang Zuping, and Xi Shiyiuan. "The Segmental Distribution of the Afferent Neurons of the 'Zusanli' Point and the Stomach-HRP Method." *The Second National Symposium on Acupuncture and Moxibustion and Acupuncture Anesthesia*, Beijing: Foreign Languages Printing House, 1984a, 491.

Tao Zhili, Wang Liangpei, Zhang Zuping, and Li Cuihong. "Application of the HRP Method to Explore the Segmental Distribution of the Sympathetic Afferent of the Stomach (Anterior Wall, Posterior Wall, Pylorus and Cardia)." *The Second National Symposium on Acupuncture and Moxibustion and Acupuncture Anesthesia*, Beijing: Foreign Languages Printing House, 1984b, 489.

Tao, Z., and R. Li. "The Segmental Distribution of Sympathetic Afferent Neurons of the Heart, Cardiac Nerve, and Projection of the Cardiac Nerve to the Central Nervous System." *Zhen Ci Yan Jiu [Acupuncture Research]* 18 (4) (1993): 257–61. (Chinese)

Tao, Z., Z. Jin, and W. Ren. "Segmental Distributions of Sensory Neurons of the 'Ganshu', 'Pishu', 'Liangmen,' 'Qimen' Points and the Gallbladder." *Zhen Ci Yan Jiu [Acupuncture Research]* 16 (1) (1991): 61–5. (Chinese)

Tao, Z. L., G. Q. Xu, and R. W. Li. "The Sensory Neurons and their Connections with the Point of 'Sibai'." *Selections from Article Abstracts on Acupuncture and Moxibustion*, Beijing: November 22–26, 1987, 479.

Thorwald, Jurgen. *Science and Secrets of Early Medicine.* Richard and Clara Winston, trans. New York: Harcourt, Brace & World, Inc., 1962.

Tominaga, K., K. Honda, A. Akahoshi, Y. Makino, T. Kawarabayashi, Y. Takano, and H. Kamiya. "Substance P Causes Adhesion of Neutrophils to Endothelial Cells Via Protein Kinase C." *Biological and Pharmaceutical Bulletin* 22 (11) (November 1999): 1,242–5.

Trafton, J. A., C. Abbadie, S. Marchand, P. W. Mantyh, and A. I. Basbaum. "Spinal Opioid Analgesia: How Critical is the Regulation of Substance P Signaling?" *Journal of Neuroscience* 19 (21) (November 1, 1999): 9,642–53.

Travell, Janet G., and David G. Simons. *Myofascial Pain and Dysfunction: The Trigger Point Manual.* London, Los Angeles, Sydney: Williams & Wilkins, Baltimore, 1983.

Ulett, G. A., J. Han, and S. Han. "Traditional and Evidence-Based Acupuncture: History, Mechanisms, and Present Status." *Southern Medical Journal* 91 (12) (December 1998): 1,115–20.

Unschuld, Paul U. *Chinese Medicine.* Brookline, Massachusetts: Paradigm Publications, 1998.

Veith, Ilza. *Huang Ti Nei Ching Su Wen: The Yellow Emperor's Classic of Internal Medicine, new edition.* Los Angeles and Berkley: University of California Press, 1949; 1966.

Veronesi, B., D. M. Sailstad, D. L. Doerfler, and M. Selgrade. "Neuropeptide Modulation of Chemically Induced Skin Irritation." *Toxicology and Applied Pharmacology* 135 (2) (December 1995): 258–67.

Von Banchet, G. S., and H. G. Schaible. "Localization of the Neurokinin 1 Receptor on a Subset of Substance P-Positive and Isolectin B4-Negative Dorsal Root Ganglion Neurons of the Rat." *Neuroscience Letters* 274 (3) (October 29, 1999): 175–8.

Walker, K., M. Perkins, and A. Dray. "Kinins and Kinin Receptors in the Nervous System." *Neurochemistry International* 26 (1) (January 1995): 1–16; discussion 17–26.

Wallengren, J. "Vasoactive Peptides in the Skin." *Journal of Investigative Dermatology, Symposium Proceedings* 2 (1) (August 1997): 49–55.

Wang Chi Min. "China's Contribution to Medicine of the Past." *Annals of Medical History* 7 (1926): 192–201.

Wang, S. Y. *Pulsology and Symptomatology in Chinese Medicine, Vol. 1.* Taichung, Taiwan: University of Chinese Medicine, 1988. (Chinese)

Wang Zhaopu. *Acupressure Therapy: Point Percussion Treatment of Cerebral Birth Injury, Brain Injury and Stroke.* London: Churchill Livingstone, 1991.

Wang Guocai, Fan Yali, and Guan Zheng. *Chinese Massage.* Zhang Enqin, ed. Shanghai: Publishing House of Shanghai College of Traditional Chinese Medicine, 1990.

Wang, K. M., S. M. Yao, Y. L. Xian, and Z. L. Hou. "A Study on the Receptive Field of Acupoints and the Relationship Between Characteristics of Needling Sensation and Groups of Afferent Fibers." *Science Sinica, Series B* 28 (9) (September 1985): 963–71.

Wang Zhuoqun, Zhao Lingzi, and Wang Ruyao. "The Segmental Distribution of Sympathetic Postganglionic Neurons in Rabbit Heart." *The Second National Symposium on Acupuncture and Moxibustion and Acupuncture Anesthesia,* Beijing: Foreign Languages Printing House, 1984, 486.

Wang Zhuoqun, Zhao Lingzi, Wang Ruyao, and Zhou Sishun. "The Segmental Distribution of Sympathetic Preganglionic Neurons in Rabbit Medulla Spinalis after Injection of Horseradish Peroxidase in Postcervical Ganglion." *The Second National Symposium on Acupuncture and Moxibustion and Acupuncture Anesthesia,* Beijing: Foreign Languages Printing House, 1984a, 487.

Wang Zhuoqun, Zhao Lingzi, Wang Ruyao, and Zhou Sishun. "The Segmental Distribution of Afferent Neurons in Point Neiguan." *The Second National Symposium on Acupuncture and Moxibustion and Acupuncture Anesthesia,* Beijing: Foreign Languages Printing House, 1984b, 492.

Wang Zongxue, Xu Pingnan, and Wang Xinhua. "Clinical Observation on the Relationship Between the Pericardium Meridian of Hand-Jue Yin and Arrhythmia." *The Second National Symposium on Acupuncture and Moxibustion and Acupuncture Anesthesia,* Beijing: Foreign Languages Printing House, 1984, 4.

Wells, J. Vivian, and Christopher S. Henney. "Immune Mechanisms in Tissue Damage." In *Basic and Clinical Immunology* 4th ed. Daniel P. Stites, John D. Stobo, H. Hugh Fudenberg, and J. Vivian Wells, eds. Los Altos, Calif: Lange Medical Publications, 1982, 136–155.

Wendeng Central Hospital Cholelithiasis Treating Group [Shangdong, China]. "Electric Needling and Magnesium Sulfate Administration for Cholelithiasis." *Advances in Acupuncture and Acupuncture Anesthesia,* Beijing: Foreign Languages Printing House, June 1–5, 1979, 5.

Weng Jiaying, Peng Guichen, Yuang Huazhang, Mao Suhua, and Zhang Huqin. "The Morphological Investigation of the Correcting Abnormal Fetus Position by Acupuncture, Moxibustion and Laser Irradiation in the Point Zhiyin." *The Second National Symposium on Acupuncture and Moxibustion and Acupuncture Anesthesia,* Beijing: Foreign Languages Printing House, 1984, 494.

Weng, T., M. Lu, X. Lu, and W. Lu. "Studies on the Phenomenon of Latent Propagated Sensation Along Channel (LPSC) by Combining Applied Knocks, Measurement of Resistance and Record Electric Current." *Zhen Ci Yan Jiu [Acupuncture Research]* 15 (1) (1990): 82–4. (Chinese)

Wenngren, B. I., J. Pedersen, P. Sjolander, M. Bergenheim, and H. Johansson. "Bradykinin and Muscle Stretch Alter Contralateral Cat Neck Muscle Spindle Output." *Neuroscience Research* 32 (2) (October 1998): 119–29.

Werb, Zena, and Ira M. Goldstein. "Phagocytic Cells: Chemotaxis and Effector Functions of Macrophages and Granulocytes." In *Basic and Clinical Immunology* 4th ed. Daniel P. Stites, John D. Stobo, H. Hugh Fudenberg, and J. Vivian Wells, eds. Los Altos, Calif.: Lange Medical Publications, 1982, 109–123.

Wieger, L. *Chinese Characters: Their Origin, Etymology, History, Classification and Signification.* New York: Paragon Book Reprint Corp. and Dover Publications, Inc., 1965.

Willis, W. D. Jr. "Dorsal Root Potentials and Dorsal Root Reflexes: A Double-Edged Sword." *Experimental Brain Research* 124 (4) (February 1999): 395–421.

Windhorst, U., and T. Kokkoroyiannis. "Interaction of Recurrent Inhibitory and Muscle Spindle Afferent Feedback During Muscle Fatigue." *Neuroscience* 43 (1) (1991): 249–59.

Wu, B. H., and X. L. Hu. "Studies on the Mechanism Underlying the Blocking of the Propagated Sensation Along Channels by Local Cooling." *Zhen Ci Yan Jiu [Acupuncture Research]* 12 Supplement 2 (1987): 21–5, 66. (Chinese)

Wu, B., X. Hu, J. Xu, B. Yang, W. Li, and B. Li. "Localization of the Meridian Track Over Body Surface by the Method of Blocking the Acupuncture Effect with Mechanical Pressure." *Zhen Ci Yan Jiu [Acupuncture Research]* 18 (2) (1993a): 114, 128–31. (Chinese)

Wu, B., X. Hu, B. Yang, J. Xu, W. Li, B. Li, J. Chen, and L. Chen. "The Influence of Pressing the Meridian Course on Electroretinogram During Acupuncture." *Zhen Ci Yan Jiu [Acupuncture Research]* 18 (2) (1993b): 132–6. (Chinese)

Wu, B., J. Xu, X. Hu, B. Yang, and B. Li. "Observation on the Functional Characteristics of Cortical Somatosensory Area During the Advance of the Propagated Sensation Along Meridians." *Zhen Ci Yan Jiu [Acupuncture Research]* 18 (2) (1993c): 123–7. (Chinese)

Wu Dingzong, Yang Liping, Deng Chunlei, and Shi Peifeng. "Effect of Acupuncture on Urinary Bladder Contraction." *The Second National Symposium on Acupuncture and Moxibustion and Acupuncture Anesthesia*, Beijing: Foreign Languages Printing House, 1984, 537.

Xi Shiyuan, and Tao Zhili. "The Parasympathetic Afferent Neurons of Different Portions of the Stomach Distributed in the Nodular Ganglions of the Vagus." *The Second National Symposium on Acupuncture and Moxibustion and Acupuncture Anesthesia*, Beijing: Foreign Languages Printing House, 1984, 489.

Xie, Y., H. Li, and W. Xiao. "Neurobiological Mechanisms of the Meridian and the Propagation of Needle Feeling Along the Meridian Pathway." *Science in China, Series C: Life Sciences* 39 (1) (February 1996): 99–112.

Xiu, R. J. "Microcirculation and Traditional Chinese Medicine." *Journal of the American Medical Association* 260 (12) (September 23–30, 1988): 1,755–7.

Xu, N. "Effect of Electroacupuncture at 'Taixi' Point on Plasma Thromboxane A2 and Prostacyclin in the Rabbit with Renal Ischemia." *Zhen Ci Yan Jiu [Acupuncture Research]* 18 (3) (1993): 240–2. (Chinese)

Xu, F., and R. Chen. "Reciprocal Actions of Acupoints on Gastrointestinal Peristalsis During Electroacupuncture in Mice." *Journal of Traditional Chinese Medicine* 19 (2) (June 1999): 141–4.

Xu Guansun, and Wang Keming. "Double Modulated Effects of Acupuncture on Electrogastrogram (EGG) in the Normal and Patients with Certain Gastric Diseases." *The Second National Symposium on Acupuncture and Moxibustion and Acupuncture Anesthesia*, Beijing: Foreign Languages Printing House, 1984, 55.

Xu, J., X. Huang, B. Wu, and X. Hu. "Influence of Mechanical Pressure Applied on the Stomach Meridian upon the Effectiveness of Acupuncture of Zusanli." *Zhen Ci Yan Jiu [Acupuncture Research]* 18 (2) (1993): 137–42. (Chinese)

Xu, R., D. Guo, H. Qin, and X. Guan. "Electroacupuncture Along Meridians Activating Subcutaneous Primary Afferents in Acupoints—CB-HRP Tracing Study." *Zhen Ci Yan Jiu [Acupuncture Research]* 21 (4) (1996): 54–8. (Chinese)

Xu Shaofen, Zhao Delu, Jiang Yanfeng, Zhang Lingmei, Xu Weimin, and Lu Yanyan. "Acupuncture Analgesia and Stress Analgesia." *The Second National Symposium on Acupuncture and Moxibustion and Acupuncture Anesthesia*, Beijing: Foreign Languages Printing House, 1984, 426.

Xu, X., J. Z. Liao, and S. R. Wang. "Relation Between Traditional Chinese Medicinal Syndrome Differentiation and Blood Platelet Function in 310 Cases of Blood Stasis." *Zhongguo Zhong Xi Yi Jie He Za Zhi [Chinese Journal of Integrated Chinese and Western Medicine]* 13 (12) (December 1993): 718–21, 707. (Chinese)

Xu Xiangcai, You Ke, Kang Kai, Bao Xuequan, and Lu Yubin, eds. *Orthopedics and Traumatology, The English–Chinese Encyclopedia of Practical Traditional Chinese Medicine, Volume 14.* Beijing: Higher Education Press, 1992.

Xu Xiangcai, You Ke, Kang Kai, Bao Xuequan, and Lu Yubin, eds. *The Chinese Materia Medica, The English–Chinese Encyclopedia of Practical Traditional Chinese Medicine, Volume 2.* Beijing: Higher Education Press, 1994a.

Xu Xiangcai, You Ke, Kang Kai, Bao Xuequan, and Lu Yubin, eds. *Pharmacology of Traditional Chinese Medical Formulae, The English–Chinese Encyclopedia of Practical Traditional Chinese Medicine, Volume 3.* Beijing: Higher Education Press, 1994b.

Xu Xiangcai, You Ke, Kang Kai, Bao Xuequan, and Lu Yubin, eds. *Tuina Therapeutics, The English–Chinese Encyclopedia of Practical Traditional Chinese Medicine, Volume 7.* Beijing: Higher Education Press, 1994c.

Xu Xiangcai, You Ke, Kang Kai, Bao Xuequan, and Lu Yubin, eds. *Medical Qigong, The English–Chinese Encyclopedia of Practical Traditional Chinese Medicine, Volume 8.* Beijing: Higher Education Press, 1994d.

Xu Xiangcai, You Ke, Kang Kai, Bao Xuequan, and Lu Yubin, eds. *Commonly Used Chinese Patent Medicines, The English–Chinese Encyclopedia of Practical Traditional Chinese Medicine, Volume 5.* Beijing: Higher Education Press, 1994e.

Yaksh, Tony L. ed. *Spinal Afferent Processing*. New York: Plenum Press, 1986.

Yamada, K., and T. Hoshino. "An Examination of the Close Relationship Between Lymphatic Vessels and Nerve Fibers Containing Calcitonin Gene-Related Peptide and Substance P in Rat Skin." *Nagoya Journal of Medical Science* 59 (3–4) (December 1996): 143–50.

Yan, J. Q., K. M. Wang, and Z. L. Hou. "The Observation on the General Properties of the Acupoint Muscle Action Potential." *Zhen Ci Yan Jiu [Acupuncture Research]* 12 (2) (1987): 138, 144–5. (Chinese)

Yang, B., W. Li, X. Hu, B. Wu, B. Li, L. Li, J. Chen, L. Chen, D. Zhang, and W. Xu. "Observation on the Phenomenon of Propagated Sensation Along Meridians in Youngsters." *Zhen Ci Yan Jiu [Acupuncture Research]* 18 (2) (1993): 159–62. (Chinese)

Yeo, I. S., and S. I. Hwang. "A Historical Study on the Introduction and Development of Anatomy in Japan." *Ui Sahak* 3 (2) (1994): 208–19. (Korean).

You, Z. "Preliminary Observation on the Relation Among Needling Sensation, Propagated Sensation Along Meridian (PSM), and Acupuncture Effect when Acupuncture Neiguan." *Zhen Ci Yan Jiu [Acupuncture Research]* 17 (1) (1992): 75–8. (Chinese)

You, Z. Q., B. H. Wu, K. Wang, X. L. Hu, J. W. Meng, W. Zhang, and Y. Z. Lin. "Influence of Perceptible and Latent Propagated Sensation Along Channels on the Effectiveness of Acupuncture." *Zhen Ci Yan Jiu [Acupuncture Research]* 12 Supplement 2 (1987a): 45–51. (Chinese)

You, Z. Q., B. H. Wu, K. Wang, X. L. Hu, W. Zhang, J. W. Meng, and Y. Z. Lin. "The Effects of Manifest and Latent Propagated Sensation Along the Channel on the Acupuncture Regulation of Cardiac Function." *Journal of Traditional Chinese Medicine* 7 (3) (September 1987b): 195–8. (Chinese)

Yu, A. "Observation on the Microstructure of Sanyinjiao Acupoint." *Zhen Ci Yan Jiu [Acupuncture Research]* 21 (2) (1996): 36–8. (Chinese)

Yu Yingao. "Two Celebrated Medical Works." *Ancient China's Technology and Science.* Beijing: Foreign Languages Press, 1983, 337–344.

Yu Fengsheng, Gong Shan, and Yin Qizhang. "Effects of Microinjection of Kainic Acid into Nucleus Raphe Dorsalis on Acupuncture, Stress and Morphine Analgesia." *The Second National Symposium on Acupuncture and Moxibustion and Acupuncture Anesthesia*, Beijing: Foreign Languages Printing House, 1984, 436.

Yu, S. Z., M. Zhang, S. An, S. Y. Yang, S. Y. Zhang, Z. X. Zhu, and Q. N. He. "Studies on the Phenomenon of Latent Propagated Sensation Along the Channels. II. Investigation on the Lines of LPSC on the Twelve Main Channels." *American Journal of Chinese Medicine* 9 (4) (Winter 1981): 291–7.

Yu, X., L. Song, H. Ma, and H. Gao. "Difference between the Discharges from the Postganglionic Fibers of the Celiac Ganglion Induced by Electroacupuncture at Zusanli and Yanglingquan." *Zhen Ci Yan Jiu [Acupuncture Research]* 21 (1) (1996): 49–51. (Chinese)

Yu Zhishun, Yu Yuecai, Shun Sentian, Jiang Shonglin, Zhu Chengxian, and Wang Xinmei. "The Effect of Needling Rabbit 'Zusanli' on the Small Intestine Mobility with Different Twisting Strengths." *The Second National Symposium on Acupuncture and Moxibustion and Acupuncture Anesthesia,* Beijing: Foreign Languages Printing House, 1984, 531.

Yukizaki, H., S. Nakajima, L. Nakashima, Y. Yamada, and T. Sato. "Electroacupuncture Increases Ipsilateral Tooth Pain Threshold in Man." *American Journal of Chinese Medicine* 14 (1986): 68–72.

Yun, M., G. W. Kai, and M. L. Qiu. "X-Ray Observation of the Effect of Acupuncture on the Function of the Biliary Tract." *Advances in Acupuncture and Acupuncture Anesthesia*, Beijing: Foreign Languages Printing House, June 1–5, 1979, 59.

Zaslawski, C., C. Rogers, M. Garvey, D. Ryan, C. X. Yang, and S. P. Zhang. "Strategies to Maintain the Credibility of Sham Acupuncture used as a Control Treatment in Clinical Trials." *Journal of Alternative and Complementary Medicine* 3 (3) (Fall 1997): 257–66.

Zhang Enqin, Lu Wenhai, Cai Jianqian, Nie Qingxi, Sun Xigang, and Yin Hongan, eds. *Rare Chinese Materia Medica*. Shanghai: Publishing House of Shanghai College of Traditional Chinese Medicine, 1990a.

Zhang Enqin, Zhao Lanfeng, Wang Jian, Zuo Lianjun, and Dong Xuemei, eds. *Highly Efficacious Chinese Patent Medicines.* Shanghai: Publishing House of Shanghai College of Traditional Chinese Medicine, 1990b.

Zhang Jianqiu, Zhang Shimei, Kang Shanzhu, and Shun Guizhen. "Influence of Needling Different Acupoints on Gallbladder Constrictive Function." *Selections from Shanghai Journal of Acupuncture and Moxibustion (1982–1984)*, 1983, 155.

Zhang, M. W., and X. Y. Sun. *Chinese Qigong Therapy.* Jinan, China: Shandong Science and Technology Press, 1988.

Zhang Wengao, Jia Wencheng, Li Shupei, Zhang Jing, Ou Yangbing, and Xu Xuelan. *Chinese Medicated Diet.* Zhang Enqin, ed. Shanghai: Publishing House of Shanghai College of Traditional Chinese Medicine, 1990.

Zhang Zhigang. *Bone-Setting Skills in Traditional Chinese Medicine.* Shandong, China: Shandong Science and Technology Press, 1996.

Zhou Zhongfu, Xuan Yuting, and Han Jisheng. "Further Investigation on Electroacupuncture Analgesia in Rabbits: The Effect of Different Strength of Electric Stimulation." *Acupuncture Research*, Beijing: Foreign Languages Printing House, 1985, 187.

Zhou Zhongfu, Xuan Yuting, Wu Wenyin, and Han Jisheng. "Electroacupuncture Tolerance in Rabbits and its Cross Tolerance to Morphine." In *Acupuncture Research*, Beijing: Foreign Languages Printing House, 1985, 127.

Zhu, C. H. *Clinical Handbook of Chinese Prepared Medicines.* Brookline, Mass.: Paradigm Publications, 1989.

Zhu, Z. X. "Research Advances in the Electrical Specificity of Meridians and Acupuncture Points." *American Journal of Acupuncture* 9 (1981): 203–216.

Zhu, Z., and R. Xu. "Morphometric Observation on the Mast Cells under the Acupuncture Meridian Lines." *Zhen Ci Yan Jiu [Acupuncture Research]* 15 (2) (1990): 157–8. (Chinese)

Zhu, Z. X., Z. Q. Yan, S. Z. Yu, R. X. Zhang, J. Y. Wang, Y. M. Liu, J. K Hao, X. L. Zhang, S. L. Yu, Q. N. He, and Z. W. Meng. "Studies on the Phenomenon of Latent Propagated Sensation along the Channels. I. The Discovery of a Latent PSC and a Preliminary Study of its Skin Electrical Conductance." *American Journal of Chinese Medicine* 9 (3) (Autumn 1981): 216–24.

Zmiewski, Paul, ed. *Georges Soulié de Morant, Chinese Acupuncture (L'acuponcture Chinoise).* Lawrence Grinnell, Claudy Jeanmougin, and Maurice Leveque, trans. Brookline, Mass.: Paradigm Publications, 1994.

Zmiewski, Paul, and Richard Feit. *Acumoxa Therapy: A Reference and Study Guide.* Brookline, Mass.: Paradigm Publications, 1989.

Index

A

B

E

F

G

H

I

J

N

V

Index to *Neijing* Citations

Neijing Lingshu (NJLS)

Neijing Suwen (NJSW)